K

EATING DISORDERS IN WOMEN AND CHILDREN

PREVENTION, STRESS MANAGEMENT, AND TREATMENT

CRC SERIES IN MODERN NUTRITION

Edited by Ira Wolinsky and James F. Hickson, Jr.

Published Titles

Manganese in Health and Disease, Dorothy J. Klimis-Tavantzis

Nutrition and AIDS: Effects and Treatments, Ronald R. Watson

Nutrition Care for HIV-Positive Persons: A Manual for Individuals and Their Caregivers,
Saroj M. Bahl and James F. Hickson, Jr.

Calcium and Phosphorus in Health and Disease, John J.B. Anderson and
Sanford C. Garner

Edited by Ira Wolinsky

Published Titles

Handbook of Nutrition in the Aged, Ronald R. Watson

Practical Handbook of Nutrition in Clinical Practice, Donald F. Kirby
and Stanley J. Dudrick

Handbook of Dairy Foods and Nutrition, Gregory D. Miller, Judith K. Jarvis,
and Lois D. McBean

Advanced Nutrition: Macronutrients, Carolyn D. Berdanier

Childhood Nutrition, Fima Lifschitz

Nutrition and Health: Topics and Controversies, Felix Bronner

Nutrition and Cancer Prevention, Ronald R. Watson and Siraj I. Mufti

Nutritional Concerns of Women, Ira Wolinsky and Dorothy J. Klimis-Tavantzis

Nutrients and Gene Expression: Clinical Aspects, Carolyn D. Berdanier

Antioxidants and Disease Prevention, Harinda S. Garewal

Advanced Nutrition: Micronutrients, Carolyn D. Berdanier

Nutrition and Women's Cancers, Barbara Pence and Dale M. Dunn

Nutrients and Foods in AIDS, Ronald R. Watson

Nutrition: Chemistry and Biology, Second Edition, Julian E. Spallholz,
L. Mallory Boylan, and Judy A. Driskell

Melatonin in the Promotion of Health, Ronald R. Watson

Nutrition and the Eye, Allen Taylor

Laboratory Tests for the Assessment of Nutritional Status, Second Edition,
H.E. Sauberlich

Advanced Human Nutrition, Robert E.C. Wildman and Denis M. Medeiros

Handbook of Dairy Foods and Nutrition, Second Edition, Gregory D. Miller,
Judith K. Jarvis, and Lois D. McBean

Nutrition in Space Flight and Weightlessness Models, Helen W. Lane
and Dale A. Schoeller

*Eating Disorders in Women and Children: Prevention, Stress Management, and
Treatment*, Jacalyn J. Robert-McComb

Forthcoming Titles

Child Nutrition: An International Perspective, Noel W. Solomons

Childhood Obesity: Prevention and Treatment, Jana Parizkova and Andrew Hills

Alcohol and Substance Abuse in the Aging, Ronald R. Watson

Nutritional Anemias, Usha Ramakrishnan

Advances in Isotope Methods for the Analysis of Trace Elements in Man, Malcolm Jackson and Nicola Lowe

Advanced Nutrition: Macronutrients, Second Edition, Carolyn D. Berdanier

Handbook of Nutrition for Vegetarians, Joan Sabate and Rosemary A. Ratzin-Tuner

Tryptophan: Biochemicals and Health Implications, Herschel Sidransky

Coenzyme Q: From Molecular Mechanisms to Nutrition and Health, Valerian E. Kagan and Peter J. Quinn

Nutraceuticals and Functional Foods, Robert E. C. Wildman

The Mediterranean Diet, Antonia L. Matalas, Antonios Zampelas, Vasilis Stavrinos, and Ira Wolinsky

Handbook of Nutrition and the Aged, Third Edition, Ronald R. Watson

Handbook of Nutraceuticals and Nutritional Supplements and Pharmaceuticals, Robert E. C. Wildman

Inulin and Oligofructose: Functional Food Ingredients, Marcel B. Roberfroid

Micronutrients and HIV Infection, Henrik Friis

Vegetables, Fruits, and Herbs in Health Promotion, Ronald R. Watson

Nutrition and AIDS, 2nd Edition, Ronald R. Watson

Nutrition Gene Interactions in Health and Disease, Niama M. Moussa and Carolyn D. Berdanier

EATING DISORDERS IN WOMEN AND CHILDREN
PREVENTION, STRESS MANAGEMENT, AND TREATMENT

EDITED BY

JACALYN J. ROBERT-McCOMB

CRC Press
Boca Raton   London   New York   Washington, D.C.

Library of Congress Cataloging-in-Publication Data

Eating disorders in women and children — prevention, stress management, and treatment / edited by Jacalyn J. Robert-McComb.
    p. ; cm. — (CRC series in modern nutrition)
Includes bibliographical references and index.
ISBN 0-8493-2027-5 (alk. paper)
1. Eating disorders. 2. Eating disorders in children. 3. Women—Mental health.
4. Children—Mental health. 5. Stress management. I. Robert-McComb, Jacalyn J.
II. Modern nutrition (Boca Raton, Fla.)
[DNLM: 1. Eating Disorders—prevention & control—Child. 2. Eating
Disorders—prevention & control. 3. Stress, Psychological—therapy—Child.
4. Stress, Psychological—therapy. 5. Women. WM 175 M2667 2000]
RC552.E18 M365 2000
616.85′26—dc21

00-039759
CIP

SERIES PREFACE FOR MODERN NUTRITION

The CRC Series in Modern Nutrition is dedicated to providing the widest possible coverage of topics in nutrition. Nutrition is an interdisciplinary, interprofessional field par excellence. It is noted by its broad range and diversity. We trust the titles and authorship in this series will reflect that range and diversity.

Published for a scholarly audience, the volumes in the CRC Series in Modern Nutrition are designed to explain, review, and explore present knowledge and recent trends, developments, and advances in nutrition. As such, they will also appeal to the educated layman. The format for the series will vary with the needs of the author and the topic, including, but not limited to, edited volumes, monographs, handbooks, and texts.

Contributors from any bona fide area of nutrition, including the controversial, are welcome.

We welcome the contribution *Eating Disorders in Women and Children: Prevention, Stress Management, and Treatment,* edited by Jacalyn J. Robert-McComb. This a very timely topic and a very important one.

Ira Wolinsky, Ph.D.
University of Houston
Series Editor

Preface

> ... *studies of women have repeatedly shown disturbing patterns: lack of self-esteem, an inability to feel powerful or in control of one's life, a vulnerability to depression, a tendency to see oneself as less talented, less able than one really is. The myriad studies that have been done over the years give the distinct impression of constriction, a crippling, a sense of being somehow not quite as good, not quite as bright, not quite as valuable as men .... Certainly there are many women who have escaped that blight, who have lived full and happy lives, but when you leaf through the studies you can sense, floating in the air, ghosts of unborn dreams, unrealized hopes, undiscovered talents. The tragedies are the "might have beens" and they are the most poignant.*
>
> — Carl Rivers, Rosalind Barnett, and Grace Baruch in *Beyond Sugar and Spice*

Women with eating disorders have that feeling of *"being not quite as good, not quite as bright, not quite as valuable"* as others. *Eating Disorders in Women and Children: Prevention, Stress Management, and Treatment* is designed to teach professionals how to help women become all they can be and avoid the tragedy of *"what might have been."* Even though eating disorders have most commonly been reported for women between the ages of 18 and 25, these disorders are not limited to one particular age category. Research indicates that fear of fatness, restrained eating, and binge eating are common among girls by age 10. In addition, reports of eating disorders are becoming more common in the elderly. Disordered eating is often an unhealthy attempt at coping with stress. Although young girls and women may use the eating disorder as a method of coping, they soon are caught in a negative cycle, increasingly using ineffective behaviors in an attempt to cope with stress. The eating disorder becomes more severe as stress levels, particularly interpersonal stress levels, increase.

Eating Disorders in Women and Children: Prevention, Stress Management, and Treatment is specifically designed to teach professionals how to help young girls and women target the interpersonal stress that contributes to disordered eating. It develops a broader understanding of eating disorder etiology and provides an application of the knowledge for practitioners to use in their particular work settings, whether in physical education classes, health classes, or support groups for athletes. This book is written for the practitioner; it is the only book on the market that covers stress management techniques specifically for eating disorder symptomatology.

Each chapter of the text is organized under the following main headings: (a) learning objectives, (b) research background, and (c) application of research question. Actual case studies are presented when deemed appropriate. This organization allows the reader to understand how the information can be applied. Throughout each chapter, the reader will be referred to supplemental material included in the appendices.

Each chapter refers to supplemental materials included in the appendices. The materials are intended to help victims of eating disorders increase personal introspection and decrease interpersonal stress. Young girls and women with eating disorders often have trouble expressing their feelings. Varied teaching tools such as movement improvisation exercises (body movements often express the essential self more deeply than words) are included in the appendix for the practitioner to use in his or her particular work setting. The appendix also includes cognitive paper and pencil exercises to help young girls and women increase personal introspection.

Eating Disorders in Women and Children: Prevention, Stress Management, and Treatment is a resource tool for professionals who are exposed to women who exhibit symptoms of disordered eating and for anyone who is experiencing the stress of an eating disorder, personally or in a friend or loved one. Because of the multidisciplinary nature of this treatment approach, varied professionals will gain the expertise to implement the knowledge contained in this text. Examples of professionals who may find this text useful are university personnel responsible for the preparation of teachers, health educators, fitness professionals and coaches; allied health professionals including therapeutic recreation specialists, occupational therapists, physical therapists, and nurses; the counseling profession, sociologists, educational psychologists, social workers, and clinical psychologists; individuals in the field of human development and family studies; and teachers, health educators, fitness professionals, and coaches in the school or community setting.

Editor

Jacalyn J. Robert-McComb, Ph.D., is an associate professor in the Department of Health at Texas Tech University Physical Education and Recreation. She also serves as adjunct professor in the Department of Physiology at the Texas Tech University Health Science Center and is the director of the Texas Tech Center for Sports Health and Human Performance. Dr. Robert-McComb has been certified by ACSM as an Exercise Test Technologist and Exercise Specialist, as well as by the American Council of Exercise as an Aerobics Instructor. She was an intercollegiate athlete in gymnastics at Southeast Missouri State University and a professional water-skier at Cypress Gardens, Florida. Dr. Robert-McComb understands the demands and stress associated with a sports culture that emphasizes maintaining a certain ideal body weight and shape for optimal performance. She is dedicated to educating young girls, coaches, teachers, and health care professionals about the importance of accepting oneself through nurturing activities and the management of stress in one's life.

Contributors

Marcia Abbott, Ph.D.
Clinical Psychologist
Private Practice
Lubbock, Texas

Yvonne Caldera, Ph.D.
Associate Professor
Department of Human Development
Texas Tech University
Lubbock, Texas

James R. Clopton, Ph.D.
Professor
Department of Psychology
Texas Tech University
Lubbock, Texas

Stephen Cook, Ph.D.
Associate Professor
Department of Psychology
Texas Tech University
Lubbock, Texas

**Lucy Ramsey DuBose, M.A.,
MSSW, DTR**
LMSW-ACP Registered Dance Therapist
Artist-in-Education/ Arkansas Arts Council
Little Rock, Arkansas

**Annette Gary, R.N., C.S., Ph.D.,
CNAA, CFNP**
Associate Dean for Practice
    and Assistant Professor
School of Nursing
Texas Tech University
    Health Science Center
Lubbock, Texas

Robert W. Grant, Ed.D.
Assistant Professor
Department of Neuropsychiatry
Texas Tech University
    Health Science Center
 Lubbock, Texas

Heather L. Haas, M.A.
Ph.D. Student in Clinical Psychology
Department of Psychology
Texas Tech University
Lubbock, Texas

Jan Hamilton, Ph.D., R.D., L.D., C.N.S.
Private Practice
Nutritional Biomedicine
Plainview, Texas

Elizabeth Jambor, Ed.D.
Texas State Government
Austin, Texas

Teddy L. Jones, R.N., C.S., Ph.D.
Professor/Family Nurse Practitioner
School of Nursing Wellness Center
Texas Tech University
    Health Science Center
Lubbock, Texas

Susan Kashubeck-West, Ph.D.
Associate Professor
Department of Psychology
Texas Tech University
Lubbock, Texas

Jan S. Kent, Ph.D.
Clinical Psychologist
Herndon Snider and Associates
Joplin, Missouri

Jeromi Kummell, B.S.
M.S. Student in Sports Health
Department of Health, Physical Education,
    and Recreation
Texas Tech University
Lubbock, Texas

Adwoa Lemieux, M.A., DTR
Registered Dance/Movement Therapist
Naropa University
University of Colorado
Boulder, Colorado

Leslie Lewis, Chaplain
Associate Chaplain
Covenant Hospital System
Lubbock, Texas

Marilyn S. Massey-Stokes,
Ed.D., CHES
Assistant Professor of Health
Department of Health, Physical Education,
  and Recreation
Texas Tech University
Lubbock, Texas

Robert Saar McComb, B.S.
Engineer and Technical Artist
Chapel Hill, North Carolina

Michelle Pettus, M.S.
Health Educator
Student Health Services
Texas Tech University
Lubbock, Texas

Jan S. Richter, Ed.D., CHES
Associate Professor
Department of Kinesiology
  and Health Studies
University of Central Oklahoma
Edmond, Oklahoma

Jacalyn J. Robert-McComb, Ph.D.
Associate Professor and Director
  of the Center for Sports Health
  and Human Performance
Department of Health, Physical
  Education, and Recreation
Texas Tech University
Adjunct Professor
Department of Physiology
Texas Tech Health Science Center
Lubbock, Texas

John Rohwer, Ed.D.
Professor
Department of Health
  and Physical Education
Bethel College
St. Paul, Minnesota

Kendra Saunders, M.A.
Ph.D. Student in Counseling Psychology
Department of Psychology
Texas Tech University
Lubbock, Texas

Anna Tacón, Ph.D.
Assistant Professor of Health
Department of Health, Physical Education,
  and Recreation
Texas Tech University
Lubbock, Texas

Cathy Thompson, M.A.
Ph.D. Student in Clinical Psychology
Department of Psychology
Texas Tech University
Lubbock, Texas

Contents

Part I

The Constitution of
Eating Disorders

1

Eating Disorders

Jacalyn J. Robert-McComb

CONTENTS

1.1   LEARNING OBJECTIVES

After reading this chapter you should be able to:

- Understand the varying types of eating disorders;
- Understand the risk factors contributing to an eating disorder;
- Recognize differentiating and similar signs and symptoms of each disorder;
- Use assessment tools to help identify eating disorder symptomatology.

1.2   Research Background

Eating disorders are typically those compulsive eating behaviors that can be life threatening. Eating disorders of any degree can have adverse health consequences, with morbidity and risks of mortality increasing with the extent of the self-destructive behavior. Females, more often than males, are affected by these disorders; however, the number of males experiencing these disorders is increasing.[1] Eating disorders appear to be prevalent among white upper-middle and middle-class women;[2] however, increasing numbers are being seen among minorities and females of all ages, even young children.[3] Disordered eating is often an unhealthy attempt at coping with stress. Research shows that females with eating disorders report higher levels of stress than a non-disordered eating group.[4]

The primary types of eating disorders are anorexia nervosa and bulimia nervosa. Two additional categories of eating disorders have recently been added by the *Diagnostic and Statistical Manual of Mental Disorders* (DSM-IV).[5] These disorders are termed eating disorders not otherwise specified and binge-eating disorders. This chapter will define, in detail, these four areas of inappropriate behavior, including the DSM-IV diagnostic criteria for each disorder, specific risk factors contributing to each disorder, the signs and symptoms of specific eating disorders, and practical tools for the assessment of eating disorder symptomatology.

1.2.1   Anorexia Nervosa

The DSM-IV[5] diagnostic criteria for anorexia nervosa are outlined in the following section.

1. Refusal to maintain body weight at or above a minimally normal weight for age and height (e.g., weight loss leading to maintenance of body weight less than 85% of that expected; or failure to make expected weight gain during period of growth, leading to body weight less than 85% of that expected).
2. Intense fear of gaining weight or becoming fat, even though underweight.
3. Disturbance in the way in which body weight or shape is experienced, undue influence of body weight or shape on self-evaluation, or denial of the current low body weight.

4. In postmenarcheal females, amenorrhea, i.e., the absence of at least three consecutive menstrual cycles. (A woman is considered to have amenorrhea if her periods occur only following hormone, e.g., estrogen, administration.)

The specific types of anorexia nervosa according to DSM-IV are as described below.

1. Restricting: During the current episode of anorexia nervosa, the person has not regularly engaged in binge-eating or purging behavior (i.e., self-induced vomiting or the misuse of laxatives, diuretics, or enemas).

2. Binge-Eating/Purging: During the current episode of anorexia nervosa, the person has regularly engaged in binge-eating or purging behavior (i.e., self-induced vomiting or the misuse of laxatives, diuretics, or enemas).

Individuals with anorexia nervosa may move back and forth between the two types of subgroups since the subgroups have similar characteristics.[6,7] The restricting subtype (AN-R) accomplishes weight loss through dieting, fasting, and excessive exercise. The bulimic subtype (AN-B) purges after binge eating, or even after the consumption of a small amount of food, through self-induced vomiting or the misuse of laxatives, diuretics, or enemas. AN-B victims tend to be heavier than AN-R victims, have more impulse-control problems, experience more mood swings, and be more sexually active.[8,9]

In order to determine the values for criterion A (< 85% of ideal body weight) as listed by the DSM-IV, the professional can use pediatric and adolescent growth guidelines (see Appendix 1-A) and height and weight tables (see Appendix 1-B). A simpler formula that can be used to roughly determine ideal weight for a young woman of average bone size is to take 100 pounds and to add 4 pounds for every inch over 5 feet in height. For a very slight bone size, add only 3 pounds for every inch over 5 feet.

The criteria established by the DSM-IV for anorexia nervosa serve only as one guideline. There are other established guidelines in addition to the ones listed by the DSM-IV. The *International Classification of Diseases* diagnostic criteria for research[10] require that an individual have a body mass index (BMI) equal to or below $17.5 \, kg/m^2$ for anorexia nervosa. These criteria can be calculated from the graph in Figure 1.1. The ranges for a normal BMI can be found in Table 1.1.

1.2.1.1 Risk Factors Contributing to Anorexia Nervosa

The mean age at onset of anorexia nervosa is 17 years, with some data suggesting the peak years are between 13 to 18 years (bimodal 13 to 14 years and 17 to 18 years). The exact cause of anorexia is unknown; however, there are predisposing risk factors associated with this disorder. Some of these factors are (a) perfectionist behavior; (b) low self-esteem; (c) a preoccupation with becoming thin; (d) dieting practices such as skipping meals; and (e) an over-concern for body weight and appearance.

Adolescence is a particularly vulnerable time period for the development of this disorder because of the pubertal changes that accompany the passage of childhood into adulthood. The preoccupation with thinness and the physical changes associated with sexual maturity, such as the increase in body fat and hip width, increases adolescent frustration.

Furthermore, participation in certain types of sports that promote as part of their culture an emphasis on maintaining a certain ideal body weight and shape for optimal performance is consistent with a predisposition to eating disorders.[11] Risk factors for the development of an eating disorder for athletes have been found to be (a) dieting at an early age; (b) unsupervised dieting (coach says you have to lose weight or be thin); (c) restrictive diets and weight cycling in association with energy deprivation; (d) reaching menarche too soon emotionally (the weight associated with maturity

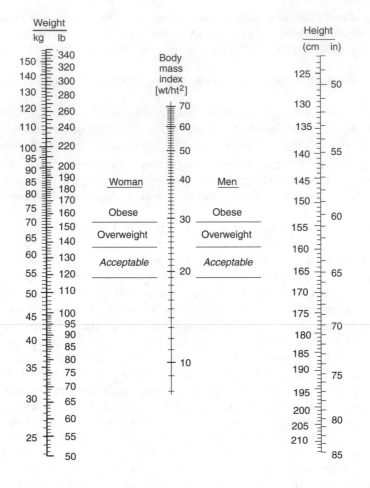

FIGURE 1.1
Nomogram for body mass index (BMI). From Bray, A., *International Journal of Obesity,* 2(2), 1978. With permission.

TABLE 1.1

Ranges for Normal Body Mass Indexes

Classification	Men	Women
Normal	24–27	23–26
Moderately obese	28–31	27–32
Severely obese	>31	>32

Source: From *The Surgeon General's Report on Nutrition and Health,* 1988, p. 284.

decreases effective performance); and (e) choosing a sport to participate in before the body matures or choosing a sport incompatible with body type.[12]

1.2.1.2   Signs and Symptoms of Anorexia Nervosa

Some of the behaviors and attitudes associated with anorexia nervosa are (a) fear of eating in public; (b) feelings of ineffectiveness; (c) need to control the environment; (d) inflexible thinking; (e) limited social spontaneity; and (f) overly restrained emotional expression.[5] The individual with anorexia nervosa does not have a loss of appetite as the term implies but rather views her body as a tool that she uses to feel in control of

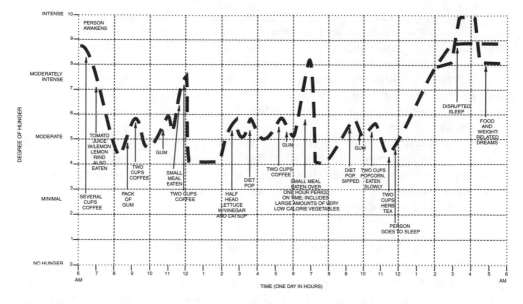

FIGURE 1.2

Typical hunger and food intake pattern of a person with anorexia nervosa. From Reiff, D. W., *Eating Disorders: Nutrition Therapy in the Recovery Process*, Aspen Publishers, Inc., 1992. With permission.

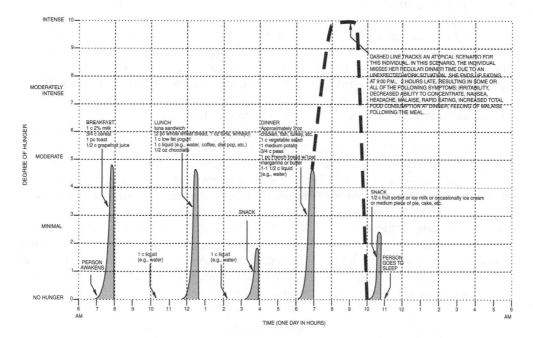

FIGURE 1.3

Normal hunger and food-intake pattern. From Reiff, D. W., *Eating Disorders: Nutrition Therapy in the Recovery Process*, Aspen Publishers, Inc., 1992. With permission.

her life. Weight loss is a sign of mastery in her life; weight gain is akin to failure. She ignores hunger pains, substituting normal food intake with low-calorie alternative choices such as coffee, gum, etc. Figure 1.2 depicts a typical hunger and food-intake pattern of a person suffering from anorexia nervosa. Her diet consists of "safe" foods; these are foods that she can eat and not gain weight such as lettuce, green beans, carrots, etc. Compare this with a normal hunger and food-intake pattern (Figure 1.3).

Obsessive compulsive features are often prominent, both related and unrelated to food.[5] Because individuals with anorexia nervosa are starving their bodies, they obsess about food constantly and have general signs of malnutrition such as depression, fatigue, and the absence of regular menstrual periods. Cessation of menstruation is correlated with bone thinning and decreased bone mass.[13] Because anorexia is more predominant during the teens and twenties or during the formation of peak bone mass, anorexics are particularly vulnerable to osteoporosis that may result in fractures later in life.

Individuals with anorexia nervosa also have a distorted body image. Again, the issue of control is dominant in their distorted body image. A thinner body is viewed as more beautiful, better than other normal female figures, and serves to reinforce their low self-esteem. Researchers have found that self-concept deficiency may contribute significantly to distortions in body image.[14]

1.2.1.3   Practical Tools to Assess the Symptoms Associated with Anorexia Nervosa

Early detection is essential in the prevention of more serious health consequences associated with eating disorders. A valid, objective, and economical instrument for evaluating symptoms frequently observed in anorexia nervosa is the Eating Attitudes Test, often seen in the literature as EAT.[15] This is a self-report inventory that may be used as a screening instrument for identifying symptoms associated with anorexia nervosa (see Appendix 1-C).

Many times there is vacillation between the behaviors associated with anorexia nervosa and bulimia. An individual may suspect that she has an eating disorder but is not sure if she has more of a tendency toward anorexia nervosa or bulimia nervosa. Another instrument that may be helpful to assess tendencies toward a specific subtype of eating disorders is a questionnaire entitled "Are You Dying To Be Thin?" This instrument is found in Appendix 1-D.

Since individuals with anorexia nervosa have a distorted body image and have even lost touch with bodily sensations, a simple exercise that can be used to heighten body awareness is body scanning. Body scanning is a form of meditation that brings one's attention to the individual body parts in succession, beginning with the feet and ending with the face and head.[16] This exercise may appeal to a particular subgroup of female athletes (dancers, gymnasts, figure skaters, and synchronized swimmers) who are especially vulnerable to the development of eating disorders.[17]

These tools are designed to gain insight into signs and symptoms of an eating disorder. These instruments do not have as their objective a formal diagnosis of an eating disorder. If an eating disorder is suspected through the use of screening instruments such as those listed in this chapter, the most appropriate method for forming a diagnosis is a clinical interview with a trained professional.

1.2.2   Bulimia Nervosa

Bulimia nervosa is more common than anorexia nervosa.[18] The DSM-IV[5] diagnostic criteria for bulimia nervosa are in the following section.

1. Recurrent episodes of binge eating. An episode of binge eating is characterized by both of the following:

    (a) eating in a discrete period of time (e.g., within any 2-hour period) an amount of food that is definitely larger than most people would eat during a similar period of time and under similar circumstances

    (b) a sense of lack of control over eating during the episode (e.g., a feeling
        that one cannot stop eating or control what or how much one is eating)

 2. Recurrent inappropriate compensatory behavior in order to prevent weight
    gain, such as self-induced vomiting; misuse of laxatives, diuretics, enemas,
    or other medications; fasting; or excessive exercise.

 3. The binge eating and inappropriate behaviors both occur, on average, at
    least twice a week for 3 months.

 4. Self-evaluation is unduly influenced by body shape and weight.

 5. The disturbance does not occur during episodes of anorexia nervosa.

Types of bulimia nervosa are described below.

 1. Purging: During the current episode of bulimia nervosa, the person has
    regularly engaged in self-induced vomiting or the misuse of laxatives,
    diuretics, or enemas.

 2. Nonpurging: During the current episode of bulimia nervosa, the person
    has used other inappropriate compensatory behaviors, such as fasting or
    excessive exercise, but has not engaged in self-induced vomiting or the
    misuse of laxatives, diuretics, or enemas.

1.2.2.1   Risk Factors Contributing to Bulimia Nervosa

Since bulimia nervosa is predominantly a female disorder, socio-cultural values specific to the idea of femininity, such as thinness, physical attractiveness, and beauty for
women in that particular culture or society, set the stage for this disorder. Today's
society values attractiveness and thinness. This ideal female stereotype is reflected in
the media through thin and beautiful celebrities, models, and actresses in magazines,
television, and films.

In early childhood, girls learn that being attractive is interwoven with pleasing and
serving others and will become one of the means they use to secure love.[19] Young girls
are more focused on their looks than boys; even their choice of toys reflects aesthetic
adornment. Heterosexual relationships, in part, are formed through being popular
and attractive (i.e., thin).

Adolescence is a particularly vulnerable period for the development of bulimia.
During adolescence, males and females alike are achieving a new sense of physical
self, establishing heterosexual relationships, and developing independence. Adolescent girls often begin to feel confused, insecure, and inadequate because their own
personal values differ from the views of society. Adolescent girls view dependence as
a positive attitude in a society that urges independence. All of these changes during
adolescence may make them feel out of control; however, they can control their
weight through dieting.

To add to their frustration, adolescents are beginning to gain sex-specific fat during
puberty. This is stressful for girls who have internalized society's values (thinness),
particularly females who are involved in activities that reward thinness or where
being svelte increases performance, such as gymnastics, dance, figure skating, and
distance running.

Through adulthood, women are continually struggling with the concepts of self-
image, interpersonal relationships, and dependence/independence. Characteristics
that have been found in bulimic women are (a) a strong need for social approval;
(b) conflict avoidance; (c) inability to identify and assert personal needs; (d) inadequate coping skills; and (e) high distress levels.[9,20]

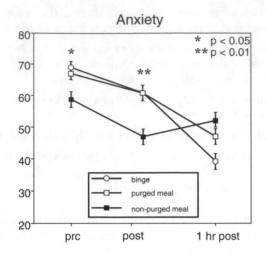

FIGURE 1.4
Anxiety levels before and after abnormal eating behaviors. From Hetherington, M., M., Altemus, M., Nelson, M. L., Bernat, A., S., and Gold, P. W., *American Journal of Clinical Nutrition*, 60, 864, 1994. With permission.

Additionally, the role of the family must be considered when discussing risk factors for bulimia. Contributing family dynamics are (a) a heavy emphasis on thinness in the family; (b) enmeshment; (c) overprotectiveness; and (d) lack of conflict resolution.[21]

It is also important to examine biological and genetic factors in the pursuit of understanding risk factors. Clinical and empirical evidence exists showing that women who are heavier through genetic endowment, and who have internalized the idea of thinness and beauty, are more likely to develop bulimia.[19,22] Also, women who have engaged in repeated dieting practices without success and who have decreased their basal metabolic rates through unhealthy practices will be vulnerable to purging as an attempt to control weight.[23]

1.2.2.2   Signs and Symptoms of Bulimia Nervosa

Bulimic women are usually within the normal weight range for their age and height. The most distinguishing characteristic of bulimia nervosa is the activity of binge eating, i.e., eating a relatively large amount of food in a discrete period of time. Since bulimics are concerned about their weight, self-induced vomiting may follow a binge. Anxiety levels are usually higher before eating a purged meal relative to a nonpurged meal, both before and after the binge. However, 1 h after purging, the anxiety is lower for those who binged and did not purge (see Figure 1.4). Researchers have also found that relief from negative mood states can be achieved, at least in the short term, by binge eating and purging. Yet, increased shame and guilt and anger have been found after binge eating and purging. It appears that any positive effect associated with binge eating appears to be short-lived.[24]

A feeling of loss of control occurs during a binge. Many times it takes place after a period of food deprivation. This vicious cycle of binge, purge, guilt, and restraint of food, followed by another binge, keeps repeating itself. Hetherington[25] found no predictable "bulimic eating style," though most eating episodes are associated with purging, perhaps stemming from the fear of being fat. Binge foods tend to be sweet, high-fat foods such as ice cream, doughnuts, puddings, chocolate, cookies, and cakes. The list is not limited to these foods. Other common foods are breads and pastas, cheeses, meats, and salty snack foods such as peanuts, popcorn, corn, and potato chips.

TABLE 1.2

Eating Episodes of Bulimic Women over a 7-Day Period

Bulimic subjects	Number of eating episodes	Meals and snacks (not purged)[a]	Binges[a]	Meals and snacks (purged)[a]
001	28	2 (7)	7 (25)	19 (68)
002	15	0	15 (100)	0
003	35	6 (17)	13 (37)	16 (46)
004	24	16 (67)	7 (29)	1 (4)
005	36	1 (3)	22 (61)	13 (36)
006	26	13 (50)	5 (19)	8 (31)
007	27	7 (26)	12 (44)	8 (30)
008	26	7 (27)	9 (35)	10 (38)
009	42	21 (50)	9 (21)	12 (29)
010	28	1 (4)	10 (35)	17 (61)
± SEM	28.7 ± 2.3	7.2 ± 2.2	10.9 ± 1.5	10.4 ± 2.0

[a] Percentage of the time that the behavior occurred in relation to eating episodes is listed in parentheses
Source: From Hetherington, M., M., Altemus, M., Nelson, M. L., Bernat, A., S., and Gold, P. W. *American Journal of Clinical Nutrition,* 60, 864, 1994. With permission.

Researchers have theorized that bulimic females are less capable of self-control and are not focused on hunger and satiety cues. They have learned to ignore hunger and fullness. These characteristics, in combination with a preoccupation with weight and body shape, contribute to uncontrolled eating episodes followed by purging behavior. Research on eating habits details the caloric cost of binging. In a study by Kaye,[24] it was found that normal-weight bulimic women averaged 7101-kcal ± 9546 kcal daily during a binging episode. Compare this figure to the amount of energy consumed daily by healthy control women: 1844 ± 518 kcal. Hetherington[25] observed and recorded 10 bulimic individuals' eating behaviors over 7 consecutive days. Bulimic patients demonstrated chaotic eating patterns, with an average daily intake of 10,034 ± 2701 kcal per day compared to 1924 ± 102 kcal for normal controls (see Table 1.2).

1.2.2.3 Practical Tools to Assess the Symptoms Associated with Bulimia Nervosa

Although binge eaters share some common symptoms with anorexics, they differ in many ways. A self-rating scale for bulimia that is easy to administer, acceptable to subjects, and easy to score is the BITE designed by Henderson and Freeman.[26] This scale measures both the symptomatology and the severity of bulimia nervosa. The average time for the completion of the questionnaire is less than 10 min. The BITE scale also appears to be sensitive to changes both in symptoms and behavior before and after treatment. Another instrument that has been used widely in the research literature is the BULIT-R.[27] This instrument is also a practical screening tool for the behaviors associated with bulimia nervosa (see Appendix 4-A).

1.2.3 Eating Disorder Not Otherwise Specified

This category is for eating disorders that meet some but not all of the specific criteria for anorexia or bulimia nervosa. The DSM-IV[5] diagnostic criteria for eating disorder not otherwise specified are described accordingly.

1. For females, all of the criteria for anorexia nervosa are met, except that the individual has regular menses.

2. All of the criteria for anorexia nervosa are met except that, despite significant weight loss, the individual's current weight is in the normal range.

3. All of the criteria for bulimia nervosa are met, except that the binge eating and inappropriate compensatory mechanisms occur at a frequency of less than twice a week or for a duration of less than 3 months.

4. The regular use of inappropriate compensatory behavior by an individual of normal body weight after eating small amounts of food (e.g., self-induced vomiting after consumption of two cookies).

5. Repeatedly chewing and spitting out, but not swallowing, large amount of food.

6. Binge-eating disorder involves recurrent episodes of binge eating in the absence of the regular use of inappropriate compensatory behaviors characteristic of bulimia nervosa.

1.2.3.1   Risk Factors Contributing to Eating Disorder Not Otherwise Specified

The risk factors associated with the classification of this particular disorder are similar if not identical to the risk factors associated with anorexia and bulimia nervosa. The severity of the symptoms may not be as severe, however.

Individuals engaging in unhealthy dieting practices such as skipping meals, fasting, using diet pills or laxatives are at a greater risk of developing an eating disorder not otherwise specified than those who do not engage in unhealthy eating habits. Once again, females are more likely than males to show greater concern for their weight and appearance and engage in these unhealthy dieting practices.[28] The significance of body weight and shape in their self-evaluations is distorted: low self-esteem, high stress levels, and mood disturbances are also common in these individuals.

Adolescents who engage in high-intensity sports that glorify leanness as part of their subculture may not exhibit all of the symptoms associated with anorexia or bulimia nervosa and would fall in this category. Whether participation in these sports is a consequence of pre-existing problems or participation is causally related to the onset of eating disorders has not been established conclusively.[29]

1.2.3.2   Signs and Symptoms of Eating Disorder Not Otherwise Specified

The signs and symptoms of these disorders are also similar to those of anorexia nervosa, except for regular occurrence of menses and weight within the normal range or age and height. If the individual is exhibiting signs of bulimia, the compensatory behaviors such as purging occur less frequently than two times a week, or she may purge after eating small amounts of food. Both anorexic and bulimic individuals have an intense preoccupation with food and engage in severe food restriction. Anorexic individuals are usually withdrawn, asexual, prone to depression, and have obsessional fears. Bulimic individuals are more outgoing and usually sexually active. They feel guilty about their binge-and-purge impulsive behaviors and may experience alcohol-drug addictions and depression. In severe cases even suicide may be attempted.

1.2.3.3   Practical Tools to Assess the Symptoms of Eating Disorder Not Otherwise Specified

The same instruments used for anorexia or bulimia nervosa can be used for this category as well. Another instrument that is also widely seen in the research literature is the Eating Disorder Inventory (EDI).[30] This inventory is more time consuming than those previously mentioned in this chapter. The inventory consists of 64 items that generate eight subscales and three provisional subscales. The eight subscales are (a) drive for thinness; (b) bulimia; (c) body dissatisfaction; (d) ineffectiveness; (e) perfectionism; (f) interpersonal distrust; (g) interoceptive awareness; and (h) maturity fears. The three provisional subscales are (a) asceticism; (b) impulse regulation; and (c) social insecurity. Numerical norms are given for specific populations for each of these subscales. This instrument provides standardized measurement of the depth or symptomatology along several dimensions that are relevant to eating disorders. You may direct your questions concerning this assessment instrument to Psychological Assessment Resources, 1-800-331-TEST.

1.2.4 Binge-Eating Disorder

Professionals have proposed categorization of binge-eating disorder as a distinct diagnosis. The proposal has not yet been formalized. Binge eating now falls under the eating-disorder-not-otherwise-specified category in the DSM-IV. More definitive future research as to the causes and diagnosis of this disorder needs to be carried out. The term 'compulsive overeating' has also been used to identify binge eating in the absence of self-induced vomiting or purgative abuse. The term *compulsive* may be misleading and obscures the fact that overeating may be explained in most instances by a long history of excessive dieting. The DSM-IV[5] diagnostic criteria for binge-eating disorder are outlined in the following section.

1. Recurrent episodes of binge eating. An episode of binge eating is characterized by both of the following:
   (a) eating, in a discrete period of time (e.g., within any 2-hour period), an amount of food that is definitely larger than most people would eat in a similar period of time under similar circumstances;
   (b) a sense of lack of control over eating during the episode (e.g., a feeling that one cannot stop eating or control what or how much one is eating).
2. The binge-eating episodes are associated with three (or more) of the following:
   (a) eating much more rapidly than normal;
   (b) eating until feeling uncomfortably full;
   (c) eating large amounts of food when not feeling physically hungry;
   (d) eating alone because of being embarrassed by how much one is eating;
   (e) feeling disgusted with oneself, depressed, or very guilty after overeating.
3. Marked distress regarding binge eating is present.
4. The binge eating occurs, on average, at least 2 days a week for 6 months. *Note:* The method of determining frequency differs from that used for bulimia nervosa; future research should address whether the preferred method of setting frequency threshold is counting the number of days on which binges occur or counting the number of episodes of binge eating.
5. The binge eating is not associated with the regular use of inappropriate compensatory behaviors (e.g., purging, fasting, excessive exercise) and does not occur exclusively during the course of anorexia nervosa or bulimia nervosa.

1.2.4.1 Risk Factors Contributing to Binge Eating Disorder

Since research to date on this disorder is limited, many of these statements are speculative at best. Once again, there seem to be more women experiencing this disorder than men. Individuals with binge-eating disorder are concerned with their weight and appearance.

Dieting plays an important role in the cause of binge eating. There are three harmful ways binge eaters diet. The first is by avoiding eating; these individuals may not eat all day and then binge when famished in the evening. The second is restricting the amount eaten to an unhealthy low amount, < 1200 calories. The third type of harmful dieting practices is avoiding certain types of foods. They view these tasty foods as "bad" or "forbidden" foods. It is easy to see the risk involved in these behaviors. The mood is set for a binge.

People with binge-eating disorder also seem to have low self-esteem and to have problems with assertiveness. Other common characteristics are (a) mood swings; (b) perfectionism; (c) all-or-nothing thinking; and (d) high anxiety levels.[31]

1.2.4.2   *Signs and Symptoms of Binge-Eating Disorder*

The signs and symptoms of this disorder are recurrent episodes of binge eating. It is suggested that the number of days when a binge occurs be counted rather than each binge separately. Binge episodes must occur 2 days a week on the average for at least 6 months.

Central to a binge is the feeling of loss of control. During the binge, the first few moments may seem pleasurable; however, as the individual begins to feels out of control she eats very rapidly until she is uncomfortably full. Many times binge eaters eat alone because of embarrassment over how much they are eating. Anxiety levels are high both during the binge and after; they feel disgust, guilt, and worry about the long-term effect on their body weight and shape.

There are varying forms of obesity with this disorder. Some individuals with this eating pattern are not overweight or only mildly overweight, although, on average, these individuals are more obese and have more of a marked weight fluctuation than individuals who do not exhibit this eating pattern. Most have a history of dieting efforts with repeated failures; some continue to restrict calories; some simply give up dieting altogether.

1.2.4.3   *Practical Tools to Assess the Symptoms Associated with Binge-Eating Disorder*

Self-inventory instruments designed to increase awareness of the attitudes and behaviors associated with a binge-eating disorder can be found in Appendices 1-E and 1-F. These instruments are adapted from a book on binge eating entitled *Body and Soul*.[32]

1.3   Application of Research Question

Even though eating disorders have many similar symptoms, there are distinguishing characteristics for each diagnosis. Eating disorders are multifaceted, and assessment of the disorder is a complex task. The importance of an accurate diagnosis lies in the treatment options. An individual may even vacillate between specific symptoms associated with each disorder. Multiple assessments are needed in order to provide the best possible treatment. In addition, the severity of the disorder can also be far reaching. Individuals with relatively uncomplicated eating disorders can be found in younger age groups and in college environments; however, patients seeking treatment at tertiary psychiatric treatment centers are far more complex. Early detection of the disorder is important in the recovery process. A diet and eating history question-naire that allows coding of behaviors that could suggest an eating disorder appears below. Coding instructions are included.

Dieting and Eating History*

Coding Instructions: Eating disorders exhibit similar behaviors and symptoms. Many of the responses have multiple diagnoses associated with them. To differentiate between the diagnoses, you must look at the composite of behaviors. This instrument serves only as a screening tool of eating order symptomatology; it does not serve as a formal diagnosis. Responses that may signify a specific eating disorder have been coded as follows:

AN: Anorexia Nervosa

ANR: Anorexia Nervosa, Restricting

ANBP: Anorexia Nervosa, Binge Eating/Purging

BN: Bulimia Nervosa

BNP: Bulimia Nervosa, Purging

BNN: Bulimia Nervosa Nonpurging

NOS: Eating Disorder not Otherwise Specified

BED: Binge Eating Disorder

Weight History:

Current weight_____ lb.

Current height _____ in.

Desired weight_____ lb.

[For AN, current weight is 85% of that expected.]

Have you ever been on a strict diet (fewer than 1200 calories a day)?

____ Yes   ____ No

[AN, BN, NOS, BED]

How long have you been concerned about your body weight and/or shape?

_____ years _____ months _____ days

[AN and BN, at least 3 months; NOS, < 3 months; BED, at least 6 months]

How long have you been exercising for weight control?

_____ years _____ months _____ days

[AN and BN, at least 3 months; NOS, < 3 months; BED, at least 6 months]

How long have you been fasting for weight control?

_____ years _____ months _____ days

[AN and BN, at least 3 months; NOS, < 3 months; BED, at least 6 months]

* From Kent, J.S. (1991). Bulimic women's perceptions of their family relationships. Unpublished dissertation, Texas Tech University, Lubbock, Texas. With permission.

How long have you used diuretics for weight control?

_____ years _____ months _____ days

[AN and BN, at least 3 months; NOS, < 3 months; BED, at least 6 months]

What has prevented you from seeking treatment for your eating difficulties? Check all that apply.

____ I don't have eating difficulties.

____ My eating difficulties are not severe enough for treatment.

____ Financial considerations.

____ I don't know where to obtain help.

____ I am concerned that others may learn of my eating difficulties.

____ Other (please explain).

[AN, BN, NOS, or BED; denial is a component of all four]

Have you ever received counseling or therapy for:

_____ Anorexia _____ Bulimia _____ Other

[AN, BN, NOS, BED]

Please describe the nature of counseling received:

What aspects of your difficulties do your family members know about?

On a scale of 1 (very underweight) to 10 (very overweight), where do you rank yourself compared to other women your age?

1 __ 2 __ 3 __ 4 __ 5 __ 6 __ 7 __ 8 __ 9 __ 10 __

[Very underweight: AN; average: BN, NOS, BED; very overweight: BED]

How long have you followed strict diets due to concern about your body size or weight?

____ Years

____ Months

____ Days

____ I don't restrict my food intake.

[AN and BN, at least 3 months; NOS, < 3 months; BED, at least 6 months]

Please give an example of a typical diet you follow to control your weight.

[Caloric restriction is severe in all four disorders. A diet below 1200 calories per day means avoidance of foods with high fat contents ("forbidden foods"). "Safe" foods like vegetables are allowed. The diet is unsustainable.]

Have you ever had an episode of eating a large amount of food in a short space of time (an eating binge)?

____ Yes   ____ No

[ANBP, BN, NOS, BED]

How long have you been binge eating?

_____ Years   _____ Months

_____ Days   _____ I don't binge eat.

[ANBP and BN at least 3 months, NOS < 3 months, BED at least 6 months]

On average, how often do you binge eat?

_____ Never   _____ Once a month [NOS]

_____ 2–4 times a month [NOS]   _____ 2 times a week [ANBP, BN, BED]

_____ 3–5 times a week   _____ Once a day [ANBP, BN, BED]
       [ANBP, BN, BED]

Have you been binge eating at least two times a week for the past three months?

_____ Yes [ANBP, BN, BED]   _____ No

How often do you feel out of control when you binge eat?

_____ Never   _____ Rarely [NOS]

_____ Sometimes [NOS]   _____ Often

_____ Always [ANBP, BN, BED]   _____ I don't binge eat.

Have you ever made yourself vomit after eating to get rid of the food eaten?

_____ Yes [ANBP, BNP, NOS]   _____ No

How long have you been using self-induced vomiting?

_____ Days   _____ Months

_____ Years   _____ I don't induce vomiting.

[ANBP and BNP at least 3 months; NOS < 3 months]

Have you ever used laxatives to control your weight or get rid of food?

_____ Yes [ANBP, BNP, NOS]

_____ No

_____ I don't use laxatives for weight control.

How long have you been using laxatives for weight control?

_____ Days   _____ Months

_____ Years

[ANBP and BNP at least 3 months; NOS < 3 months]

On the average, how often do you engage in the following behaviors? Check one.
Strict Dieting (under 1200 calories per day)

_____ Never   _____ Once a month

_____ 2–4 times a month   _____ 2 times a week

_____ 3–5 times a week   _____ Once a day

[All responses except "Never" could suggest any of the eating disorders.]

Fasting (skipping meals for entire day)

____ Never   ____ Once a month

____ 2–4 times a month   ____ 2 times a week

____ 3–5 times a week   ____ Once a day

____ More than once a day

[All responses except "Never" could suggest any of the eating disorders.]

Vigorous exercise (at least 20 minutes of aerobic exercise — jogging, walking, swimming, bicycling)

____ Never   ____ Once a month

____ 2–4 times a month   ____ 2 times a week

____ 3–5 times a week   ____ Once a day

____ More than once a day [AN, ANR, BNN, NOS]

[Be alert to other signs.]

Use of diuretics (water pills)

____ Never   ____ Once a month

____ 2–4 times a month   ____ 2 times a week [ANBP, BNP]

____ 3–5 times a week   ____ Once a day [ANBP, BNP]

[ANBP, BNP]

____ More than once a day [ANBP, BNP]

Laxative use

____ Never   ____ Once a month

____ 2–4 times a month   ____ 2 times a week [ANBP, BNP]

____ 3–5 times a week   ____ Once a day (ANBP, BNP)

[ANBP, BNP]

____ More than once a day [ANBP, BNP)]

Vomiting

____ Never   ____ Once a month

____ 2–4 times a month   ____ 2 times a week [ANBP, BNP]

____ 3–5 times a week   ____ Once a day [ANBP, BNP]

[ANBP, BNP]

____ More than once a day [ANBP, BNP]

Are any of your family members aware of your eating difficulties?

____ Yes

____ No

____ I don't have eating difficulties

If you answered yes to the preceding question, which family members are aware of your eating difficulties?

Since high school, have you stolen anything?

____ Yes   ____ No

If yes, please describe types of items stolen:

[Impulse control disorders are common in BN]

Menstrual History

Age at onset of menses (mark 0 if you have never had a period) ____

How regular are your cycles?

____ Fairly regular (same number of days +3)

____ Somewhat irregular (variation of 4–10 days)

____ Very irregular (variation greater than 10 days) [Be alert to other signs associated with AN.]

____ Never menstruated [AN]

How many time have you skipped periods for 3 months or more when you were not pregnant? [One or more, AN]

If an eating disorder is suspected, the individual should be encouraged to seek professional guidance and counseling. Trained professionals should attempt at the onset to build trust, establish mutual respect, and establish a caring relationship. Initial assessment generally includes (a) a longitudinal history regarding lifetime actual and desired weight in relation to height; (b) onset and patterns of menstruation; (c) food restriction and avoidance; (d) frequency and extent of binge eating; (e) self-induced vomiting and spontaneous vomiting; (f) use of laxatives, diuretics, diet pills, and ipecac; and (g) body image and self-image disturbances. An example of a questionnaire that could be used in a clinical setting can be found in Appendix 1-G.

References

1. Romeo, F., Adolescent boys and anorexia nervosa, *Adolescence*, 29(115), 643–647, 1994.
2. Kendler, K. S., MacLean, C., Neale, M., Kessler, R., Heath, A., and Eaves, L., The genetic epidemiology of bulimia nervosa, *American Journal of Psychiatry*, 148, 1627–1637, 1991.
3. American Psychiatric Association, Practice guidelines for eating disorders, *American Journal of Psychiatry*, 150(2), 207–225, 1993.
4. Soukup, V. M., Beiler, M. E., and Terrell, F. Stress, coping style, and problem-solving ability among eating-disordered inpatients, *Journal of Clinical Psychology*, 46(5), 592–599, 1990.
5. American Psychiatric Association, *Diagnostic and Statistical Manual of Mental Disorders IV*, Washington, D.C.: 1994, 539–555, 729.
6. Welch, G., Hall, A., Renner, R., and Norring, The factor structure of the eating disorders inventory, *International Journal of Eating Disorders*, 9, 79–85, 1990.
7. Russel, G. F. M., Bulimia nervosa: an ominous variant of anorexia nervosa, *Psychological Medicine*, 9, 429–448, 1979.
8. Haimes, A. L., and Katz, J. L., Sexual and social maturity versus social conformity in restricting anorectic, bulimic, and borderline women, *International Journal of Eating Disorders*, 7, 331–334, 1988.

9. Laessle, R. G., Beumont, P. J., Butow, P., Lennerts, W., O'Conner, M., Pirke, K. M., Touyz, S. W., and Waadt, S., A comparison of nutritional management with stress management in the treatment of bulimia nervosa, *British Journal of Psychiatry*, 159, 250–261, 1991.

10. U. S. Department of Health and Human Services, Health Care Financing Administration, *International Classification of Diseases* (9th revision, clinical modification), Washington, D.C.: Office of Research and Demonstrations, 1984.

11. French, S. A., Perry, C. L., Leon, G. R., and Fulkerson, J. A., Food preferences, eating patterns, and physical activity among adolescents: correlates of eating disorder symptoms, *Journal of Adolescent Health*, 15, 286–294, 1993.

12. Sundgot-Borgen, J., Risk and trigger factors for the development of eating disorders in female elite athletes, *Medicine and Science in Sports and Exercise*, 26(4), 414–419, 1994.

13. Dalsky, G. P., Effect of exercise on bone: permissive influence of estrogen and calcium, *Medicine and Science in Sports and Exercise*, 22(3), 281–285, 1990.

14. Strauss, J. and Ryan, R. M., Autonomy disturbances in subtypes of anorexia nervosa, *Journal of Abnormal Psychology*, 96, 254–258, 1987.

15. Garner, D. M. and Garfinkel, P. E., The eating attitudes test: an index of the symptoms of anorexia nervosa, *Psychological Medicine*, 9, 273–279, 1979.

16. Roth, B. and Creaser, T., Mindfulness meditation-based stress reduction: experience with a bi-lingual inner-city program, *The Nurse Practitioner*, 22(3), 150–176, 1997.

17. Johnson, M., Disordered eating in active and athletic women, *The Athletic Woman*, 13(2), 355–369, 1994.

18. Whitaker, A., Johnson, J., Schaffer, D., Rapoport, J. L. Kalikow, K., Walsh, B. T., Davies, M., Braiman, S., and Dolinsky, A., Uncommon troubles in young people: Prevalence estimates of selected psychiatric disorders in a nonreferred adolescent population, *Archives of General Psychiatry*, 47, 487–496, 1990.

19. Striegel-Moore, R. H., Silberstein, L. R., and Rodin, J., Toward an understanding of risk factors for bulimia, *American Psychologist*, 41(3), 246–263, 1986.

20. Neckowitz, P. and Morrison, T. L. Interactional coping strategies of normal-weight bulimic women in intimate and nonintimate stressful situations, *Psychological Reports*, 69, 1167–1175, 1991.

21. Kent, J.S. and Clopton, J. R., Bulimic women's perceptions of their family relationships, *Journal of Clinical Psychology*, 48, 281–292, 1992.

22. Yager, J. Landsverk, J. Lee-Benner, K., and Johnson, C., The continuum of eating disorders: An examination of diagnostic concerns based on a national survey. Unpublished manuscript, Neuropsychiatric Institute, University of California, Los Angeles, 1985.

23. Polivy, J. and Herman, C. P., Dieting and binging: A causal analysis, *American Psychologist*, 40, 193–201, 1985.

24. Kaye, W., H., Weltzin, T., E., McKee, M., McConaha, C., Hansen, D., and Hsu, L., K., G., Laboratory assessment of feeding behavior in bulimia nervosa and healthy women: methods for developing a human feeding laboratory, *American Journal of Clinical Nutrition*, 55, 372–380, 1992.

25. Hetherington, M., M., Altemus, M., Nelson, M. L., Bernat, A., S., and Gold, P. W., Eating behavior in bulimia nervosa: multiple meal analysis. *American Journal of Clinical Nutrition*, 60, 864–873, 1994.

26. Henderson, M. and Freeman, C. P., A self-rating scale for bulimia: the BITE, *British Journal of Psychiatry*, 150, 18–24, 1987.

27. Thelan, M., BULLIT-R, *Journal of Consulting and Clinical Psychology*, 52, 863–872.

28. Kirkley, B. G. and Burge, J. C., Dietary restriction in young women: issues and concerns. *Annals of Behavioral Medicine*, 11, 66–72, 1989.

29. Kirk, S., Nutritional counseling in bulimia nervosa. A case study, *Journal of Human Nutrition and Dietetics*, 6, 57–61, 1993.

30. Garner, D., *Eating Disorder Inventory 2*, Psychological Resources, Inc., Odessa, TX, 1990, chap. 2–3.

31. Fairburn, C., *Overcoming Binge Eating*, New York, Guilford Press, 1995, chap. 2.

32. Meltsner, S., *Body and Soul*, Hazelden Educational Materials, Center City, MN, 1993, chap. 1, 4.

Appendix 1-A: Rules of Thumb for Growth and Weight by Age Percentiles Graph for Girls

Weight

1. Weight loss in first few days: 5–10% of birth weight
2. Return to birth weight: 7–10 days of age
   Double birth weight: 4–5 mo
   Triple birth weight: 1 yr
   Quadruple birth weight: 2 yr
3. Average weights: 3.5 kg at birth
                        10 kg at 1 yr
                        20 kg at 5 yr
                        30 kg at 10 yr
4. Daily weight gain: 20–30 g for first 3–4 mo
                        15–20 g for rest of the first yr
5. Average annual weight gain: 5 lb between 2 yr and puberty (spurts and plateaus may occur)

Height

1. Average length: 20 in. at birth, 30 in. at 1 yr
2. At age 3 yr, the average child is 3 ft tall
3. At age 4 yr, the average child is 40 in. tall (double birth length)
4. Average annual height increase: 2–3 in. between age 4 yr and puberty

Head Circumference (HC)

1. Average HC: 35 cm at birth (13.5 in.)
2. HC increases: 1 cm/mo for first yr (2 cm/mo for first 3 mo, then slower)
                  10 cm for rest of life

Source: From Behrman, R. E., and Kliegman, R. M., *Nelson's Essentials of Pediatrics*, 3rd ed., W. B. Saunders, 1998. With permission.

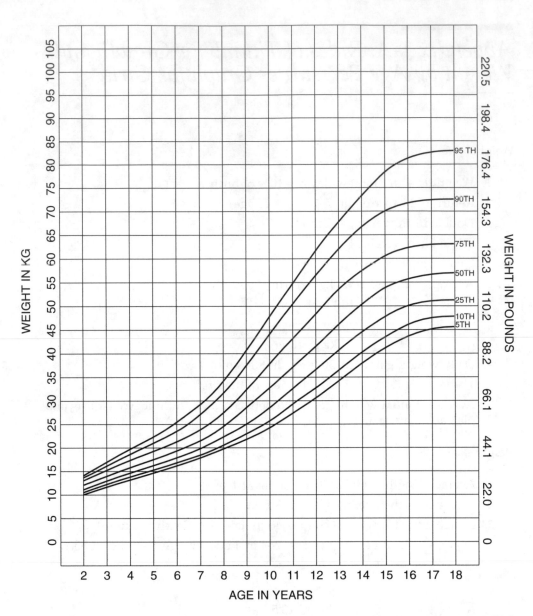

Source: From Hamill, P.V.V., Drizd, T.A., and Johnson, C.L., et al., *Am. J. Clin. Nutr.*, 32, 607, 1979. With permission.

Appendix 1-B: Metropolitan Life Insurance Companies' Height and Weight Tables

How to approximate frame size: Extend patient's arm and bend forearm upward at 90° angle. With fingers straight, turn inside of wrist toward body. Place your thumb and index finger on the prominent bones on either side of elbow. Measure space between thumb and forefinger against ruler or tape measure. Compare with measurements listed on chart, which indicates elbow widths for medium framed men and women. Measurements lower than those listed indicate small frame. Higher measurements indicate a large frame.

Men		Women	
Height in 1" heels	Elbow Breadth	Height in 1" heels	Elbow Breadth
5'2"–5'3"	2 1/2"–2 7/8"	4'10"–4'11"	2 1/4"–2 1/2"
5'4"–5'7"	2 5/8"–2 7/8"	5'0"–5'3"	2 1/4"–2 1/2"
5'8"–5'11"	2 3/4"–2"	5'4"–5'7"	2 3/8"–2 5/8"
6'0"–6'3"	2 3/4"–3 1/8"	5'8"–5'11"	2 3/8"–2 5/8"
6'4"	2 7/8"–3 1/4"	6'0"	2 1/2"–2 3/4"

Ideal Weight[a]

Men				Women			
Height	Small Frame	Medium Frame	Large Frame	Height	Small Frame	Medium Frame	Large Frame
5'2"	128–134	131–141	138–150	4'10"	102–111	109–121	118–131
5'3"	130–136	133–143	140–153	4'11"	103–113	111–123	120–134
5'4"	132–138	135–145	142–156	5'0"	104–115	113–126	122–137
5'5"	134–140	137–148	144–160	5'1"	106–118	115–129	125–140
5'6"	136–142	139–151	146–164	5'2"	108–121	118–132	128–143
5'7"	138–145	142–154	149–168	5'3"	111–124	121–135	131–147
5'8"	140–148	145–157	152–172	5'4"	114–127	124–138	134–151
5'9"	142–151	148–160	155–176	5'5"	117–130	127–141	137–155
5'10"	144–154	151–163	158–180	5'6"	120–133	130–144	140–159
5'11"	146–157	154–166	161–184	5'7"	123–136	133–147	143–163
6'0"	149–160	157–170	164–188	5'8"	126–139	136–150	146–167
6'1"	152–164	160–174	168–192	5'9"	129–142	139–153	149–170
6'2"	155–168	164–178	172–197	5'10"	132–145	142–156	152–173
6'3"	158–172	167–182	176–202	5'11"	135–148	145–159	155–176
6'4"	162–176	171–187	181–207	6'0"	138–151	148–162	158–179

[a] Weights at ages 25 to 59 based on lowest mortality. Source of basic data: 1979 Build Study, Society of Actuaries and Association of Life Insurance Medical Directors of America, 1980.

Appendix 1-C: Eating Attitude Test

Please place an (X) under the column which applies best to each of the numbered statements. All of the results will be *strictly* confidential. Most of the questions directly relate to food or eating, although other types of questions have been included. Please answer each question carefully. Thank you.

Answer Key:　A=Always　V=Very Often　O=Often　S=Sometimes　R=Rarely　N=Never

A　V　O　S　R　N

( )( )( )( )( )(X)[†] 1. Like eating with other people.

( )( )( )( )( )( ) 2. Prepare foods for others but do not eat what I cook.

(X)( )( )( )( )( ) 3. Become anxious prior to eating.

(X)( )( )( )( )( ) 4. Am terrified about being overweight.

(X)( )( )( )( )( ) 5. Avoid eating when I am hungry.

(X)( )( )( )( )( ) 6. Find myself preoccupied with food.

(X)( )( )( )( )( ) 7. Have gone on eating binges where I feel that I may not be able to stop.

(X)( )( )( )( )( ) 8. Cut my food into small pieces.

(X)( )( )( )( )( ) 9. Aware of the calorie content of foods that I eat.

(X)( )( )( )( )( ) 10. Particularly avoid foods with a high carbohydrate content (e.g. bread, potatoes, rice, etc.).

(X)( )( )( )( )( ) 11. Feel bloated after meals.

(X)( )( )( )( )( ) 12. Feel that others would prefer if I ate more.

(X)( )( )( )( )( ) 13. **Vomit after I have eaten.

(X)( )( )( )( )( ) 14. Feel extremely guilty after eating.

(X)( )( )( )( )( ) 15. **Am preoccupied with a desire to be thinner.

(X)( )( )( )( )( ) 16. Exercise strenuously to burn off calories.

(X)( )( )( )( )( ) 17. **Weigh myself several times a day.

( )( )( )( )( )(X) 18. #Like my clothes to fit tightly.

( )( )( )( )( )(X) 19. Enjoy eating meat.

(X)( )( )( )( )( ) 20. Wake up early in the morning.

A　V　O　S　R　N

( )( )( )( )( )( ) 21. Eat the same foods day after day.

( )( )( )( )( )(X) 22. Think about burning up calories when I exercise.

( )( )( )( )( )(X) 23. Have regular menstrual periods.

(X)( )( )( )( )( ) 24. Other people think that I am too thin.

(X)( )( )( )( )( ) 25. Am preoccupied with the thought of having fat on my body.

(X)( )( )( )( )( ) 26. Take longer than others to eat my meals.

( )( )( )( )( )( ) 27. Enjoy eating at restaurants.

(X)( )( )( )( )( ) 28. **Take laxatives.

(X)( )( )( )( )( ) 29. Avoid foods with sugar in them.

(X)( )( )( )( )( ) 30. Eat diet foods.

(X)( )( )( )( )( ) 31. Feel that food controls my life.

(X)( )( )( )( )( ) 32. Display self-control around food.

(X)( )( )( )( )( ) 33. Feel that others pressure me to eat.

(X)( )( )( )( )( ) 34. Give too much time and thought to food.

(X)( )( )( )( )( ) 35. *Suffer from constipation.

(X)( )( )( )( )( ) 36. Feel uncomfortable after eating sweets.

(X)( )( )( )( )( ) 37. Engage in dieting behavior.

(X)( )( )( )( )( ) 38. Like my stomach to be empty.

( )( )( )( )( )(X) 39. Enjoy trying rich foods.

(X)( )( )( )( )( ) 40. Have the impulse to vomit after meals.

The 'X' represents the most 'symptomatic' response and would receive a score of 3 points.
* $P < 0.05$, *t*-test.　** $P < 0.01$, *t*-test.　# $P < 0.05$, *t*-test.
For all remaining items, group means differed at the $P < 0.001$ level of confidence with a *t*-test.

Scoring the EAT

The 'X' represents the most 'symptomatic' response and receives a score of 3 points, while the adjacent alternatives receive scores of 2 points and 1 point, respectively. Mean EAT Scores and SD are given for specific groups.

Anorexia nervosa	(N = 33)	Mean = 58.9,	SD =13.3
Normal controls	(N = 59)	Mean = 15.6,	SD = 9.3
Male controls	(N = 49)	Mean = 8.6,	SD = 5.3
Obese subjects	(N = 16)	Mean = 16.5,	SD = 9.6
Clinically recovered anorexia nervosa	(N = 9)	Mean = 11.4,	SD = 5.1

Source: From Garner, D. M., and Garfinkel, P. E., *Psychological Medicine*, 9, 273–279, 1979. With permission.

Appendix 1-D: "Are You Dying To Be Thin?" Awareness Instrument

Are You Dying To Be Thin?

Due to an increase in publicity and public awareness, anorexia nervosa (key symptom: extreme weight loss due to self-starvation accompanied by an intense fear of being fat or gaining weight) and bulimia nervosa (key symptom: binge eating — eating what the individual considers to be too much food in a way that feels out of control — followed by purging) are becoming more and more openly acknowledged.

The following questionnaire will tell you whether or not you think or behave in a way that indicates that you have tendencies toward anorexia nervosa or bulimia nervosa.

DIRECTIONS: Answer the questions below honestly. Respond as you are now, not the way you used to be or the way you would like to be. Write the number of your answer in the space at the left. Do not leave any questions blank unless instructed to do so.

_____ 1. I have eating habits that are different from those of my family and friends.
   1] Often   2] Sometimes   3] Rarely   4] Never

_____ 2. I find myself panicking if I cannot exercise as I planned because I am afraid I will gain weight if don't.
   1] Often   2] Sometimes   3] Rarely   4] Never

_____ 3. My friends tell me I am thin, but I don't believe them because I feel fat.
   1] Often   2] Sometimes   3] Rarely   4] Never

_____ 4. *(Females only)* My menstrual period has stopped or become irregular due to no known medical reasons.
   1] True   2] False

_____ 5. I have become obsessed with food to the point that I cannot go through a day without worrying about what I will or will not eat.
   1] Almost always   2] Sometimes   3] Rarely   4] Never

_____ 6. I have lost more than 15% of what is considered a healthy weight for my height (e.g., female 5'4" tall healthy weight — 122 lbs, lost 20 lbs) and currently weigh that weight or less.
   1] True   2] False

_____ 7. I would panic if I got on the scale tomorrow and found out I had gained 2 lbs.
   1] Almost always   2] Sometimes   3] Rarely   4] Never

_____ 8. I find that I prefer to eat alone or when I am sure no one will see me, thus make excuses so I can eat less and less with friends and family.
   1] Often   2] Sometimes   3] Rarely   4] Never

_____ 9. I find myself going on uncontrollable eating binges during which I consume large amounts of food to the point that I feel sick and make myself vomit.

1] Never   2] Less than 1 time per week

3] 1–6 times per week   4] 1 or more times per day

_____ 10. *(NOTE: Answer only if your answer to #9 is "1", otherwise leave blank.)* I find myself compulsively eating more than I want to while feeling out of control and/or unaware of what I am doing.

1] Never   2] Less than 1 time per week

3] 1–6 times per week   4] 1 or more times per day

_____ 11. I use laxatives or diuretics as a means of weight control.

1] Never   2] Rarely   3] Sometimes   4] On a regular basis

_____ 12. I find myself playing games with food (e.g., cutting it up into tiny pieces, hiding food so people will think I ate it, chewing it and spitting it out without swallowing it, keeping hidden stashes of food) and/or telling myself certain foods are bad.

1] Often   2] Sometimes   3] Rarely   4] Never

_____ 13. People around me have become very interested in what I eat and I find myself getting angry at them for pushing me to eat more.

1] Often   2] Sometimes   3] Rarely   4] Never

_____ 14. I have felt more depressed and irritable recently than I used to and/or have been spending an increasing amount of time alone.

1] True   2] False

_____ 15. I keep a lot of my fears about food and eating to myself because I am afraid no one would understand.

1] Often   2] Sometimes   3] Rarely   4] Never

_____ 16. I enjoy making gourmet and/or high calorie meals for others as long as I don't have to eat any myself.

1] Often   2] Sometimes   3] Rarely   4] Never

_____ 17. The most powerful fear in my life is the fear of gaining weight or becoming fat.

1] Often   2] Sometimes   3] Rarely   4] Never

_____ 18. I exercise a lot (more than 4 times per week and/or more than 4 hours per week) as a means of weight control.

1] True   2] False

_____ 19. I find myself totally absorbed when reading books or magazines about dieting, exercising and calorie counting to the point that I spend hours studying them.

1] Often   2] Sometimes   3] Rarely   4] Never

_____ 20. I tend to be a perfectionist and am not satisfied with myself unless I do things perfectly.

1] Almost always   2] Sometimes   3] Rarely   4] Never

_____ 21. I go through long periods of time without eating (fasting) or eating very little as a means of weight control.

1] Often   2] Sometimes   3] Rarely   4] Never

_____ 22. It is important to me to try to be thinner than all of my friends.

1] Almost always   2] Sometimes   3] Rarely   4] Never

Scoring

Step 1: Add scores together. **Total is** _____.

Step 2: Compare your score with the table below.

38 or less   – Strong tendencies toward anorexia nervosa.

39–50   – Strong tendencies toward bulimia nervosa.

50–60   – Weight conscious. May or may not have tendencies toward an eating disorder. Not likely to have anorexia or bulimia nervosa. May have tendencies toward compulsive eating or obesity.

Over 60   – Extremely unlikely to have anorexia or bulimia nervosa, however, scoring over 60 does not rule out tendencies toward compulsive eating or obesity.

If you scored below 50, it would be wise for you to (1) seek more information about anorexia nervosa and bulimia nervosa and (2) contact a counselor, pastor, teacher, or physician in order to find out if you have an eating disorder, and if you do, talk about what kind of assistance would be best for you.

If you scored between 50 and 60, it would be a good idea for you to talk to a counselor, pastor, teacher, or physician in order to find out if you have an eating disorder, and if you do, how to get some help.

If you scored over 60 but have questions and concerns about the way you eat and/or your weight, it would be a good idea for you to talk to a counselor, pastor, teacher, or physician in order to determine if you have an eating disorder and if you do, how to get some help.

Note! Eating disorders are potentially life-threatening disorders which can be overcome with the proper information, support, and counseling. The earlier you seek help, the better, although it is never too late to start on the road to recovery.

Source: From Reiff, D. W., *Eating Disorders: Nutrition Therapy in the Recovery Process,* Aspen Publishers, 1992. With permission.

Appendix 1-E: Attitudes and Behaviors Associated with a Binge-Eating Disorder

This tool is a self-inventory instrument designed to increase awareness of the attitudes and behaviors associated with a binge-eating disorder. Please read these questions and answer them honestly. If upon reflection, you think that you may be a victim of behaviors associated with binge eating disorders, you may want to seek help from a trained professional.

Do you worry a great deal about your weight or body size?

_____ almost always   _____ often   _____ sometimes

_____ occasionally   _____ almost never

Do you weigh yourself several times a day or repeatedly compare yourself to others and wish you could look like them?

_____ almost always   _____ often   _____ sometimes

_____ occasionally   _____ almost never

Are there a lot of frustrating shoulds and shouldn'ts where food is concerned in your life?

_____ almost always   _____ often   _____ sometimes

_____ occasionally   _____ almost never

Do you suffer from bouts of sadness or anxiety?

_____ almost always   _____ often   _____ sometimes

_____ occasionally   _____ almost never

Are you still overeating or yo-yo dieting despite one or more of the following medical complications: hypertension, arteriosclerosis, diabetes, gallbladder disease, or impaired breathing?

_____ almost always   _____ often   _____ sometimes

_____ occasionally   _____ almost never

Do you isolate yourself, staying at home or keeping an emotional distance from people because they might reject you, criticize you, try to change your eating habits, or delay or interfere with what you'd rather be doing (that is, eating or binging and purging)?

_____ almost always   _____ often   _____ sometimes

_____ occasionally   _____ almost never

Do you eat like a bird in front of others and then pig out when you're alone?

_____ almost always   _____ often   _____ sometimes

_____ occasionally   _____ almost never

Do you become defensive if anyone tries to suggest that you do something about your eating habits?

_____ almost always   _____ often   _____ sometimes

_____ occasionally   _____ almost never

Do you insist that you can get your eating, dieting excesses, or binging and purging under control whenever you make up your mind to even though it has not worked in the past?

_____ almost always   _____ often   _____ sometimes

_____ occasionally   _____ almost never

Adapted from Meltsner, S., *Body and Soul*, Hazelden Educational Materials, Center City, MN, 1993.

Appendix 1-F: What Do Food and Being Overweight Mean to You?

Please read this self-inventory and answer the questions honestly. If you find that many of these questions are true for you, you may want to further explore the meaning you assign to food and what your body image means to you.

Has food been a substitute for love?

_____ frequently _____ sometimes _____ rarely _____ never

Has food filled the void left by the absence of close relationships?

_____ frequently _____ sometimes _____ rarely _____ never

Have you nurtured yourself with food — feeding yourself when you longed for another person's care?

_____ frequently _____ sometimes _____ rarely _____ never

Have you reached for food when a deadline was approaching or a conflict was brewing?

_____ frequently _____ sometimes _____ rarely _____ never

Have you eaten out of frustration or impatience when things didn't go the way you wanted?

_____ frequently _____ sometimes _____ rarely _____ never

Have you used eating to get back at someone or prove that you weren't entirely controlled by someone who made unreasonable demands or stifled you in some other way?

_____ frequently _____ sometimes _____ rarely _____ never

Have you used food as consolation or solace for various losses or disappointments?

_____ frequently _____ sometimes _____ rarely _____ never

After making a mistake or otherwise "misbehaving" have you overeaten and then berated yourself for it?

_____ frequently _____ sometimes _____ rarely _____ never

How has food assisted you in blocking out unacceptable emotions? How often have you eaten instead of expressing or acknowledging

FEAR?	___ frequently	___ sometimes	___ rarely ___ never
HATE?	___ frequently	___ sometimes	___ rarely ___ never
ANGER?	___ frequently	___ sometimes	___ rarely ___ never
SADNESS?	___ frequently	___ sometimes	___ rarely ___ never
ANXIETY?	___ frequently	___ sometimes	___ rarely ___ never
GUILT?	___ frequently	___ sometimes	___ rarely ___ never
SEXUAL IMPULSES?	___ frequently	___ sometimes	___ rarely ___ never

Fat can be a social barrier signaling our desire to be left alone or supplying us with an excuse to avoid certain social interactions. How likely is it that you used your weight that way?

_____ very likely ___ quite likely _____ somewhat likely _____ very unlikely

Fat can be a protective barrier against unwanted sexual overtures, our own sexual impulses, and the guilt, shame, vulnerability, intimacy, or victimization that could result from either or both. How likely is it that you used your weight that way?

_____ very likely ___ quite likely _____ somewhat likely _____ very unlikely

Fat can be a handy explanation for rejection, failure, or lack of companionship. Better to be passed over for a promotion because "society discriminates against fat people" or to be dateless on a Saturday night because "men aren't interested in women who don't look like cover girls" than because of some other deficiency. How likely is it that you used your weight that way?

_____ very likely ___ quite likely _____ somewhat likely _____ very unlikely

Being fat can be a way to keep others from expecting too much of us. By taking advantage of the assumptions that fat people are lazy, undisciplined, physically unhealthy, and difficult to take seriously, we get out of anything from mowing the lawn to chairing a committee. How likely is it that you used your weight that way?

_____ very likely ___ quite likely _____ somewhat likely _____ very unlikely

Being fat can be a form of self-punishment. Suffering from low self-esteem and years of dieting failure, we hang on to our extra-large bodies as retribution for being "rotten" or "stupid." In addition, because success, serenity, and happiness are so out of sync with our internal belief system, when we sense that things are going too well, we begin to take back weight we've lost and further punish ourselves by feeling bad about it. How likely is it that you used your weight that way?

_____ very likely ___ quite likely _____ somewhat likely _____ very unlikely

Fat can help us project a more powerful physical presence and create the impression that we are stronger or more substantial than we might otherwise appear to be. In business as well as in personal relationships we can gain an advantage by intimidating others with our size. How likely is it that you used your weight that way?

_____ very likely ___ quite likely _____ somewhat likely _____ very unlikely

Finally, being overweight can be a means of expressing anger and resentment, especially toward parents, spouses, or other people who put a lot of stock in physical appearances. By keeping weight on — or even adding a few more pounds — we're able to get back at those who nag us to lose weight or insinuate that we are less lovable or capable because of it. How likely is it that you used your weight that way?

_____ very likely ___ quite likely _____ somewhat likely _____ very unlikely

Adapted from Meltsner, S., *Body and Soul*, Hazelden Educational Materials, Center City, MN, 1993.

Appendix 1-G: Personal History Questionnaire

Directions: Enter your name, the date, your age, sex, marital status, and occupation. Complete the questions on the rest of this page. Then turn to the next page and carefully follow the instructions.

Name _____   Date _____

Age_____   Sex _____   Marital status_____   Occupation _____

A. Current weight: _____ pounds
B. Height: _____ feet   _____ inches
C. Highest past weight excluding pregnancy: _____ pounds
    How long ago did you first reach this weight? _____ months
    How long did you weigh this weight? _____ months
D. Lowest weight as an adult: _____ pounds
    How long ago did you first reach this weight? _____ months
    How long did you weigh this weight? _____ months
E. What weight have you been at for the longest period of time? _____ pounds
    At what age did you first reach this weight? _____ years old
F. If your weight has changed a lot over the years, is there a weight that you keep coming back to when you are not dieting? _____ Yes _____ No
    If yes, what is this weight? _____ pounds
    At what age did you first reach this weight? _____ years old
G. What is the most weight you have ever lost? _____ pounds
    Did you lose this weight on purpose? _____ Yes _____ No
    What weight did you lose to? _____ pounds
    At what age did you reach this weight? _____ years old
H. What do you think your weight would be if you did not consciously try to control your weight? _____ pounds
I. How much would you like to weigh? _____ pounds
J. Age at which weight problems began (if any): _____ years old
K. Father's occupation: _____
L. Mother's occupation: _____

The next set of questions pertain to the topic in ALL CAPS preceding the set of questions. Please answer the questions as honestly as possible. All information is confidential.

M. DIETING
    Have you *ever* restricted your food intake due to concerns about your body size or weight? _____ Yes _____ No

How old were you *the very first time* that you began to seriously restrict your food intake due to concern about your body size or weight?
_____ years old

N. EXERCISE

On average, over the *last 3 months*, how often have you exercised (including going on walks, riding a bicycle, etc.)? If you exercise more than once a day, please count the *total number of times* that you exercise in a typical week. _____ times a week

   On average, how long do you exercise each time _____ minutes

   What percentage of your exercise is aimed at controlling your weight?

   _____ 0%   _____ less than 25%   _____ 25–50%   _____ 50–75%

   _____ more than 75%   _____ 100%

O. BINGE EATING

Please remember in answering the following questions that an eating binge *only* refers to eating an amount of food that others of your age and sex regard as *unusually large*. It does *not* include times when you may have eaten a normal quantity of food which you would have preferred not to have eaten.

Have you *ever* had an episode of eating an amount of food that others would regard as *unusually large*?

_____ Yes   _____ No

If no, please skip to Question P.

How old were you when you *first* had an eating binge? _____ years old

How old were you when you began binge eating on a regular basis?
_____ years old

   During the *last 3 months*, how often have you typically has an eating binge?

   _____ I have not binged in the last 3 months.

   _____ Monthly–I usually binge _____ time(s) a month.

   _____ Weekly–I usually binge _____ time(s) a week.

   _____ Daily–I usually binge _____ time(s) a day.

At the *worst* of times, what was your average number of binges per week?
_____ binges per week

How long ago was that? _____ months ago _____ at its worst right now

If you have not binged in the last 3 months, please skip to Question P.

Do you feel out of control when you binge?
___ Never ___ Rarely ___ Sometimes ___ Often ___ Usually ___ Always

Do you feel that you can stop once a binge has started?
___ Never ___ Rarely ___ Sometimes ___ Often ___ Usually ___ Always

Do you feel that you can prevent a binge from starting in the first place?
___ Never ___ Rarely ___ Sometimes ___ Often ___ Usually ___ Always

Do you feel you can control you *urges* to eat large quantities of food?
___ Never ___ Rarely ___ Sometimes ___ Often ___ Usually ___ Always

Do you feel distressed by your binging?
___ Never ___ Rarely ___ Sometimes ___ Often ___ Usually ___ Always

Do you find binging pleasurable?
___ Never ___ Rarely ___ Sometimes ___ Often ___ Usually ___ Always

P. PURGING

Have you *ever* tried to vomit after eating in order to get rid of the food eaten?
_____ Yes _____ No
If no, please skip to Question Q.

How old were you when you induced vomiting for the first time?
_____ years old
During the *last 3 months*, how often have you typically induced vomiting?
_____ I have not vomited in the last 3 months.
_____ Monthly–I usually vomit _____ time(s) a month.
_____ Weekly–I usually vomit _____ time(s) a week.
_____ Daily–I usually vomit _____ time(s) a day.
At the *worst* of times, what was your average number of vomiting episodes per week? _____
How long ago was that? _____ months

Q. LAXATIVES

Have you ever used laxatives to control your weight or get rid of food?
_____ Yes _____ No
If no, please skip to Question R.

How old were you when you *first* took laxatives for weight control?
_____ years old
How old were you when you began taking laxatives for weight control on a regular basis? _____ years old
During the *last 3 months*, how often have you been taking laxatives for weight control?
_____ I have not taken laxatives in the last 3 months.
_____ Monthly–I usually take laxatives _____ time(s) a month.
_____ Weekly–I usually take laxatives _____ time(s) a week.
_____ Daily–I usually take laxatives _____ time(s) a day.
How many laxatives do you usually take each time? _____ laxatives
What kind of laxatives do you take? _____
*At the *worst* of times, what was the average number of laxatives that you were taking per week? _____ laxatives per week.
How long ago was that? _____ months

R. DIET PILLS
Have you ever taken diet pills? _____ Yes   _____ No
If no, please skip to Question S.

*During the last 3 months, how often have you typically taken diet pills?
_____ I have not taken diet pills in the last 3 months.
_____ Monthly–I usually take diet pills _____ times a month.
_____ Weekly–I usually take diet pills _____ times a week.
_____ Daily–I usually take _____ diet pills a day.
*At the worst of times, what was the average number of diet pills that you were taking per week? _____ diet pills per week
How long ago was that? _____ months

S. DIURETICS
Have you ever taken diuretics (water pills) to control your weight?
_____ Yes   _____ No
If no, please skip to Question T.

During the last 3 months, How often have you typically taken diuretics?
_____ I have not taken diuretics in the last 3 months.
_____ Monthly–I usually take diuretics _____ time(s) a month.
_____ Weekly–I usually take diuretics _____ time(s) a week.
_____ Daily–I usually take _____ diuretics a day.
At the worst of times, what was the average number of diuretics that you were taking per week? _____
How long ago was that? _____ months

T. MENSTRUAL HISTORY
(For females only)
Have you ever had a menstrual period? _____ Yes   _____ No
Do you have menstrual periods now? (check one)
_____ Yes, regularly every month.
_____ Yes, but I skip a month once in a while.
_____ Yes, but not very often (for example, once in 6 months).
_____ No, I have not had a period in at least 6 months.
_____ No, I am post-menopausal, have had a hysterectomy, or am pregnant.
How long has it been since your last period? _____ months
Have you ever has a period of time when you did not menstruate for 3 months or more (excluding pregnancy)? _____ Yes   _____ No
If yes, how old were you when you first missed your period for 3 months or more? _____ years old
For how many months did you miss your period? _____ months
How much did you weigh when you stopped menstruating? _____ pounds

Are you currently taking birth control pills _____ Yes _____ No

    If yes, how old were you when you first starting using the pill?

    _____ years old

U. CURRENT MEDICATION

    Are you currently taking any medication prescribed by a physician?

    _____ Yes _____ No

If yes, please list the medications you are taking.

_____

_____

_____

2

Psychology of an Eating Disorder

Heather L. Haas and James R. Clopton

CONTENTS

2.1 Learning Objectives

After completing this chapter you should be able to:

- Identify aspects of adolescence that contribute to the development of eating disorders;

- Explain why certain adolescents are more likely to develop eating disorders than others;

- Identify personality characteristics that are often associated with eating disorders, and understand how those characteristics may precipitate or perpetuate the disorder;

- Use your knowledge of the personality characteristics typically associated with eating disorders to devise the most appropriate treatment plan for eating disordered women;

- Identify reasons why ignoring comorbid personality characteristics in the treatment of eating disorders may lead to relapse or failure to recover.

2.2   Research Background

2.2.1   Adolescence

Eating disorders occur most often during adolescence, with estimates that up to 20% of high-school and college-aged women have eating disorders, and that more than 50% of women in this age group are dissatisfied with their body size and shape.[1] The high rates of disturbed eating behaviors and attitudes that prevail among adolescents seem even more pronounced when compared to the estimated 1 to 3% prevalence rate of eating disorders in the general population.[2] Symptoms of eating disorders are most common during adolescence and decrease in frequency following the adolescent stage of development.[3]

While there is consensus that eating disorders generally increase during ages 15 to 19, there is less understanding as to why such an increase occurs and whether disordered eating patterns are present before adolescence. The bulk of the research on eating disorders has been conducted with adolescent girls or young women, but several studies have focused on children. The groundwork for the development of eating disorders appears to be laid when children learn to equate "fat" with "bad" several years before reaching adolescence. Young children believe being fat is bad, but they do not yet associate thinness with attractiveness.[4] Thus, while it is evident that some characteristics related to eating disorders begin in childhood, it appears that events and issues specific to the age of adolescence are responsible for fueling the fire of disturbed eating attitudes and behaviors. The actual process of going through puberty can serve as one of the major catalysts in the development of an eating disorder.[5] Thus, in order to better understand and help eating-disordered women, it is imperative to gain an understanding of important issues and events that often serve as precipitating factors in the development of eating disorders during adolescence.

2.2.1.1   *Physical and Mental Changes*

The period of adolescence is a difficult one, which few adults would care to repeat. Many of us can all too clearly remember the upheaval and confusion associated with the time when our bodies and minds experienced a bewildering metamorphosis. Adolescence is a developmental period when young girls go through substantial physiological and biochemical changes, during which their bodies alter from those of children to those of young women in a relatively short period of time.[5] Society asks that adolescents rapidly learn to behave and think like adults rather than like children. There is evidence that the onset of adolescence is occurring earlier and earlier, implying that children are being asked to transform to adulthood at an even earlier mental and emotional age, possibly before they are able to handle the transition.[6] In terms of physical change, girls gain a marked amount of body fat during this period. It is not uncommon for a young girl to go shopping for clothes with her mother one summer, complaining that all the pants and skirts are too big in the hips, while the next summer, the same girl's clothing will not fit over her newly developed hips. As with the mental and emotional leaps to adulthood, young girls may also be unprepared to cope adequately with the physical changes of adolescence.

Many physical and mental changes that occur during the shift from childhood to adulthood may contribute to the onset of eating disturbances and eventually clinical eating disorders. Young women may find themselves struggling with the natural changes their bodies are experiencing and as a result they try to control the physical changes through maladaptive thoughts and behaviors such as fasting or purging. While pre-adolescent females typically exhibit healthy views of themselves and their bodies, by the time they reach the end of adolescence, they have more negative body images, are more dissatisfied with their bodies, and are preoccupied with dieting in attempts to control their body shapes.[5] These characteristics are found for nearly all adolescent women, not just those with eating disorders. This finding of a decrease in body satisfaction is especially alarming, since both bulimia nervosa and anorexia nervosa are defined in part by disturbance in and preoccupation with body image. During adolescence, changes in attitudes and behaviors related to body size and body image may encourage women in an unrealistic pursuit of thinness, which has been found to be the most important factor in predicting dietary restraint, and subsequent eating disorders.[5]

2.2.1.2 Importance of Appearance and Social Acceptance

In addition to substantial physical changes that occur during this time, adolescence is also a period in which acceptance via physical appearance becomes especially important. Appearance ranks among the most desirable traits when adolescents are asked to identify traits evident in the most popular people at school.[6] To adolescents, being attractive is essential for being well liked, or for becoming a member of a popular clique. For women in Western culture, being attractive and being thin are now synonymous. Women are judged as attractive when they are slender.[7] Thus, a teenage girl can easily begin to believe that the weight she is gaining in adolescence is not acceptable if she is to be attractive. The rapid weight gain and body changes seen in adolescence, along with the importance placed on attractiveness and thinness in order to be liked, may culminate in providing an arena in which adolescents become suddenly more concerned with body weight, size, image and, as a result, take extreme measures to control body size.[5]

In addition to attractiveness, social approval is reported by teenagers to be the most important quality for determining self-esteem.[6] Many people with eating disorders share a fear that they will be rejected by others and exhibit a marked sensitivity to the approval of others. It is important to keep in mind that fear of rejection and desire for social approval are not just traits common to eating-disordered women, but are also common among adolescents.[8,9] In fact, self-esteem both in adolescents without eating disorders and in women with eating disorders is defined by attractiveness and social approval.[7] To avoid the discomfort that results from being rejected or not enjoying social approval, adolescents may rush into accepting ready-made values and trends.[10] It seems that a young woman will examine her surroundings to determine how attractiveness is defined, and if her surroundings indicate that the ideal is thinness, then the adolescent will strive toward thinness. She begins to feel that to be attractive in a socially acceptable way, she must emulate a thinness ideal that is approved of by peers and by society. An adolescent may feel that if losing some weight elicits approval, acceptance, and compliments from others, losing a much larger amount of weight will elicit even greater approval from peers.[8] The adolescent may feel lonely and alienated, and may believe that if she were only thin and attractive, she would have more friends or gain more approval from peers. She may feel encouraged to embark on extreme means of weight control in order to become more attractive to peer groups and, more specifically, to men. In fact, about 25% of adolescents report believing that being thinner would help them to have more dates.[11] It quickly becomes clear that a need for approval from others may prompt adolescents to engage in eating-disordered activities in an effort to meet a socially approved ideal of thinness.

2.2.1.3   Expression of the Disorder

Now that several characteristics of adolescence and eating disorders have been examined, the question remains: Why do eating disorders develop in some adolescents but not in others? Our society is one that places excessive value upon being thin and attractive, while being overweight is highly stigmatized.[12] All women in Western society confront the same social pressures, yet only some of them develop eating disorders in response to social pressures. Most adolescents seem to determine their self-worth by their perceived attractiveness among and approval from others during that time of substantial physical change, yet not all adolescents develop eating disorders.

2.2.1.4   Stressful Life Events

One of the most influential theories used to explain why some people are more susceptible to social pressures equating thinness with attractiveness focuses on stressful life events.[13] A person may be predisposed to developing an eating disorder in adolescence, and stressful events may trigger that disorder, whereas others who do not experience stressful events do not exhibit any symptoms. For example, Humpty Dumpty may have had a predisposition, such as a fragile shell, but he did not break his shell until he experienced a stressful event, in his case, falling off the wall.[14] Stressful life events have been shown to have a strong association with the occurrence of eating disorders and other psychological disorders in adolescence.[15] The stressful events associated with eating disorders may be related to a conflict between premature exposure to the adult world and a fear of that world.[13] Remember that the shift from childhood to young adulthood occurs quite rapidly, and in some individuals, the shift may happen before the child is psychologically ready. Research has shown that people with eating disorders report feeling forced into an exaggerated style of feminine behavior by family and friends.[13] Possibly, before a girl is mentally ready to begin becoming a woman, family and friends may make adult or womanly demands of her. Women with eating disorders also commonly report feeling that they must follow their parents' ambitions rather than follow their own.[13] Parents may expect an adolescent to be able to achieve things much as adults do, before she is ready. This pressure may force the adolescent into unhealthy coping responses such as eating disorders.

2.2.1.5   Degree of Need for Social Approval

Another explanation of why only a portion of women develop eating disorders has to do with their degree of need for social approval. While most adolescents exhibit great needs to experience social approval, some women adopt personality styles that are even more highly sensitive to social approval than others. Thus, while adolescents in general strongly associate their self-worth with acceptance, some women derive their self-worth almost entirely from public approval.[12] Women with eating disorders have been shown to place less emphasis on assertiveness, autonomy, and self-approval than other women in their age group.[12] Women who report that they often compare their bodies to the bodies of other women are more likely to be concerned with body image and dieting and are more likely to exhibit abnormal dieting extensions such as eating disorders.[11]

Knowing about the implications of stressful life events and varying degrees of need for attractiveness and approval may serve as important aspects for therapeutic intervention.[13] A therapist, teacher, or parent could spend hours lecturing a young woman on the horrible and life-threatening physical consequences of self-starvation or purging, but never get through to her because of a failure to understand and incorporate

TABLE 2.1

Psychological Characteristics Associated with Eating Disorders

Alexythymia	Lack of social support
Borderline personality disorder	Low self-esteem
Concern over body image	Need for control
Depression	Need to be accepted
Difficulty coping with physical changes	Need to be attractive
Distorted body image	Negative thought patterns
Eating attitudes	Obsessiveness
Family variables	Perfectionism
Fear of fatness/gaining weight	Poor communication skills
Impulsivity	Self-criticism
Inadequate coping skills	Stressful life events
Internalizing sociocultural ideals	

the deep-seated needs of the young woman to be attractive and to be accepted. With additional understanding of these issues, a therapist or other adult may be able to help an eating-disordered woman find other ways of feeling attractive, or help her become less reliant on the perceived approval of her peers. A greater understanding of the issues associated with adolescence may greatly benefit young women in the struggle to treat and prevent eating disorders.

2.2.2   Psychological Characteristics

Considering personality characteristics is critically important when attempting to understand and treat eating disorders.[16] Some researchers suggest that while maladaptive eating patterns stem from concerns about body image and attractiveness, full-blown clinical eating disorders occur only when body concerns co-exist with other psychopathology.[17] That is, an adolescent may experience all of the abovementioned pressures related to needs for attractiveness and needs for acceptance, but when those pressures co-exist with other maladaptive thoughts and behavior patterns, eating disorders are more likely to appear. Studies have shown a variety of personality traits to be associated with eating disorders, the most common having to do with obsessiveness, perfectionism, need for control, and depression.[18] In addition to understanding the issues and events related to adolescence, it is important to have some knowledge about other personality characteristics associated with anorexia and bulimia when trying to develop a better grasp of the complexities of eating disorders. This need is especially important since these characteristics appear to exist before an eating disorder develops and often persist even after recovery from the disorder.[16] The discussion of personality traits in this chapter is not exhaustive. Several other personality traits in addition to those explained here have been associated with eating disorders, and a knowledge of these traits is of great importance in understanding and treating eating disorders. For a more extensive list of personality characteristics associated with eating disorders, see Table 2.1.

2.2.2.1   *Obsessiveness*

Obsessiveness is a common trait among women with eating disorders and is characterized by persistent and obtrusive thoughts or ideas.[19] For example, women with eating disorders are often plagued by persistent thoughts that they are overweight or that any food they eat will lead to weight gain. Over 35% of women with anorexia are comorbid for obsessive-compulsive disorders. It is likely that many more women with anorexia may not fully meet clinical criteria for such disorders, but may still have obsessive thinking patterns that are associated with their eating disorders.[20] Being obsessive appears to be a premorbid characteristic of eating disorders, as it has been shown that obsessive thinking predates eating disorders by approximately 5 years.[20] Thus, the adolescent who obsessively counted her books and dolls when she was a young child may find that ruminating about calories, body size, or the possibility of gaining weight is an appropriate way of focusing an obsessive style. Recognizing the degree to which an obsessive style perpetuates the course of an eating disorder may be essential in thinking of ways to treat the disorder. For example, a woman with anorexia who is obsessed with counting calories consumed and burned may be directed to avoid such obsessions, or to use her obsessive thinking in healthier ways, such as working on math homework or solving crossword puzzles. Whatever the method, it appears that correcting or redirecting obsessiveness is imperative when working with young women with obsessive traits.

2.2.2.2   *Perfectionism*

Perfectionism involves the development of exceptionally high, and possibly unreasonable, performance standards.[21] There are multiple dimensions to perfectionism, one of which involves setting exceedingly high standards for the self. A perfectionist with extremely high personal standards may be likely to view even minor faults as monumental. For example, she may have aspirations of following her diet perfectly so that eating an extra bowl of popcorn one day, or failing to exercise for an entire hour, would be seen as complete failure, instead of just a small deviation from her diet. A perfectionist with high self-standards is also very likely to have many doubts about her actions.[22] She may spend a significant amount of time mulling over whether she exercised hard enough that day, or planned her food intake properly. Additionally, this dimension of perfectionism is related to inability to admit imperfection.[23] For example, a young girl may not realize she has not been perfect in doing schoolwork because she is so busy exercising, or she may not admit that her health is far from perfect due to her self-starvation. Another dimension of perfectionism has to do with holding high and unrealistic expectations for others to live up to.[21] An eating-disordered woman with this type of perfectionistic trait may, for example, be convinced that her mother and sister should also be able to attain unrealistic weights so that they too may be perfect.

The other dimension of perfectionism seems to be the one that women with eating disorders are most likely to show: socially prescribed perfectionism.[21] That is, they are likely to feel a strong need to strive toward standards that they perceive others maintain for them, or to appear "perfect" in the eyes of others. A woman with an eating disorder often feels as though her self-worth and success are defined by whether she meets external standards, such as living up to a thin ideal.[21] While she may not be as driven by personal goals, a woman with an eating disorder is likely to be extremely sensitive to the opinions of others, even when those opinions express goals that are unrealistic, such as striving for extreme weight loss. The act of setting unrealistic weight-loss goals will inevitably lead to failure, in much the same way that attempting repeatedly to stretch oneself will fail to help a person to become taller. Continuing to fail in meeting unrealistic expectations she believes others have for her may discourage a young woman, and force her to feel worse about herself, or to try even harder to meet perceived expectations. Setting lower or more reasonable goals may create a situation where she is less likely to fail, and thus more likely to maintain self-worth. While helping young women to establish more realistic weight-loss goals may be important in treatment, of equal importance for these women is to help them become less reliant on others' perceived opinions. Helping a young woman to come to a point where she can create more of her own goals, and rely less on the goals she believes others have for her, may help to discourage unhealthy dieting behaviors.

Several other aspects of perfectionism are characteristic of women with eating disorders. Perfectionists are often extremely rigid or inflexible in their thinking.[23] What may be an acceptable deviation from a diet to most, such as going out to eat on one's birthday when one has been faithful to a diet thus far, would be completely unacceptable to a perfectionist. Perfectionists allow no flexibility to their diets or exercise plans, as they are either perfect or imperfect. In addition to being inflexible, thinking is often unrealistic, with the obvious example being that women with eating disorders may believe they should be able to attain a weight that is much lower than that which is natural for their frame and genetic make up.[24] Perfectionists are also likely to be quite meticulous and ritualistic about how they plan their day, in ways related to how and when they exercise, binge, or purge. The aspects of perfectionism that may be the most devastating to women with eating disorders are the tendencies to be more socially introverted while also being restrained in an ability to express emotions.[7] Women may find themselves struggling with a serious eating disorder, yet have no social support system to turn to because of a history of avoiding social contact or shying away from developing close relationships. Very often, even when perfectionistic women are able to sustain social relationships, they will be unwilling to divulge or express any emotions to friends, and, as a result, will neglect to use friends as a much-needed social support.

2.2.2.3 Need for Control

A preoccupation with control is pervasive in the lives of women with eating disorders and is also an essential feature of obsessive thinking.[10] Women with eating disorders often report feeling that although they can no longer control friendships, grades, or other areas of their lives, the one area where they do have control is in what they put into and take out of their bodies. A woman with anorexia typically shows her strong need for control by strictly monitoring the amount of food she eats. She may come to feel "special" because she has the will power to abstain from food that others do not have.[8] However, women with bulimia also exhibit their own version of control. The woman with bulimia may lose control while consuming food, yet she may feel she regains control through such behavior as self-induced vomiting, laxative use, large periods of food restriction, or excessive exercise.

Women with eating disorders often feel compelled to stay in control where weight is concerned, or to regain control as quickly as possible when they sense a loss of control over their eating or weight. To lose that control, say, by eating what the nutritionist advises, or by not purging following a binge, can cause intense fear in an eating-disordered woman. Unfortunately, the young woman with an eating disorder, though convinced she has mastered this area of her life, has actually lost a great deal of control by virtue of the fact that she is now obsessed with weight, and has allowed that area to dominate everything else. The control that is so hoped for to gain attractiveness, acceptance, and ultimate success leads only to failure — failure to lose weight, failure to stay healthy, failure in interpersonal relationships, and very often, failure to stay out of the hospital as well.[10]

2.2.2.4 Depression

Clinical depression has been found in 45% of eating-disordered patients, and it is likely that many more women with eating disorders, although not clinically depressed, may experience symptoms of depression.[25] Symptoms of depression are commonly seen in women with eating disorders, but it is unclear whether eating disorders cause depression, depression causes eating disorders, or depression and eating disorders are both caused by some third factor.[26] It is clear, however, that depression is a significant problem for eating-disordered women before and after the onset of the eating problems, and demands attention in the course of treatment.

While symptoms of depression can vary from person to person, several symptoms are more common in women with eating disorders. These women have been shown to have greater negative affect and less positive affect than other women.[16] Negative thoughts and feelings are not limited to issues of weight and body image. Women with eating disorders frequently report feeling generally sad and hopeless about life, and they often show other characteristics of depression, such as withdrawing from others. Women with anorexia tend to become more socially withdrawn, and may not see any problem in their behavior. As a result, women with anorexia often have little social support and also may be hard to engage in therapy. By contrast, women with bulimia do not become as withdrawn, and because they realize that their behavior is abnormal, they may be more likely to respond positively to therapy.[8] Developing a strong social support system is important in the treatment of many psychological disorders, but the support system is likely to be especially important for women with anorexia, since they may have withdrawn to a point where they have very few friends. Another important characteristic seen both in depression and eating disorders is dichotomous thinking. A young woman is likely to see everything in terms of stark contrasts; things are either wonderful or horrible. She may feel that since one friend rejected her, everyone will always hate her, or she may act as though gaining 1 pound is equivalent to gaining 100.[8]

The co-existence of eating disorders and depressive symptoms has significant implications for the diagnosis and treatment of these disorders.[25] The knowledge that depressive symptoms may exist in eating-disordered women can be of great help, since it has been shown that treating depressive symptoms, either with medication or psychotherapy, often helps to alleviate eating disorder symptoms.[26] Evidence also suggests that depressive symptoms can remain even after eating symptoms dissipate. This clearly indicates a need to help young women prepare to cope with future depressive symptoms and monitor future feelings of depression in order to prevent relapses.

2.2.3 Conclusion

Adolescence is a time when young women are easily influenced by parents, teachers, and peers. As a result, others may be able to help women with eating disorders by discouraging extreme weight-control measures, modifying social attitudes, and lending support. Friendships may enhance or diminish the importance of thinness and dieting, and therefore, peers may exert a positive influence on eating-disordered women, countering the assumption that peer influence is always negative for women with eating disorders.[11] Adolescence is a period when one's sense of attractiveness, need for acceptance, and self-image are still evolving, which is encouraging to those involved in the lives of eating-disordered women, who may be able to change maladaptive attitudes and behaviors to more healthy ones.[4]

Long-term follow-up studies have shown that 30% of eating-disordered women relapse, and up to 40% still show symptoms of disturbed eating thoughts and behaviors even after improvement in treatment.[25] Looking at other psychological characteristics that go hand in hand with eating disorders, such as obsessiveness, perfectionism, need for control, and depression, may be essential to truly helping women with eating disorders to recover.

2.3 Application of Research Question

The importance of assessing related characteristics among women with eating disorders should by now be clear. Clinicians have found that dealing with characteristics that co-exist with eating disorders greatly complicates the treatment of the disorders but, at the same time, can greatly improve the quality of these women's lives and reduce the likelihood that eating disorders will recur.[2] Several instruments have been developed to assess for various psychological characteristics associated with eating disorders. The use of such instruments can greatly enhance clinicians' abilities to determine the most important psychological characteristics exhibited by young women and, in addition, can help them to develop the most effective treatment plans.

Several measures can assist with the assessment of comorbid personality characteristics of eating disorders. For example, the Beck Depression Inventory (BDI) is a 21-item forced-choice measure of the cognitive, motivational, and physiological symptoms of depression.[28] The Maudsley Obsessional-Compulsive Inventory is a 30-item true-false measure of obsessive symptoms.[27] The Multidimensional Perfectionism Scale is a 45-item measure of perfectionism containing three subscales: (a) self-oriented, (b) other-oriented, and (c) socially-prescribed perfectionism.[29]

References

1. Sands, R., Tricker, J., Sherman, C., Armatas, C., and Maschette, W., Disordered eating patterns, body image, self-esteem, and physical activity in preadolescent school children, *International Journal of Eating Disorders*, 21, 159, 1997.
2. Wakeling, A., Epidemiology of anorexia nervosa, *Psychiatry Research*, 62, 3, 1996.
3. Stienhausen, H. C., Winkler, C., and Meier, M., Eating disorders in adolescence in a Swiss epidemiological study, *International Journal of Eating Disorders*, 22, 147, 1997.
4. Smolak, L. and Levine, M. P., Toward an empirical basis for primary prevention of eating problems with elementary school children, *Eating Disorders*, 2, 293, 1994.
5. De Castro, J. M. and Goldstein, S. J., Eating attitudes and behaviors of pre- and post-pubertal females: clues to the etiology of eating disorders, *Physiology and Behavior*, 58, 15, 1995.
6. Cole, M. and Cole, S. R., *The Development of Children*, 2, Scientific American Books, New York, 1993, 567.
7. Beren, S. E. and Chrisler, J. C., Gender role, need for approval, childishness, and self-esteem: markers of disordered eating, *Research Communications in Psychology, Psychiatry and Behavior*, 15, 183, 1990.
8. Peters, C., Swassing, C. S., Butterfield, P., and McKay, G., Assessment and treatment of anorexia nervosa and bulimia in school age children, *School Psychology Review*, 13, 183, 1984.
9. Steiger, H., Leung, F. Y., Puentes-Neuman, G., and Gottheil, N., Psychosocial profiles of adolescent girls with varying degrees of eating and mood disturbances, *International Journal of Eating Disorders*, 11, 121, 1992.
10. Rothenberg, A., Adolescence and eating disorder: the obsessive-compulsive syndrome, *Adolescence: Psychopathology, Normality, and Creativity*, 13, 469, 1990.
11. Paxton, S. J., Prevention implications of peer influences on body image dissatisfaction and disturbed eating in adolescent girls, *Eating Disorders*, 4, 334, 1996.
12. Pike, K., Bulimic symptomatology in high school girls, *Psychology of Women Quarterly*, 19, 373, 1995.

13. Horesh, N., Apter, A., Ishai, J., Danziger, Y., Miculincer, M.,Stein, D., Lepkifker, E., and Minouni, M., Abnormal psychosocial situations and eating disorders in adolescence, *Journal of the American Academy of Child and Adolescent Psychiatry*, 35, 921, 1996.

14. Holmes, D. S., *Abnormal Psychology*, 3, Longman, New York, 1997, 315.

15. Goodyer, I. M., Recent stressful life events: their long term effects, *European Journal of Child and Adolescent Psychiatry*, 2, 1, 1993.

16. Pryor, T. and Wiederman, M. W., Measurement of nonclinical personality characteristics of women with anorexia nervosa or bulimia nervosa, *Journal of Personality Assessment*, 67, 414, 1996.

17. Garner, D. M., Olmsted, M. P., Polivy, J., and Garfinkel, P. E., Comparison between weight-preoccupied women and anorexia nervosa, *Psychosomatic Medicine*, 46, 255, 1984.

18. Vitousek, K. and Manke, F., Personality variables and disorders in anorexia nervosa and bulimia nervosa, *Journal of Abnormal Psychology*, 103, 137, 1994.

19. American Psychiatric Association, *Diagnostic and Statistical Manual of Mental Disorders IV*, Washington, D.C., 1994, 393.

20. Thornton, C. and Russell, J., Obsessive compulsive comorbidity in the dieting disorders, *International Journal of Eating Disorders*, 21, 83, 1997.

21. Pliner, P. and Haddock, G., Perfectionism in weight-concerned and unconcerned women: an experimental approach, *International Journal of Eating Disorders*, 19, 381, 1996.

22. Srinivasagam, N. M., Kaye, W. H., Plotnicov, K. H., Greeno, C., Weltzin, T. E., and Rao, R., Persistent perfectionism, symmetry, and exactness after long-term recovery from anorexia nervosa, *American Journal of Psychiatry*, 152, 1630, 1995.

23. Hewitt, P. L., Flett, G. L., and Ediger, E., Perfectionism traits and perfectionistic self-presentation in eating disorder attitudes, characteristics, and symptoms, *International Journal of Eating Disorders*, 18, 317, 1995.

24. Davis, C., Normal and neurotic perfectionism in eating disorders: an interactive model, *International Journal of Eating Disorders*, 22, 421, 1997.

25. Zerbe, K. J., Marsh, S. R., and Lolafay, C., Comorbidity in an inpatient eating disordered population: clinical characteristics and treatment implications, *The Psychiatric Hospital*, 24, 3, 1991.

26. Fava, M., Abraham, M., Clancy-Colecchi, K., Pava, J. A., Matthews, J., and Rosenbaum, J., Eating disorders symptomatology in major depression, *The Journal of Nervous and Mental Disorders*, 185, 140, 1997.

27. Hodgson, R. A. and Rachman, S., Obsessional compulsive complaints, *Behavior, Research, and Therapy*, 15, 389, 1977.

28. Beck, A. T., Ward, C. H., Mendelson, M., Mock, J., and Erbaugh, J., An inventory for measuring depression, *Archives of General Psychiatry*, 4, 561, 1961.

29. Hewitt, P. L. and Flett, G. L., Perfectionism in the self and social contexts: conceptualization, assessment, and association with psychopathology, *Journal of Personality and Social Psychology*, 60, 456, 1991.

3

The Pathophysiology of Eating Disorders

Annette Gary

CONTENTS

3.1 Learning Objectives

After completing this chapter, the reader should be able to:

- Discuss physiological signs and symptoms of anorexia nervosa and bulimia nervosa;
- Discuss eating disorder-related changes in physiological parameters such as the electrocardiograph (EKG), blood pressure, body fat percentage, heart rate, and metabolic rate;
- Identify abnormal laboratory values associated with eating disorders;
- State potential long-term physiological consequences of eating disorders.

3.2 Research Background

Diagnostic criteria for anorexia nervosa and bulimia nervosa have in common an intense preoccupation with body weight, and individuals with these disorders also exhibit a variety of behaviors that contribute to the physical signs and symptoms found during examination. Physical abnormalities evidenced in individuals with anorexia nervosa generally occur secondary to disturbed eating patterns, dietary restrictions, and starvation. Physical abnormalities found in individuals with bulimia nervosa are usually a result of purging behaviors. Up to 50% of individuals with anorexia nervosa are also believed to engage in purging behaviors such as vomiting, laxative and diuretic abuse, and/or excessive exercise,[1] further compounding symptomatology and contributing to serious physical problems in these individuals.

Physical complications from an eating disorder may increase a person's sense of vulnerability or personal inadequacy and lead to an increase in psychological symptoms such as increased anxiety or a depressed mood. Some physical manifestations may be life-threatening and lead the individual to seek medical attention. Although adolescent and young adult women constitute the majority of those who are most often affected by eating disorders, increasing numbers of males, minorities, and women of other age groups are also developing these disorders.

This chapter will discuss the physical signs and symptoms of eating disorders. Since behaviors such as calorie restriction or purging frequently occur to varying degrees in each disorder, the information presented is linked to causative factors such as starvation, which occurs primarily in anorexia, or vomiting and laxative/diuretic abuse, which occur primarily in bulimia, rather than to the specific disorders themselves.

3.2.1 Physiological Signs and Symptoms

Eating disorders create numerous physiological signs and symptoms and, in many cases, symptoms of both anorexia nervosa and bulimia nervosa exist to some degree in the same person. Physiological complications of eating disorders are serious and may be life-threatening. In addition to severe weight changes, individuals with eating disorders may experience fluid and electrolyte disturbances, as well as cardiovascular, gastrointestinal, endocrine, central nervous system, and other abnormalities. A summary of signs and symptoms specific to each disorder is provided in Tables 3.1 and 3.2.

3.2.1.1 *Weight Changes*

Individuals diagnosed with either anorexia or bulimia have an intense preoccupation with body weight. The individual may practice numerous behaviors focused on weight control, such as calorie restriction, excessive exercise, and purging behaviors such as vomiting and laxative or diuretic abuse. The body weight of the individual with anorexia nervosa generally reflects the degree of calorie restriction, as well as the amount of exercise engaged in by the individual. Patients diagnosed with anorexia nervosa generally evidence severe weight loss and may be described as thin or emaciated, having lost as much as 50% of their ideal body weight for a body mass index (BMI) of 10 or below (23 to 26 is considered normal for adult females). Table 1.1 in Chapter 1 categorizes ranges of BMI from normal to severely obese. (See Figure 1.1 in Chapter 1 in order to determine BMI.) By contrast, individuals with bulimia nervosa may be below, at, or above ideal body weight, reflecting a balance among dieting, binging, vomiting, and use of cathartics and other substances for weight control.[2]

3.2.1.2 *Fluid and Electrolyte Abnormalities*

Individuals with eating disorders frequently develop disturbances in body fluid and electrolyte levels related to prolonged malnutrition and dehydration. Fluid and

TABLE 3.1

Common Signs and Symptoms of Anorexia Nervosa

Cardiovascular	Gastrointestinal
Bradycardia	Abdominal discomfort
Tachycardia	Bloating/feeling of fullness
Hypotension	Constipation
Arrhythmias	Delayed gastric emptying
Prolonged QT intervals	Decreased gastric and intestinal motility
ST-T wave changes	Pancreatitis
ST segment depression	Sore throat
U waves	Gastroesophageal reflux

Endocrine	Integumentary
Amenorrhea	Dry, flaky/scaly, yellow skin
	Decreased body fat
Oligomenorrhea	Lanugo (fine facial and body hair)
Anovulation	Thinning hair
Cold sensitivity	Pruritus
	Brittle nails

Hematologic	Central Nervous System
Anemia	Poor problem-solving skills and memory
Leukopenia	Decreased concentration and attention
Thrombocytopenia	Depressed mood

TABLE 3.2

Common Signs and Symptoms of Bulimia Nervosa

Cardiovascular	Gastrointestinal
Arrhythmias	Dyspepsia and dysphagia
Hypotension	Esophageal rupture or ulcers
Mitral valve prolapse	Esophagitis
Cardiomyopathy	Hematemesis
Heart failure	Sore throat
Palpitations	Cheilosis
	Dental caries
	Dental abscesses
	Constipation
	Diarrhea
	Pancreatitis

Endocrine	Metabolic
Anovulation	Alkalosis
	Acidosis

Integumentary	Musculoskeletal
Pruritis	Muscle cramps
Dry, flaky skin	Tetany
Calluses on back of hand and fingers	Weakness

electrolyte disturbances may be even more serious when an individual also engages in vomiting and laxative or diuretic abuse. Dehydration may result from inadequate fluid intake and/or excess fluid loss during purging. Dehydration leads to increased blood levels of urea, urate, and creatinine and may result in decreased urine volume and renal failure. A rebound peripheral edema may also occur and can contribute to a dramatic increase in body weight (5 to 20 kg). Metabolic acidosis may result from vomiting and loss of stomach acid and sodium bicarbonate. If the individual also

engages in laxative abuse, the loss of alkaline bowel fluids may result in metabolic acidosis.[3] Individuals who abuse laxatives are four times more likely to suffer serious
medical complications than non-laxative abusers.[4]

3.2.1.3   Cardiovascular Abnormalities

Probably the most serious and life-threatening complication of an eating disorder
results from a compromise of the cardiovascular system. Individuals with eating
disorders frequently develop a number of serious cardiac abnormalities which, if not
recognized and treated, may result in death. Frequently, these individuals present
with mottled or cyanotic hands and feet and complain of palpitations. Prolonged starvation leads to decreased sympathetic tone in the heart and blood vessels. The heart's
ability to pump and the vessels' ability to transport blood may be altered, resulting in
bradycardia or tachycardia and orthostatic hypotension.[5] Tachycardia can occur
when the circulating fluid volume decreases as a result of dehydration, and the heart
is forced to pump faster to compensate for the decrease. Bradycardia is believed to
occur due to a starvation-induced metabolic decrease controlled by circulating catecholamines and a change in thyroid hormone levels.[6] Studies have shown that 91% of
the subjects with anorexia nervosa have pulse rates less than 60 beats per minute,[7] and
up to 85% of patients with anorexia nervosa also have hypotension, with blood pressures below 90/60.[8]

Purging behaviors lead to a loss of body fluids and electrolytes that are essential for
muscle contraction and conduction of nerve impulses in the cardiovascular system.
Electrolyte loss contributes to the development of severe arrhythmias with prolonged
QT intervals[9] and nonspecific ST-T wave changes, including ST segment depression.[5]
U-waves may also be visible when serum potassium and magnesium levels drop
below normal levels. Individuals with anorexia nervosa have been found to have
higher incidences of mitral valve abnormalities and left ventricular dysfunction than
individuals who do not have eating disorders.[10] The use of ipecac to induce vomiting
may contribute to the occurrence of cardiomyopathies or peripheral muscle weakness[11]
hastening cardiovascular compromise. All of these factors contribute to a significant
risk of sudden death due to cardiovascular problems in this population.[12,13]

3.2.1.4   Endocrine Abnormalities

Eating disorders have been linked to numerous endocrine system effects, including
dysfunction of the hypothalamus, the pituitary gland, the adrenal glands, and the
gonads. Individuals with anorexia nervosa, in particular, are known to have alterations in the neuroendocrine mechanisms, but the relationship between various
behaviors and these alterations is unclear. Research indicates that changes in the
hypothalamic-pituitary-adrenal axis, result in hypercortisolemia and increased cerebrospinal fluid (CSF) levels of corticotropin-releasing hormones. Since the hypothalamus controls the pituitary gland, pituitary function is also inhibited, resulting
in alterations in the normal circulating levels of gonadotropins, cortisol, growth
hormone, and thyroid hormones. As a result, prepubertal patients may have altered
sexual maturation and arrested physical development and growth patterns.[14]

Patients with anorexia nervosa frequently display a range of menstrual cycle abnormalities which have been linked to starvation and extreme weight loss. In approximately 30 to 50% of the women with anorexia nervosa, there are menstrual cycle
disruptions ranging from anovulation to oligomenorrhea to amenorrhea.[2,15] Individuals with bulimia nervosa frequently demonstrate menstrual cycle abnormalities,
particularly when they engage in extreme dieting or other caloric and nutritional

restrictions. Starvation and weight loss are known to create hypothalamic abnormalities that profoundly affect other organs within the endocrine system. A chain of interrelated events begins when the hypothalamus fails to signal the release of gonadotropin-releasing hormones from the pituitary. The absence of this signal causes a decrease in luteinizing hormone (LH) and follicular-stimulating hormone (FSH) levels and inhibits the positive feedback mechanism to the ovaries. Consequently, the ovaries do not release estrogen or progesterone in normal amounts, which further inhibits the pituitary gland. Ovarian and uterine volume are decreased and the vaginal mucosa becomes atrophic.[5]

Although eating disorders are rare in males and comprise only about 10% of the cases, male anorexia nervosa is also characterized by alterations in normal hormonal mechanisms. Studies have found low testosterone levels, decreased testicular volume, oligospermia, and diminished sexual functioning in subjects with eating disorders.[16]

Normal functioning of the thyroid gland is also disrupted in individuals who have eating disorders. Individuals with anorexia nervosa frequently demonstrate thyroid abnormalities as a result of decreased calorie intake and starvation. Free thyroxine (free T4) decreases to low normal levels, whereas triiodothyronine (T3) levels decrease to abnormally low levels in proportion to the degree of weight loss,[5] and thyroid-stimulating hormone (TSH) levels are usually within normal range.[17] The resting bradycardia, hypotension, and decreased metabolic rate observed in some patients with eating disorders may actually reflect decreased sympathetic and thyroid activity.[18]

3.2.1.5   Gastrointestinal Abnormalities

Individuals with anorexia nervosa frequently describe mealtime as an uncomfortable experience associated with symptoms of anxiety such as sweating and increased pulse and respiratory rates. Occasionally, when the patient is required to eat more than a small amount, bloating occurs, due primarily to delayed gastric emptying.[19] Delayed gastric emptying is a common occurrence taking place in approximately 80% of patients with anorexia nervosa[20] and similarly in patients with bulimia nervosa.[21] As poor nutrition and caloric restriction continue, individuals develop gastrointestinal motility disturbances, hypothermia, and other evidence of hypometabolism. Complaints of chronic constipation and abdominal pain are common in individuals who present themselves for evaluation.[22]

If an individual engages in bulimic behaviors such as vomiting, esophageal irritation and bleeding may occur. Complaints may include a sore throat, difficulty swallowing or eating, spontaneous reflux of gastric contents into the lower esophagus, and the presence of blood in the vomitus.[23] Prolonged vomiting may result in esophageal rupture (Boerhaave's syndrome), a potentially life-threatening occurrence with an overall mortality rate of 20%.[22]

Vomiting may also lead to several severe dental problems. When stomach acid is repeatedly regurgitated over the tooth, the surface becomes smooth, dull, and yellow, and abscesses eventually form due to the loss of protective enamel.[19] The teeth may appear chipped and jagged, and the patient may complain of tooth sensitivity to heat or cold.

Vomiting-related parotid gland enlargement also is found in 25% of patients with bulimia,[24] but the mechanism underlying the occurrence is not known. The enlarged glands can be seen on the individual's face, in the area immediately in front of and slightly below the ears just above the jawbone. Parotid gland enlargement is usually accompanied by elevated salivary amylase levels, which are generally related to the degree of vomiting engaged in by the patient.[21]

Due to malnutrition[22] and repeated episodes of binge eating,[25] pancreatitis is a common occurrence in patients with eating disorders. Patients with pancreatitis may complain of steady and intense, upper abdominal pain which may diffuse to the back, chest, or lower abdomen. Numerous mechanisms have the potential to cause pancreatitis, including a sudden increase in calorie intake after malnutrition or the ingestion of various medications including laxatives and diuretics, used in purging.[21]

3.2.1.6   Central Nervous System Abnormalities

Disruptions in neuroendocrine and neurotransmitter systems are prevalent in patients with eating disorders. Studies have found increased levels of beta endorphin and norepinephrine and decreased plasma norepinephrine and CSF homovanillic acid, a metabolite of dopamine. Altered levels of cholecystokinin found in patients with bulimia nervosa suggest a disruption in the post-satiety mechanism[26] which may be linked to binging engaged in by these patients.

Severe starvation has been linked to depressed mood, decreased concentration and attention, and poor problem-solving skills and memory. These factors may contribute to poor judgment about the severity of the illness and, therefore, hamper the individual's recognition of the need for treatment.[19]

Structural changes in the brain have been demonstrated in both anorexia nervosa and bulimia nervosa patients. Changes include widening of the sulcal spaces and cerebroventricular enlargement[27] and reductions in the size of the pituitary.[28] Patients with anorexia nervosa demonstrate increased metabolism in the cortex and caudate nucleus;[29] by contrast, patients with bulimia nervosa demonstrate differences in right- and left-brain hemisphere activity.[30] Refeeding and reversal of starvation are not known to correct these problems.

3.2.1.7   Hematologic and Immunologic Abnormalities

Hematologic and immunologic abnormalities are often found in patients with eating disorders. Poor nutrition with severe weight loss often results in dramatic decreases in red blood cells, white blood cells, and platelets. Often, these effects can be corrected with nutritional improvement and refeeding. Impairment of the immune system has also been found and is believed to be a consequence of hypercortisolism. All of these factors promote the development of other medical complications.[31]

3.2.1.8   Integumentary Abnormalities

Patients with eating disorders demonstrate changes in skin and tissues that appear to be directly related to malnutrition, loss of body fat, and dehydration. Frequently, the skin is dry, scaly, and covered with lanugo, a fine, downy hair resembling that of newborn babies. Fingernails and hair are brittle, and hair loss may occur in patches or uniformly over the scalp and other body areas.[32] Rarely, petechiae may occur on the extremities. Scars or calluses on the dorsum of the hand (Russell's Sign) may also be seen in individuals with purging behavior, due to contact with the teeth when the fingers are used to induce vomiting.[14] A yellowish discoloration of the skin occurs in approximately 80% of patients with anorexia nervosa.[33]

3.2.2   Laboratory Findings

The initial evaluation of an individual with an eating disorder must include a comprehensive physical exam and health history to rule out existing physiological

TABLE 3.3

Normal and Abnormal Values Resulting from Eating Disorders

Laboratory Test	Normal Value	Effect
Red blood cells	4.2–5.4 million/mm^3	low
White blood cells	5000–10000/mm^3	low
Platelets	150,000–400,000/mm^3	low
Blood urea nitrogen	10–20 mg/dL	increase
Serum magnesium	1.2–2.0 mEq/L	low
Serum sodium	40–229 mEq/L	increase
Serum chloride	90–110 mEq/L	low
Serum potassium	3.5–5.0 mEq/L	low
Serum amylase	56–190 IU/L	increase
Thyroxine	5–12 ug/dL	increase or normal

pathology. Several lab tests including a complete blood count; full blood chemistry, electrolyte profile, liver and function tests, and urinalysis should also be performed. An EKG is essential to evaluate the cardiovascular system and to rule out potentially life-threatening arrhythmias. A chest X-ray may be performed to evaluate heart size and placement.[34] Table 3.3 summarizes lab findings often found in patients with eating disorders.

Numerous lab abnormalities may be found in patients with eating disorders; however, research findings indicate that laboratory results may be normal even in the presence of profound malnutrition. Over 60% of patients with anorexia nervosa have leukopenia (a reduction in the number of leukocytes in the blood) believed to be due to bone marrow hypoplasia and decreased neutrophil (a granular leukocyte having a nucleus of three to five lobes) lifespan.[33] Leukopenia accompanied by a relative lymphocytosis has also been reported.[35] Normochromic, normocytic anemia and thrombocytopenia have been found in approximately one third of patients with anorexia nervosa. Hypoglycemia, hypercortisolemia, hypercholesterolemia, low serum zinc levels, and various other electrolyte disturbances such as decreased levels of potassium, chloride, and magnesium may be found, depending upon the degree of dehydration. Thyroid function tests reveal low T3 levels in proportion to weight loss (which are generally reversible with weight restoration), low normal T4 levels,[5] and decreased metabolic rates.[18]

3.2.3 Long-Term Complications

A number of long-term complications may result from the prolonged and severe malnutrition that often accompanies an eating disorder. Medical complications can be expected to progress as long as the individual continues to exercise without proper nutritional intake.[2] Without early, aggressive intervention, the prognosis for patients with eating disorders is poor. Remission is difficult to achieve, and at 5- to 10-year follow-up, the remission rate is only approximately 40%.[36] Recent long-term follow-up studies reveal a mortality rate of 18%, with the majority of deaths related to medical complications of the disorders.

Long-term complications of an eating disorder may involve any of the body's systems; however, the bones and teeth are two areas that are significantly affected. Since puberty and adolescence are critical times for skeletal development, eating disorders which occur during this developmental period may interfere with the development of peak bone mass and, therefore, produce permanent long-term skeletal effects.[19] Decreased bone density is known to be particularly prevalent in individuals with anorexia nervosa who have been severely emaciated for a prolonged period of time.[37-39] Fractures of the long bones, vertebrae, and sternum have been reported in individuals with anorexia nervosa who have been amenorrheic for as short a period as 1 year.[35] In a recent long-term study of 103 patients with anorexia, osteoporosis with multiple fractures and terminal renal deficiency accounted for the most severe disabilities experienced by subjects.[40] Bone loss, osteopenia (decrease in bone mass), and associated stress fractures have been linked to endocrine disturbances that alter normal hormonal mechanisms and lead to oligomenorrhea and amenorrhea.[41] Dietary deficiency, low circulating estrogen levels, hypercortisolism, laxative misuse, and disturbed acid-base balance are also believed to be responsible,[34] but the exact mechanism underlying this process is unknown.

Dental complications are prevalent in patients who engage in repeated vomiting as a method of purging unwanted calories. Repeated vomiting contributes to erosion of tooth enamel particularly in patients who vomit regularly or at least four times per week.[42] The lingual (inner) surface of the teeth is affected more than the outside and fillings/amalgams may project above the surface of the teeth.[35]

Skeletal and dental problems can be minimized or prevented by early recognition and intervention. Long-term complications can be expected to occur and progress as long as an individual continues to exercise without proper nutritional intake.[2]

3.3 Application of Research Question

Individuals with eating disorders frequently lack insight into and deny the existence of problems related to eating. They are often reluctant to seek help from friends, family members, or health professionals. When they do seek help on their own, it may be due to severe distress over physical or psychological issues that occur as a result of or in conjunction with the eating disorder. In an attempt to conceal their disorders from health professionals, individuals who have eating disorders may try to hide signs of these disorders or provide inaccurate information to the clinician.

Prevention is critical. Health professionals must be educated about the dangers and warning signs of eating disorders to promote early recognition, evaluation, and treatment. Parents, teachers, and coaches who recognize common signs should express their concerns to these individuals and encourage further evaluation. Individuals often develop an eating disorder in the aftermath of a diet. Overweight individuals should be encouraged to lose weight through nutritionally balanced meals and exercise rather than by strict dieting that can trigger binging and cyclic eating behaviors.[22] Health professionals must develop realistic attitudes toward body weight and shape in order to communicate information and focus on preventive efforts appropriate for the promotion of health.

References

1. Fairburn, C. G., Physiology of anorexia nervosa, in *Eating Disorders and Obesity: A Comprehensive Handbook*, Brownell, K. D. and Fairburn, C. G., Eds., Guilford Press, New York, 1995, chap. 27.
2. Katz, J. L., Eating disorders, in *Women and Exercise: Physiology and Sports Medicine*, Shangold, M. and Mirkin, G., Eds., F. A. Davis Company, Philadelphia, 1994, chap. 17.

3. Mitchell, J. E., Hatsukami, D., Pyle, R. L., Ekert, E. D., and Boutacoff, L. I., Metabolic acidosis as a marker for laxative abuse in patients with bulimia, *International Journal of Eating Disorders*, 6, 557, 1987.

4. Mitchell, J. E., Boutacoff, L. I., Hatsukami, D., Pyle, R. L., and Eckert, E. D., Laxative abuse as a variant of bulimia, *Journal of Nervous and Mental Disorders*, 174(3), 174, 1986.

5. Yager, Joel, Eating disorders: guide to medical evaluation and treatment, *Psychiatric Clinics of North America*, 19(4), 657, 1996.

6. Hall, R. C. W., Hoffman, R. S., Beresford, T. P., Wooley, B., Hall, A. K., and Kubasak, L., Physical illness encountered in patients with eating disorders, *Psychosomatics*, 30(2), 174, 1989.

7. Fohlin, L., Body composition, cardiovascular and renal function in adolescent patients with anorexia nervosa, *Acta Paediatrica Scandinavia Supplement*, 268, 1, 1977.

8. Warren, M. P. and Vande Wiele, R. L., Clinical and metabolic features of anorexia nervosa, *American Journal of Obstetrics and Gynecology*, 117(3), 435, 1973.

9. Cooke, R. A., Chambers, J. B., Singh, R., Todd, G., Smeeton, N. C., Treasure, J. L., and Treasure, T., The QT interval in anorexia nervosa, *British Heart Journal*, 72(1), 69, 1994.

10. De Simone, G., Scalfi, L., Galderisi, M., Celentano, A., Di Biase, G., Tammaro, P., Garofalo, M., Mureddu, G. F. De Divitiis, O., and Contaldo, F., Cardiac abnormalities in young women with anorexia nervosa, *British Heart Journal*, 71(3), 287, 1994.

11. Palmer, E. P. and Guay, A. T., Reversible myopathy secondary to use of ipecac in patients with eating disorders, *New England Journal of Medicine*, 313(3), 1457, 1985.

12. Hall, R. C. W. and Beresford, T. P., Medical complications of anorexia and bulimia, *Psychiatric Medicine*, 7(4), 165, 1989.

13. Schocken, D. D., Holloway, J. D., and Powers, P. S., Weight loss and the heart: effects of anorexia nervosa and starvation, *Archives of Internal Medicine*, 149, 877, 1989.

14. American Psychiatric Association, Practice guidelines for eating disorders, *American Journal of Psychiatry*, 150(2), 212, 1993.

15. Stewart, D. E., Robinson, E., Goldbloom, D. S., and Wright, C., Infertility and eating disorders, *American Journal of Gynecology and Obstetrics*, 163(87), 1196, 1990.

16. Andersen, A. E., Wirth, J. B., and Strahlman, E. F., Reversible weight-related increase in plasma testosterone during treatment of male and female patients with anorexia nervosa, *International Journal of Eating Disorders*, 1, 74, 1982.

17. Schwabe, A. D., Lippe, B. M., Chang, R. J., Pops, M. A., and Yager, J., Anorexia nervosa, *Annals of Internal Medicine*, 94(3), 371, 1981.

18. Obarzanek, E., Lesem, M. D., Goldstein, D. S., and Jimerson, D. C., Reduced metabolic rate in patients with bulimia nervosa, *Archives of General Psychiatry*, 48, 712, 1991.

19. Treasure, J. and Szmukler, G., Medical complications of chronic anorexia nervosa, in *Handbook of Eating Disorders: Theory, Treatment and Research*, Szmukler, G., Dare, C., and Treasure, J., Eds., Wiley & Sons, New York, 1995, chap. 11.

20. Kiss, A., Bergmann, H., Abatzi, T. A., Schneider, C., Wiesnagrotzki, S., Hobart, J., Steiner-Mittelbach, G., Gaupmann, G., Kugi, A., Stacher-Janotta, G., Steinringer, H., and Stacher, G., Esophageal and gastric motor activity in patients with bulimia nervosa, *Gut*, 31(3), 259, 1990.

21. McClain, C. J., Humphries, L. L., Hill, K. K., and Nickl, N. J., Gastrointestinal and nutritional aspects of eating disorders, *Journal of American College of Nutrition*, 12(4), 466, 1993.

22. Rock, C. L. and Zerbe, K. J., Keeping eating disorders at bay, *Patient Care*, 11, 78, 1995.

23. Mehler, P. S., Eating disorders: 1. Anorexia nervosa, *Hospital Practice*, 31(1), 109, 1996a.

24. Riad, M., Barton, J. R., Wilson, J. A., Freeman, C. P. and Maran, A. G., Parotid salivary secretion pattern in bulimia nervosa, *Acta Otolaryngology*, 111(2), 392, 1991.

25. Gavish, D., Eisenerg, S., Berry, E. M., Kleinman, Y., Witztum, E., Norman, J., and Leitersdorf, E., Bulimia: an underlying behavioral disorder in hyperlipidemic pancreatitis: a prospective multidisciplinary approach, *Archives of Internal Medicine*, 147(4), 705, 1987.

26. Haller, E., Eating disorders: a review and update, *Western Journal of Medicine*, 157(6), 658, 1992.

27. Palazidou, E., Robinson, P., and Lishman, W. A., Neuroradiological and neuropsychological assessment in anorexia nervosa, *Psychological Medicine*, 20, 521, 1990.
28. Husain, M. M., Black, K. J., Doraiswamy, P. M., Shah, S. A., Rockwell, W. J. K., Ellinwood, E. H., and Krishnan, K. R., Subcortical brain anatomy in anorexia and bulimia, *Biology of Psychiatry*, 31(7), 735, 1992.
29. Kreig, J. C., Holthoff, V., Schreiber, W., Pirke, K. M., and Herholz, K., Glucose metabolism in the caudate nuclei of patients with eating disorders, measured by PET, *European Archives of Psychiatry and Clinical Neuroscience*, 240(6), 331, 1991.
30. Wu, J. C., Hagman, J., Buchsbaum, M. S., Blinder, B., Derrfler, M., Tai, W. Y., Hazlett, B. S., and Sicotte, N., Greater left cerebral hemispheric metabolism in bulimia assessed by positron emission tomography, *American Journal of Psychiatry*, 147(3), 309–312, 1990.
31. Mehler, P. S., Eating disorders: 2. Bulimia nervosa, *Hospital Practice*, 31(2), 107, 1996b.
32. Schwartz, D. M. and Thompson, M. G., Do anorexics get well? *American Journal of Psychiatry*, 138(3), 319, 1981.
33. Sharp, C. W. and Freeman, C. P. L., Medical complications of anorexia nervosa, *British Journal of Psychiatry*, 162, 452, 1993.
34. Garner, D., Pathogenesis of anorexia nervosa, *Lancet*, 341(8861), 1631, 1993.
35. Mitchell, J. E., Medical complications of anorexia nervosa and bulimia, *Psychological Medicine*, 1(3), 229, 1983.
36. Brotman, A. W., Rigotti, N. A., and Herzog, D. B., Medical complications of eating disorders, *Comprehensive Psychiatry*, 26(3), 258, 1985.
37. Kiriike, N., Iketani, T., Nakanishi, S., Nagata, T., Inoue, K., Okuno, M., Ochi, H., and Kawakita, K., Reduced bone density and major hormones regulating calcium metabolism in anorexia nervosa, *Acta Psychiatrica Scandinavia*, 86(5), 358, 1992.
38. Hay, P. J., Delahunt, J. W., Hall, A., Mitchell, A. W., Harper, G., and Salmond, C., Predictors of osteopenia in premenopausal women with anorexia nervosa, *Calcified Tissue International*, 50(6), 498, 1992.
39. Biller, B. M. K, Saxe, V., Herzog, D. B., Rosenthal, D. I., Holzman, S., and Klibanski, A., Mechanisms of osteoporosis in adult and adolescent women with anorexia nervosa, *Journal of Clinical Endocrinology and Metabolism*, 68(3), 548, 1989.
40. Herzog, W., Deter, H. C., Schellberg, D., Seilkopf, S., Sarembe, E., Kroger, F., Minne, H., Mayer, H., and Petzold, S., Somatic findings at 12-year follow-up of 103 anorexia nervosa patients: results of the Heidelberg-Mannheim follow-up, in *The Comprehensive Medical Text*, Herzog, W., Deter, H. C., Vandereycken, W., Eds., Springer-Verlag, Berlin, 1992.
41. Rigotti, N. A., Neer, R. M., Skates, S. J., Herzog, D. B., and Nussbaum. S. R., The clinical course of osteoporosis in anorexia nervosa: a longitudinal study of cortical bone mass, *Journal of the American Medical Association*, 265(9), 1133, 1991.
42. Simmons, M. S., Grayden, S. K., and Mitchell, J. E., The need for psychiatric-dental liaison in the treatment of bulimia, *American Journal of Psychiatry*, 143(6), 783, 1986.

4

Inventories Used to Assess Eating Disorder Symptomatology in Clinical and Non-Clinical Settings

Susan Kashubeck-West and Kendra Saunders

CONTENTS

4.1   Learning Objectives

After completing this chapter, you should be able to:

- Understand what measures of eating-disordered behavior and body image are available;
- Understand the limitations of various methods for assessing disordered eating and body image;
- Acquire knowledge of some widely used measures of disordered eating and body image.

4.2   Research Background

The purpose of this chapter is to review means for assessing the behavioral and psychological characteristics of individuals with problems suggestive of eating disorders. The most widely used instruments for assessing these constructs will be considered, including self-report inventories and structured interview methods. Psychometric data, including validity and reliability, will be discussed for each method. The reliability of an instrument refers to the degree to which a test can be repeated with the same results. Tests with high reliability yield scores that are less susceptible to insignificant or random changes in the test taker or the testing environment. The validity of a measure refers to the degree to which it measures what it is intended to measure. For example, does a measure of body dissatisfaction really assess a person's negative feelings toward her body, or does it capture some other phenomenon, such as depression or anxiety? The validity of an assessment procedure will affect the appropriateness, meaningfulness, and usefulness of the test data. Generally, the higher the reliability and validity of an instrument, the more confident one may be in the accuracy of the data.

4.2.1   Self-Report Inventories for Eating Disorder Symptomatology

Numerous self-report instruments have been created to assess symptoms related to eating disorders. By self-report, we mean paper-and-pencil measures completed by the individual. Self-report questionnaires offer several advantages. They are typically inexpensive and often require less time to administer than an interview. Furthermore, administration of a self-report questionnaire is usually simple, and such a measure can often be administered and scored by nonprofessional staff (although professionals with knowledge about eating disorders should interpret the results). In addition, self-report measures can be given to groups of individuals, making it possible to collect data from large samples. However, there are disadvantages to self-report inventories. They are vulnerable to various types of error and bias, including difficulty in distinguishing between individuals who deny the existence of psychological problems and those who are psychologically healthy.[1] People may not be truthful in completing the questions. Respondents may circle more than one answer, leave an answer blank, or pick the best answer when they do not feel they identify with the options presented.[2] Questions asked by an interviewer can often determine nuances in people's answers that are not available with a self-report measure. It may be difficult to assess complex concepts accurately with a paper-and-pencil measure. In addition, many of the self-report measures are based upon outdated diagnostic criteria for eating disorders.[3]

Because of their advantages, and despite their limitations, self-report instruments are widely used. Researchers often use them to get information from a large number of people, so that relationships between eating disorder symptomatology and other psychological or nonpsychological constructs can be determined. A clinician who suspects a client has symptoms associated with an eating disorder might ask her to fill out a self-report measure to get an initial assessment of her problem. Summaries of popular self-report inventories for the measurement of eating-disorder symptoms are described below.

4.2.1.1 *Eating Disorder Inventory (EDI) and EDI-2*

The EDI is a popular 64-item self-report measure constructed to assess the cognitive and behavioral traits found in anorexia nervosa and bulimia nervosa.[4] Although the EDI was not designed for this purpose, it has also been utilized as a screening instrument for eating disorders.[5] This measure is a paper-and-pencil test in which an individual rates his or her behavior and beliefs on a six-point scale ranging from "always" to "never." One can use scores on the eight subscales described below individually, or total the scores on the subscales for an overall score. If one's overall score is above 42, the respondent is suspected to have an eating disorder and he or she should be evaluated further.

The EDI has eight subscales that are positively correlated: (1) *Drive for Thinness* measures concern with thinness, weight, and dieting; (2) *Bulimia* measures episodes of uncontrollable overeating (binging) and the urge to engage in self-induced vomiting (purging); (3) *Body Dissatisfaction* assesses the belief that certain body parts (hips, thighs, stomach, buttocks) that change at puberty are too large; (4) *Ineffectiveness* measures feelings of insecurity, worthlessness, and inadequacy, as well as feelings of not being in control of one's life; (5) *Perfectionism* assesses the magnitude of expectations for superior achievement; (6) *Interpersonal Distrust* evaluates feelings of alienation and reluctance to form close relationships; (7) *Interoceptive Awareness* measures an individual's lack of confidence in identifying sensations of hunger or satiety and emotions; and (8) *Maturity Fears* assesses an individual's desire to return to the state of preadolescence to avoid the demands of adulthood. The first three subscales assess behaviors and attitudes toward weight, eating, and body shape, whereas the other five subscales measure general psychological characteristics associated with eating disorders.[6]

The EDI was founded on the authors' clinical experience and research with anorectic and bulimic patients. In their original report, the authors provide evidence that the EDI is generally a reliable and valid test, and that the eight subscales differentiate between patients with anorexia nervosa and females from a college comparison group.[7] In addition, Welch, Hall, and Norring[8] report that in a sample of eating-disorder patients they found an eight-factor solution that corresponded to the original eight factors proposed by the EDI authors. However, other researchers propose that many subscales of the EDI measure dimensions of general psychological disturbance and do not adequately differentiate individuals with eating disorders from individuals with other psychological disorders.[9] For example, a study by Hurley, Palmer, and Stretch[10] suggests that the Ineffectiveness, Perfectionism, Interpersonal Distrust, and Maturity Fears subscales of the EDI have no specific association with eating disorders. Furthermore, most support for the factorial integrity of the EDI was established from studies using clinical populations.[8,11] Unfortunately, studies using nonpatients have revealed that the factorial integrity and validity of the EDI may not be adequate. For example, different studies with female college students report different factor structures.[6] Such findings suggest that the EDI is not a sensitive instrument with normal populations, and some authors have proposed that the EDI should not be used for screening purposes until the validity of its use in this manner has been established.[12] Thus, controversy exists over the usefulness of the EDI, especially with non-clinical populations.

In 1991, Garner[13] introduced the Eating Disorder Inventory 2 (EDI-2), consisting of 91 self-report items that examine psychological features and behaviors commonly associated with anorexia nervosa and bulimia nervosa. The EDI-2 contains all 64 items from the original EDI (including the eight subscales described above) and 27 additional items that are classified into three subscales. The additional subscales are (1) *Asceticism*, which measures belief in self-discipline, control of bodily urges, and self-denial; (2) *Impulse Regulation*, which assesses a tendency toward impulsivity and self-destructiveness; and (3) *Social Insecurity*, an indicator of insecurity in social situations and relationships. The EDI-2 may be purchased though the publisher, Psychological Assessment Resources, Inc. (800-331-8378). Administration of the EDI-2 does not require a trained examiner, but the test interpreter should have a mental health background, plus some knowledge of the test and the intended variables of interest. The EDI-2 can be administered individually or in groups, is designed for ages 12 and older, and takes approximately 20 minutes to complete. A computerized version of the EDI-2 is also available. Examples of the Personal History Questionnaire from the EDI-2 can be found in Appendix 1-G.

The primary purpose of the EDI-2 is to assess client symptomatology and to aid in treatment planning. As Crowther and Sherwood[14] point out, the items on the EDI-2 can be used to generate a psychological profile for targeting treatment goals. Crowther and Sherwood[14] and Garner[13] also suggest that the EDI-2 may be utilized in non-clinical settings as a screening device for identifying individuals who may have eating disorders. However, Garner[13] states that the EDI-2 should not be used alone as a diagnostic instrument. Unfortunately, the new subscales of the EDI-2 have considerably lower reliability than the subscales in the original EDI.[15] In addition, the item-total correlation appears to be substantially lower for the three additional subscales. Furthermore, Eberenz and Gleaves[16] suggest that these three new subscales do not appear to measure a distinct construct and may measure a construct not intended by the developer. Clearly, more research on the psychometric properties of the EDI-2 is needed.

4.2.1.2 Eating Attitudes Test (EAT)

The EAT[17] is a widely utilized instrument that contains 40 self-rated items that assess behaviors and attitudes associated with anorexia nervosa. The scale (see Appendix 1-E) uses a 6-point, forced-choice format in which the respondent is asked to rate the occurrence of a variety of behaviors and attitudes on a scale ranging from "always" to "never." A total score of 30 or more is generally used as an indicator that the individual has symptoms of anorexia nervosa and further evaluation is needed.[17] An abbreviated 26-item version of the EAT (EAT-26) is also available, and it is highly correlated with the EAT-40.[18] Both the longer version and the EAT-26 are available free of charge from the authors.

The EAT-40 and the EAT-26 have been used as outcome measures in clinical groups to assess whether treatment has had an effect. In addition, they have been used as screening instruments in populations of high-risk people to detect individuals who may have anorexia nervosa. Although many individuals who score high on the EAT end up by not being formally diagnosed with anorexia nervosa, most are identified as having abnormal eating patterns that interfere with daily functioning.[17] However, research suggests that the EAT yields a high false positive rate for anorexia and bulimia nervosa among non-clinical samples,[19-21] and thus it should not be used as a screening device for anorexia nervosa in non-clinical samples.[18]

Both the EAT-40 and the EAT-26 have been found to be relatively valid and reliable measures.[17,18] The EAT generally appears to measure attitudes and behaviors shown by those in the anorexic population, and it discriminates between individuals with anorexia nervosa and normal control subjects. Furthermore, the EAT distinguishes individuals with bulimia nervosa from control subjects.[22] Unfortunately, there is no evidence that the EAT discriminates between individuals with anorexia nervosa and persons with bulimia nervosa. As noted by Mintz et al.,[3] the EAT items do not reflect the definition of anorexia in the *Diagnostic and Statistical Manual of Mental Disorders, Fourth Edition*[23] (DSM-IV), and many of them relate to bulimia. Thus, the EAT should be used with its limitations in mind.

4.2.1.3 Bulimia Test – Revised (BULIT-R)

The BULIT-R[24] is a frequently used self-report questionnaire developed to measure behavioral, physiological, and cognitive aspects of bulimia nervosa. Respondents answer 36 items, of which 28 are scored using a five-choice multiple-choice format. Questions on the BULIT-R investigate binge eating, purging behavior, negative affect, and weight fluctuations.[24] An individual who scores at or above a cutoff score of 104 on the BULIT-R is at risk for being diagnosed with bulimia nervosa in a subsequent interview. Consequently, the test is recommended as a screening instrument.[24] In addition, Thelen et al.[24] suggest that researchers interested in identifying individuals with problematic eating behaviors use a lower cutoff of 85 points. The BULIT-R is available free of charge from the authors. It takes approximately 10 minutes to complete and has an 11th-grade reading level.

The BULIT-R has been shown to be a reliable and valid measure for identifying individuals who may suffer from bulimia nervosa in both clinical and nonclinical populations.[25] The internal consistency is very high, and test-retest reliability over a two-month interval is very stable.[24] Furthermore, the BULIT-R consistently differentiates bulimic individuals from normal controls.[24] A recent study reported by Thelen et al.[25] indicates that the BULIT-R, which was based upon DSM-III-R criteria for bulimia, also captures DSM-IV criteria. Generally, the BULIT-R is a useful self-report inventory for the assessment of bulimia nervosa, and it has achieved increased popularity (see Appendix 4-A).

4.2.1.4 Questionnaire for Eating Disorder Diagnoses (Q-EDD)

The Questionnaire for Eating Disorder Diagnoses[3] was developed to operationalize criteria of the DSM-IV for eating disorders. In addition, the Q-EDD differentiates (a) between women who have and those who have not been diagnosed with eating disorders; (b) between women with anorexia and those with bulimia; and (c) among women with eating disorders, between those exhibit symptoms but do not meet DSM criteria, and those with no symptoms of eating disorders. The Q-EDD contains 50 self-report items (see Appendix 4-B) that provide frequency data for behaviors related to disordered eating and labels that can be used to place individuals into categories, such as eating-disordered or non eating-disordered. The items take approximately 5 to 10 minutes to complete, and scoring is conducted using a manual (available from Laurie Mintz) that contains flowchart decision rules that are easily learned.

Initial reliability and validity studies by Mintz et al.[3] indicate that the Q-EDD has strong psychometric support. Test-retest reliabilities are in the expected range, and there are significant relationships between the Q-EDD and the BULIT-R and the EAT (described above). Importantly, diagnoses based on the Q-EDD show a high correspondence with diagnoses made through clinical interviews and clinician judgments. Finally, the Q-EDD is slightly better than the BULIT-R in differentiating women with bulimia from those with anorexia, symptomatic women, and asymptomatic women.

4.2.1.5   Mizes Anorectic Cognitions Questionnaire

The Mizes Anorectic Cognitions Questionnaire (MAC) contains 33 items and is used to measure cognitive aspects of anorexia and bulimia nervosa.[26] Respondents rate items on a 5-point Likert-type scale ranging from "strongly disagree" to "strongly agree." Factor analysis reveals three factors related to cognitive distortion: rigid weight and eating regulation, self-worth based upon excessive self-control, and weight and eating as the basis for approval from others. The MAC has demonstrated high validity and reliability and accurately discriminates between clinical and normal groups.[27] However, the MAC has not been shown to discriminate between anorexic and bulimic individuals, or between individuals with eating disorders and persons with other types of psychopathology.[28] The MAC may be used for research purposes and as a screening device, but is not recommended for clinical decision making.[29] The MAC is available free of charge from the authors, takes only a short time to complete, is easy to administer, and has a sixth-grade reading level.[6]

4.2.2   Structured Interview Measures for Eating Disorder Symptomatology

Structured interviews offer a methodical way to gather information about eating-disordered behavior, thoughts, and attitudes that then can be used, along with other information, to make a diagnosis. A paramount advantage of structured interviews includes the ability to gather an abundance of information that may or may not be accessible through self-report measures. However, structured interviews also require more effort from the assessor, and often the examiner must be well trained in the administration and scoring of the interview. In addition, individuals may lie to examiners. Two structured interviews for the assessment of eating disorders are described below.

4.2.2.1   Eating Disorders Examination (EDE)

The EDE is a 62-item, semi-structured clinical interview developed to measure behavioral and cognitive features of eating disorders, including extreme concerns about weight and shape.[30] The authors designed the EDE to correct for problems found in self-report measures, such as the lack of a commonly accepted definition of the word "binge."[6] Four subscales assess pertinent aspects of eating disorders and include: *Eating Concern*, *Shape Concern*, *Dietary Restraint*, and *Weight Concern*.[31] Each variable/item features at least one mandatory question, as well as several optional questions. In addition, the interviewer is encouraged to ask further questions to obtain additional information. Most responses are rated on a seven-point scale, with four defined anchor points. In most cases, a score of zero represents the absence of the feature in question, and six represents its presence to an extreme degree. Other questions are scored in terms of frequency of occurrence of a particular behavior. The interview takes about 45 minutes, and the examiner must be trained to develop knowledge in both the techniques of interviewing and in the concepts governing the ratings of the EDE.[30]

The EDE has been revised numerous times in order in increase its reliability and validity and is now in its twelfth edition. Several studies have examined the validity and reliability of the EDE, all of which support the interview as a sound psychometric measure.[31-33] The EDE can discriminate between individuals with anorexia and individuals with bulimia, and between individuals with bulimia and individuals with restrained eating patterns.[33,34] The EDE is recommended as a measure of treatment outcome and as a measure of binge-eating and vomiting frequencies. The EDE has also been recommended for use in research on the nature and course of eating disorders, and for investigations into the effectiveness of treatment.[33] However, the EDE is not intended to be used alone to make an eating-disorder diagnosis.[30]

A self-report version of the EDE (EDE-Q) is also available.[35] The EDE-Q is a 38-item, 7-point, forced-choice questionnaire, and each question is extracted from an item on the EDE. Like the EDE, a score of 7 on an item on the EDE-Q represents increased severity or the presence of a feature. An advantage of the EDE-Q is that it can be administered and scored by nonprofessional staff. Finally, the EDE-Q has demonstrated an ability to discriminate accurately between individuals with eating disorders and controls and is recommended as a screening device for detecting the presence of eating-disorder symptoms.[36]

4.2.2.2 Structured Clinical Interview for Axis 1 DSM-IV Disorders (SCID)

The Structured Clinical Interview for Axis 1 DSM-IV Disorders (SCID) for Module H (Eating Disorders) was designed to correspond to DSM-IV criteria for eating disorders.[37] Interviewers ask questions that are based on each criterion and definitions of each criterion.[2] Test-retest reliabilities of earlier versions of the SCID for eating disorders are solid; for example, the coefficients range from .82 to .90 for the bulimia nervosa section, based on DSM-III-R criteria.[2] Similarly, studies (not looking specifically at eating-disorder diagnoses) have shown that the interrater reliability (agreement of different judges as to what the diagnosis should be) of the SCID to be high.[38] Validity studies of the SCID suggest that it provides "valid assessment of binge eating and purging relevant to the diagnosis of the eating disorders. ...[The SCID] provides the essential information for discriminating among the eating disorders, in particular"[2] (p. 323). Interviewers should have some clinical experience, be familiar with the DSM-IV, and be trained and supervised in conducting the interview appropriately. SCID materials are available from the Biometrics Research Department in New York City and from the American Psychiatric Press.

4.2.3 Self-Report Measures of Restraint

The concept of restraint postulates that the eating patterns of individuals are influenced by physiological cues that create a desire to eat, and cognitively mediated processes that inhibit the desire to eat.[39] The restraint construct has been useful in the study of eating behavior, eating disorders, and obesity.[40] Restrained eaters are aware of continuously monitoring what food they eat, whereas nonrestrained eaters seem to not be concerned with monitoring their food intake.[41] Generally, individuals who receive a high score on a restraint scale alter between periods of disinhibited eating and intense dieting in order to control body weight. Researchers have suggested that dietary restraint may be a factor in the etiology of bulimia nervosa and binge-eating disorder.[42] Three major scales have been constructed to measure restraint and are summarized below.

4.2.3.1 Dutch Restrained Eating Scale (DRES)

The DRES is a subscale of the Dutch Eating Behavior Questionnaire[43] (DEBQ) and contains 10 items that have a forced-choice Likert-style format with a 5-point scale ranging from "never" to "very often." The DRES measures the degree to which an individual eats less than what is desired in order to maintain or achieve a certain weight. A high score on the DRES indicates a high degree of restrained eating, a characteristic of bulimia nervosa.[43] The validity and reliability of the DRES have been studied and found to be moderate to high.[44,45] Gorman and Allison[41] report that the internal consistency and test-retest reliability of the DRES are high, and that the DRES does not appear to be differentially valid for obese and non-obese individuals. The DRES was printed in the Van Strien, Frijters, Bergers, and Defares[43] article and thus is easily available for no cost. Allison and Franklin[46] note that the reading level is between the fifth and eighth grades.

4.2.3.2 Restraint Scale

The Restraint Scale[47,48] (RS) is a 10-item, self-report questionnaire that investigates restraint in eating, concern about dieting, and weight fluctuation. It was developed to identify people who are chronically concerned about how much they weigh, and who try to control or lose weight by reducing food intake or dieting.[41] The RS has two subscales: Weight Fluctuation and Concern for Dieting. Generally, the RS has demonstrated moderate to high validity and reliability.[49,50] In addition, the RS has been shown to be a significantly stronger predictor of bulimic symptomatology than the Dutch Restrained Eating Scale.[39] However, the reliability of the RS has been shown to decrease when obese samples are used.[49] In addition, the factor structure of the RS appears to differ in normal-weight and overweight samples.[41] Therefore, the validity of the RS may differ for obese persons when compared to normal-weight subjects. Also, both the DRES and the RS measures do not appear to predict unrestrained eating.[39] The RS is available from the authors free of charge, takes only a short time to complete, and has been estimated to require a reading competency level of between the fourth and ninth grades.[46]

4.2.3.3 Cognitive Restraint Scale of the Three-Factor Eating Questionnaire

The Cognitive Restraint scale of the Three-Factor Eating Questionnaire[51] (TFEQ) also measures restrained eating patterns and consists of 21 items scored on a two-point scale (0 to 1). Higher scores on this scale reflect a higher degree of restrained eating. Stunkard and Messick[52] indicate that scores from 0 to 10 are low to average, from 11 to 13 are high, and 14 or more are suggestive of a clinically significant problem. As noted by Gorman and Allison,[41] there are wide differences across gender and nationality, and caution is needed in classifying individuals into low- or high-restraint groups. The TFEQ has demonstrated high reliability and validity.[50,51] Furthermore, the Cognitive Restraint scale appears to be less susceptible to dissimulation when compared to the two previously described restraint scales, indicating that scores on this scale are difficult to fake.[50] In addition, unlike the RS, the Cognitive Restraint scale does not appear to be less reliable among obese individuals.[41] The Cognitive Restraint scale is recommended for research in studying restrained eating and for the assessment of cognitive restraint. However, this scale should not be used as a diagnostic tool.[53] The TFEQ has a reading level that ranges from the sixth to the ninth grade.[41] The TFEQ has been renamed the Eating Inventory[52] and can be purchased from The Psychological Corporation (800-211-8378).

4.2.4   Assessment of Binge-Eating Disorder

Binge-eating disorder (BED) is characterized by recurrent episodes of binge eating during which an individual eats an amount of food that is larger than most people could eat in a discrete period of time.[23] During binge eating, the individual experiences a lack of control and feels that she cannot stop eating. The binge eating must occur, on average, at least twice a week for a 6-month period.[52] The following measure assesses this eating disorder.

4.2.4.1   Questionnaire of Eating and Weight Patterns – Revised (QEWP-R)

The Questionnaire of Eating and Weight Patterns[55] is a diagnostic self-report instrument used to identify individuals with BED. Initially developed in 1992, the QEWP was revised in 1993.[56] The QEWP-R contains 28 items that measure binge eating and purging behaviors and follow the diagnostic criteria for BED outlined in the DSM-IV. Individuals may be diagnosed with BED, purging bulimia, or nonpurging bulimia. The original QEWP demonstrated the ability to discriminate between clinical and nonclinical binge eaters and proved to be both reliable and valid.[54] Moreover, Nangle et al.[57] recommend the QEWP for the identification of BED, the evaluation of treatment outcome, and for use in research.

According to Pike et al.,[2] some predictive validity of the QEWP-R has been demonstrated, although there is little research on its psychometric properties. Although criticism of the QEWP is scarce, it has been suggested that its overreliance on a dichotomous, all-or-none approach may overlook some clinically significant individuals.[58] Furthermore, there appears to be a low correlation between the classification of those with BED using the QEWP, and another similar measure, the Binge-Eating Scale.[58] Gladis et al.[58] believe that this low correlation is due to differences in the way the two measures assess the critical dimensions of binge eating. The revised QEWP is available from Robert Spitzer and has been reprinted in Pike et al.[2]

4.2.5   Assessment of Body Image Disturbance

Body image disturbances have been associated with the cause and the maintenance of eating disorders. Generally, body image has been conceptualized as a person's attitudes, thoughts, feelings, and behaviors toward her body. The three components of body image disturbance that are commonly assessed include: (a) body image distortion, which occurs when one over- or underestimates current body size; (b) preference for thinness, which refers to an individual's sense of her ideal body size; and (c) body-size dissatisfaction, which is a function of the discrepancy between perceived current body size and estimate of ideal body size. Individuals with anorexia nervosa and bulimia nervosa tend to overestimate their actual body sizes, prefer to be significantly thinner, and profess larger discrepancies between perceived body size and ideal body size. For measurement purposes, researchers and clinicians have focused on two aspects of body image: a perceptual component, which assesses size-perception accuracy, and a subjective component, which assesses feelings about body size and physical appearance. The following sections describe the most commonly used assessment techniques for assessing body image disturbance, including several methods for assessing size-perception accuracy and body distortion, as well as measures that assess subjective feelings about one's body.

4.2.5.1   Body Image Detection Device (BIDD)

The BIDD[59] was created to assess body image disturbance. It consists of a measure of perceptual body image distortion (BPI) and a subjective rating of weight. For the BPI scale, the subject adjusts a single beam of light to match her estimation of the size of a certain body region.[59] This technique utilizes an overhead projector that aims a narrow, horizontal band of light onto a wall. Individuals are able to adjust the length of the light band with a template. Body image distortion is measured by the extent to which the light band exceeds the subject's actual dimensions for five body sites. The individual then gives a subjective rating (0 to 100) of the size of each body part, relative to what she thinks is average for her sex, height, and age. Zero represents the body part size of an extremely underweight person, 50 represents the body part size of a normal weight person, and 100 represents the body part size of an extremely overweight person. These subjective ratings are combined to form an overall subjective rating index.[28] The reliability of the BIDD is moderate to high.[59] However, research examining the validity of this measure has been mixed. For example, a study by Cash and Green[60] suggests that the BPI subscale of the BIDD demonstrates only a minimal correlation with other measures of body image distortion. Other studies have also questioned the validity of the BPI subscale, especially when used with a nonclinical sample, and caution using this measure is urged.[28]

4.2.5.2   Contour Drawing Rating Scale (CDRS)

The Contour Drawing Rating Scale[61] is a measure of body-size dissatisfaction that determines an individual's perceived versus ideal body size. The discrepancy between these two measures is thought to indicate level of body dissatisfaction. The scale consists of nine male and nine female schematic figures that range from underweight to overweight.[61] Unlike a number of other figural stimulus materials, the CDRS features precisely graduated increments from the smallest to largest figures.[62] Using these stimuli, individuals choose the figure they think most accurately depicts current body size, and the figure that represents ideal body size. The larger the discrepancy, the greater the presumed body dissatisfaction. The CDRS has demonstrated moderate to high reliability and high validity.[61] Consequently, the CDRS is recommended as a measure of body-size perception. The scale is available in Thompson and Gray.[61]

4.2.5.3   Body Image Testing System (BITS)

Similar to the CDRS, the Body Image Testing System[63] also involves asking individuals to judge schematic figures of the human body. The BITS is an interactive computer program that assesses body image disturbance. On the computer, individuals are able to manipulate the size of nine body parts independently until that particular individual judges that the image created matches the current instructions. Usually the instructions include creating an image that represents that individual's ideal body size and shape (the way she wishes she looked) and producing an image that represents how she perceives herself currently.[63] In addition, each participant rates her satisfaction with each body region. As with the CDRS, body image is assessed by the discrepancy between the person's perceived and ideal body sizes, and by the person's subjective satisfaction ratings. Perceptual distortion may also be assessed by measuring the discrepancy between an individual's perceived and actual body size. The BITS has demonstrated adequate reliability and validity and is suggested as a useful tool for studying body image in women, or for the experimental study of body image.[63] For availability, please contact the authors of the BITS.

4.2.5.4   *Multidimensional Body-Self Relations Questionnaire (MBSRQ)*

The MBSRQ[64,65] assesses body image attitudes and weight-related variables. The MBSRQ (see Appendix 4-C) consists of 69 items rated on a 5-point Likert-type scale that ranges from 1 "definitely disagree" to 5 "definitely agree" that comprise three special subscales: The Body-Areas Satisfaction Scale (BASS), the Overweight Preoccupation Scale, and the Self-Classified Weight Scale.[65] The BASS assesses satisfaction with specific body features, while the Overweight Preoccupations Scale assesses anxiety about fat, dieting, eating restraint, and weight vigilance, and the Self-Classified Weight Scale obtains a self-appraisal of weight from underweight to overweight.[65] In addition, the questionnaire also includes seven factor subscales: Appearance Evaluation, Appearance Orientation, Fitness Evaluation, Fitness Orientation, Health Evaluation, Health Orientation, and Illness Orientation. Generally, research has revealed that the MBSRQ has excellent psychometric characteristics, demonstrating solid reliability and validity.[64-67] An advantage of the MBSRQ is that the factor structure is the same for both males and females, allowing for the investigation of gender differences in body image attitudes. In addition, unlike other instruments, the MBSRQ assesses both affective components of body image and cognitive-behavioral or motivational aspects. The MBSRQ and a users' manual are available from Thomas F. Cash at Old Dominion University.

4.2.5.5   *Body Dissatisfaction Subscale of the Eating Disorder Inventory – 2*

One of the most popular methods for assessing body image dissatisfaction is to administer the Body Dissatisfaction Subscale from the EDI-2.[13] This scale consists of nine items that assess an individual's level of satisfaction with the shape and size of her hips, thighs, stomach, and buttocks. Higher scores represent greater dissatisfaction. The EDI-2 is described above.

4.3   Application of Research Question

Our research question is as follows: How does a clinician pick which measure to use with a client? Given the variety of measures described above, which only represent a fraction of the many measures available for use, this question is an important one. We suggest the clinician keep in mind a number of factors when deciding how to assess a client. First, the clinician needs to identify the purpose of the assessment. Is it to rule out the possibility of an eating disorder? Is it to make a diagnosis of a suspected eating disorder? If the clinician wants to rule out an eating disorder, he/she could administer several of the self-report screening measures described above. If the client scores in the normal range or not in the clinically significant range on the instruments, the clinician has evidence that suggests the client is not suffering from an eating disorder. However, it must be kept in mind that these screening measures are not 100% accurate, and it is important to obtain follow-up information through interview questions or other sources. If the clinician suspects an eating disorder and wants to make a diagnosis, then he/she ought to consider administering a self-report instrument such as the Q-EDD and conducting a structured interview such as the EDE or the SCID. It is always important to gather information from as many sources as possible, so the clinician might interview the client's friends, family, and/or teachers for their perspectives on the client's eating behaviors and symptoms. In addition, the clinician ought to send the client for a full medical check-up from a physician, given the serious nature of many eating-disorder symptoms.

Second, clinicians need to keep in mind the psychometric properties of the assessment tools they are using. As noted above, the reliability and validity of measures may vary depending on whether the client is from a non-clinical or a clinical population. It is very difficult to measure accurately such constructs as food intake, activity level, purging behavior, and obesity.[68] Third, clinicians need to keep in mind the limitations of self-report measures and interview tools. For example, few of these measures have been assessed for their psychometric utility with individuals who are not white and middle class. Finally, it is not inconceivable that the client might lie, given the secretive nature of eating disorders. Clinicians need to be prepared to handle lying so that it does not alienate the client or ignore the potential health risks inherent in continued eating-disordered behaviors.

References

1. Shedler, J., Mayman, M., and Manis, M., The illusion of mental health, *American Psychologist*, 48, 1117–1131, 1993.
2. Pike, K. M., Loeb, K., and Walsh, B. T., Binge eating and purging, in *Handbook of Assessment Methods for Eating Behaviors and Weight-Related Problems: Measures, Theory, and Research*, Allison, D.B., Ed., Sage Publications, Thousand Oaks, CA, 1995, 303–346.
3. Mintz, L. B., O'Halloran, M. S., Mulholland, A. M., and Schneider, P. A., Questionnaire for eating disorder diagnoses: reliability and validity of operationalizing DSM-IV criteria into a self-report format, *Journal of Counseling Psychology*, 44, 63–79, 1997.
4. Garner, D. M. and Olmsted, M. P., *The Eating Disorder Inventory Manual.*, Psychological Assessment Resources, Odessa, TX, 1984.
5. Raciti, M. C. and Norcross, J. C., The EAT and EDI: screening, interrelationships, and psychometrics, *International Journal of Eating Disorders*, 6, 579–586, 1987.
6. Williamson, D. A., Anderson, D. A., Jackman, L. P., and Jackson, S. R., Assessment of eating disordered thoughts, feelings, and behaviors, in *Handbook of Assessment Methods for Eating Behaviors and Weight-related Problems: Measures, Theory, and Research*, Allison, D.B., Ed., Sage Publications, Thousand Oaks, CA, 1995, 347–386.
7. Garner, D. M., Olmsted, M. P., and Polivy, J., Development and validation of a multidimensional Eating Disorder Inventory for anorexia nervosa and bulimia, *International Journal of Eating Disorders*, 2, 15–34, 1983.
8. Welch, G., Hall, A., and Norring, C., The factor structure of the Eating Disorder Inventory in a patient setting, *International Journal of Eating Disorders*, 9, 79–85, 1990.
9. Cooper, Z., Cooper, P. J., and Fairburn, C. G., The specificity of the Eating Disorder Inventory, *British Journal of Clinical Psychology*, 24, 129–130, 1985.
10. Hurley, J. B., Palmer, R. L., and Stretch, D., The specificity of the Eating Disorder Inventory: a reappraisal, *International Journal of Eating Disorders*, 9, 419–424, 1990.
11. Norring, C. E. A., The Eating Disorder Inventory: its relation to diagnostic dimensions and follow-up status, *International Journal of Eating Disorders*, 9, 685–694, 1990.
12. Klemchuk, H. P., Hutchinson, C. B., and Frank, R. I., Body dissatisfaction and eating-related problems on the college campus: usefulness of the Eating Disorder Inventory with a nonclinical population, *Journal of Counseling Psychology*, 37, 297–305, 1990.
13. Garner, D. M., *Eating Disorder Inventory-2 Professional Manual*, Psychological Assessment Resources, Inc., Odessa, TX, 1991.
14. Crowther, J. H. and Sherwood, N. E., Assessment, in *Handbook of Treatment for Eating Disorders*, 2nd ed., Garner, D.M. and Garfinkel, P.E., Eds., Guilford Press, New York, 1997, 34–49.

15. Brookings, J. B., Eating Disorder Inventory-2, in *Test Critiques*, Vol. 10, Keyser, D. J. and Sweetland, R. C., Eds., Pro-Ed, Austin, TX, 1994, 226–233.

16. Eberenz, K. P. and Gleaves, D. H., An examination of the internal consistency and factor structure of the Eating Disorder Inventory-2 in a clinical sample, *International Journal of Eating Disorders*, 16, 371–379, 1994.

17. Garner, D. M. and Garfinkel, P. E., The Eating Attitudes Test: an index of the symptoms of anorexia nervosa, *Psychological Medicine*, 9, 273–279, 1979.

18. Garner, D. M., Olmsted, M. P., Bohr, Y., and Garfinkel, P. E., The Eating Attitudes Test: psychometric features and clinical correlates, *Psychological Medicine*, 12, 871–878, 1982.

19. Carter, P. I. and Moss, R. A., Screening for anorexia and bulimia nervosa in a college population: problems and limitations, *Addictive Behaviors*, 9, 417–419, 1984.

20. Johnsone-Sabine, E., Wood, K., and Patton, G., Abnormal eating attitudes in London schoolgirls – a prospective epidemiological study: factors associated with abnormal response on screening questionnaires, *Psychological Medicine*, 18, 615–622, 1988.

21. Meadows, G. N., Palmer, R. C., Newball, E. U. M., and Kenrick, J. M. T., Eating attitudes and disorders in young women: a general practice based survey. *Psychological Medicine*, 16, 351–357, 1986.

22. Gross, J., Rosen, J. C., Leitenberg, H., and Willmuth, M. E., Validity of the Eating Attitudes Test and the Eating Disorders Inventory in bulimia nervosa, *Journal of Counseling and Clinical Psychology*, 54, 875–876, 1986.

23. American Psychiatric Association, *Diagnostic and Statistical Manual of Mental Disorders*, 4th ed., Washington, D.C., 1994.

24. Thelen, M. H., Farmer, J., Wonderlich, S., and Smith, M., A revision of the Bulimia Test. the BULIT-R, *Psychological Assessment*, 3, 119–124, 1991.

25. Thelen, M. H., Mintz, L. B., and Vander Wal, J. S., The Bulimia Test – Revised: validation with DSM-IV criteria for bulimia nervosa, *Psychological Assessment*, 8, 219–221, 1996.

26. Mizes, J. S. and Klesges, R. C., Validity, reliability, and factor structure of the anorectic cognitions questionnaire, *Addictive Behaviors*, 14, 589–594, 1989.

27. Mizes, J. S., Personality characteristics of bulimic and non-eating disordered female controls: a cognitive behavioral perspective, *International Journal of Eating Disorders*, 7, 541–550, 1988.

28. Mizes, J. S., Construct validity and factor stability of the anorectic cognitions questionnaire, *Addictive Behaviors*, 16, 89–93, 1991.

29. Nunnally, J. C., *Psychometric Theory*, McGraw-Hill, New York, 1978.

30. Cooper, Z. and Fairburn C., The Eating Disorder Examination: a semi-structured interview for the assessment of the specific psychopathology of eating disorders, *International Journal of Eating Disorders*, 6, 1–8, 1987.

31. Fairburn, C. G. and Cooper, Z., The Eating Disorder Examination (12th ed.), in *Binge Eating: Nature, Assessment, and Treatment*, Fairburn, C.G. and Wilson, G.T., Eds., Guilford Press, New York, 1993, 317–360.

32. Beglin, S. J., Eating Disorders in Young Adult Women, Unpublished doctoral dissertation, Oxford University, Oxford, U.K., 1990.

33. Wilson, G. T. and Smith, D., Assessment of bulimia nervosa: an evaluation of the Eating Disorders Examination, *International Journal of Eating Disorders*, 8, 173–179, 1989.

34. Cooper, Z., Cooper, P. J., and Fairburn, C. G., The validity of the Eating Disorder Examination and its subscales, *British Journal of Psychiatry*, 154, 807–812, 1989.

35. Fairburn, C. G. and Beglin, S. J., Assessment of eating disorders: interview or self-report questionnaire? *International Journal of Eating Disorders*, 16, 363–370, 1994.

36. Black, C. M. D. and Wilson, G. T., Assessment of eating disorders: interview versus questionnaire. *International Journal of Eating Disorders*, 20, 43–50, 1996.

37. First, M. B., Spitzer, R. L., Gibbon, R. L., Gibbon, M., and Williams, J. B. W., *Structured Clinical Interview for Axis I DSM-IV Disorders, Patient Edition (SCID-IL, Version 2.0)*, Biometrics Research Department, New York, 1994.

38. Skre, I., Onstad, S., Torgersen, S., and Kringlen, E., High interrater reliability for the Structured Clinical Interview for DSM-III-R Axis (SCID-I), *Acta Psychiatrica Scandinavica*, 84, 167–173.

39. Stice, E., Ozer, S., and Kees, M., Relation of dietary restraint to bulimic symptomatology: the effects of the criterion confounding of the restraint scale, *Behavior Research and Therapy*, 35, 145–152, 1997.

40. Ruderman, A. J., Dietary restraint: a theoretical and empirical review, *Psychological Bulletin*, 99, 247–262, 1986.

41. Gorman, B. S. and Allison, D. B., Measures of restrained eating, in *Handbook of Assessment Methods for Eating Behaviors and Weight-Related Problems: Measures, Theory, and Research*, Allison, D. B., Ed., Sage Publications, Thousand Oaks, CA, 1995, 149–184.

42. Polivy, J. and Herman, C. P., Dieting and binging: a causal analysis, *American Psychologist*, 40, 193–204, 1985.

43. Van Strien, T., Frijters, J. E. R., Bergers, G. P. A., and Defares, P. B., The Dutch Eating Behavior Questionnaire (DEBQ) for assessment of restrained, emotional, and external eating behavior, *International Journal of Eating Disorders*, 5, 295–315, 1986.

44. Van Strien, T., Frijters, J. E. R., Van Staveren, W. A., Defares, P. B., and Deurenberg, P., The predictive validity of the Dutch Restrained Eating Scale, *International Journal of Eating Disorders*, 5, 747–755, 1986.

45. Wardle, J., Eating style: A validation study of the Dutch Eating Behavior Questionnaire in normal subjects and women with eating disorders, *Journal of Psychosomatic Research*, 31, 161–169, 1987.

46. Allison, D. B. and Franklin, R. D., The readability of three measures of dietary restraint, *Psychotherapy in Private Practice*, 12, 53–57, 1993.

47. Herman, C. P. and Polivy, J., Anxiety, restraint, and eating behavior, *Journal of Abnormal Psychology*, 84, 666–672, 1975.

48. Herman, C. P. and Polivy, J., Restrained eating, in *Obesity*, Stunkard, A. J., Ed., W. B. Saunders, Philadelphia, 1980, 208–225.

49. Klem, M. L., Klesges, R. C., Bene, C. R., and Mellon, M. W., A psychometric study of restraint: the impact of race, gender, weight and marital status, *Addictive Behaviors*, 15, 147–152, 1990.

50. Allison, D. B., Kalinsky, L. B., and Gorman, B. S., A comparison of the psychometric properties of three measures of dietary restraint, *Psychological Assessment*, 4, 391–398, 1992.

51. Stunkard, A. J. and Messick, S., The three-factor eating questionnaire to measure dietary restraint, disinhibition and hunger, *Journal of Psychosomatic Research*, 29, 71–83, 1985.

52. Stunkard, A. J. and Messick, S., *The Eating Inventory*. Psychological Corporation, San Antonio, TX, 1988.

53. Collins, L. R., Lapp, W. M., Helder, L., and Saltzberg, J. A., Cognitive restraint and impulsive eating: insights from the Three-Factor Eating Questionnaire, *Psychology of Addictive Behaviors*, 6, 47–53, 1992.

54. Spitzer, R. L., Yanovski, S., Wadden, T., Wing, R., Marcus, M. Stunkard, A., Devlin, M., Mitchell, J., Hasin, D., and Horne, R. L. Binge eating disorder: its further validation in a multisite study, *International Journal of Eating Disorders*, 13, 137–153, 1993.

55. Spitzer, R. L., Devlin, M., Walsh, B. T., Hasin, D., Wing, R. Marcus, M., Stunkard, A., Wadden, T., Yanovski, S., Agras, S., Mitchell, J., and Nonas, C. Binge eating disorder: A multi-site field trial of the diagnostic criteria, *International Journal of Eating Disorders*, 13, 161–169, 1992.

56. Spitzer, R. L., Yanovski, S. Z., and Marcus, M. D., The Questionnaire on Eating and Weight Patterns – Revised (QEWP-R, 1993), New York State Psychiatric Institute, New York, 1993.

57. Nangle, D. W., Johnson, W. G., Carr-Nangle, R. E., and Engler, L. B., Binge Eating Disorder and the proposed DSM-IV criteria: psychometric analysis of the Questionnaire of Eating and Weight Patterns, *International Journal of Eating Disorders*, 16, 147–157, 1994.

58. Gladis, M. M., Wadden, T. A., Foster, G. D., Vogt, F. R., and Wingate, B. J., A comparison of two approaches to the assessment of binge eating in obesity, *International Journal of Eating Disorders*, 23, 17–26, 1998.

59. Ruff, G. A. and Barrios, B. A. Realistic assessment of body image, *Behavioral Assessment*, 8, 237–251, 1986.

60. Cash, T. F. and Green, G. K., Body weight and body image among college women: perception, cognition, and affect, *Journal of Personality Assessment*, 50, 290–301, 1986.
61. Thompson, M. A. and Gray, J. J., Development and validation of a new body-image assessment scale, *Journal of Personality Assessment*, 64, 258–269, 1995.
62. Thompson, J. K., Assessment of body image, in *Handbook of Assessment Methods for Eating Behaviors and Weight-Related Problems: Measures, Theory, and Research*, Allison, D.B., Ed., Sage Publications, Thousand Oaks, CA, 1995, 119–148.
63. Schlundt, D. G. and Bell, C., Body Image Testing System: a microcomputer program for assessing body image, *Journal of Psychopathology and Behavioral Assessment*, 15, 267–285, 1993.
64. Brown, T. A., Cash, T. F., and Mikulka, O. J., Attitudinal body-image assessment: factor analysis of the Body-Self Relations Questionnaire, *Journal of Personality Assessment*, 55, 135–144, 1990.
65. Cash, T. F., The Users' Manual for the Multidimensional Body-Self Relations Questionnaire. Unpublished manuscript, Old Dominion University, Norfolk, VA, 1994.
66. Brown, T. A, Cash, T. F., and Lewis, R. J., Body-image disturbances in adolescent female binge-purgers: a brief report of the results of a national survey in the USA, *Journal of Child Psychology and Psychiatry*, 30, 605–613, 1989.
67. Cash, T. F., Body-image affect: Gestalt versus summing the parts, *Perceptual and Motor Skills*, 69, 17–18, 1989.
68. Agras, W. S., The big picture, in *Handbook of Assessment Methods for Eating Behaviors and Weight-related Problems: Measures, Theory, and Research*, Allison, D.B., Ed., Sage Publications, Thousand Oaks, CA, 1995, 561–579.

Appendix 4-A: Bulimia Test — Revised (BULIT-R)

Answer each question by circling the appropriate response. Please respond to each item as honestly as possible; remember all of the information you provide will be kept strictly confidential.

1. I am satisfied with my eating patterns.
   1. agree
   2. neutral
   3. disagree a little
   4. disagree
   +5. disagree strongly

2. Would you presently call yourself a "binge eater"?
   +1. yes, absolutely
   2. yes
   3. yes, probably
   4. yes, possibly
   5. no, probably not

3. Do you feel you have control over the amount of food you consume?
   1. most or all of the time
   2. a lot of the time
   3. occasionally
   4. rarely
   +5. never

4. I am satisfied with the shape and size of my body.
   1. frequently or always
   2. sometimes
   3. occasionally
   4. rarely
   +5. seldom or never

5. When I feel that my eating behavior is out of control, I try to take rather extreme measures to get back on course (strict dieting, fasting, laxatives, diuretics, self-induced vomiting, or vigorous exercise).
   +1. always
   2. almost always
   3. frequently
   4. sometimes
   5. never or my eating behavior is never out of control

6. X I use laxatives or suppositories to help control my weight.
   1. once a day or more
   2. 3–6 times a week
   3. once or twice a week
   4. 2–3 times a month
   5. once a month or less (or never)

7. I am obsessed about the size and shape of my body.
   +1. always
   2. almost always
   3. frequently
   4. sometimes
   5. seldom or never

8. There are times when I rapidly eat a very large amount of food.
   +1. more than twice a week
   2. twice a week
   3. once a week
   4. 2–3 times a month
   5. once a month or less (or never)

9. How long have you been binge eating (eating uncontrollably to the point of stuffing yourself)?
   1. not applicable; I don't binge eat
   2. less than 3 months
   3. 3 months–1 year
   4. 1–3 years
   +5. 3 or more years

10. Most people I know would be amazed if they knew how much food I can consume at one sitting.
   +1. without a doubt
   2. very probably
   3. probably
   4. possibly
   5. no

11. X I exercise in order to burn calories
   1. more than 2 hours per day
   2. about 2 hours per day
   3. more than 1 but less than 2 hours per day
   4. one hour or less per day
   5. I exercise but not to burn calories or I don't exercise

12. Compared with women your age, how preoccupied are you about your weight and body shape?
   + 1. a great deal more than average
   2. much more than average
   3. more than average
   4. a little more than average
   5. average or less than average

13. I am afraid to eat anything for fear that I won't be able to stop.
   + 1. always
   2. almost always
   3. frequently
   4. sometimes
   5. seldom or never

14. I feel tormented by the idea that I am fat or might gain weight.
   +1. always
   2. almost always
   3. frequently
   4. sometimes
   5. seldom or never

15. How often do you intentionally vomit after eating?

    +1. 2 or more times a week   4. once a month

     2. once a week   5. less than once a month or never

     3. 2–3 times a month

16. I eat a lot of food when I'm not even hungry.

    +1. very frequently   4. sometimes

     2. frequently   5. seldom or never

     3. occasionally

17. My eating patterns are different from the eating patterns of most people.

    +1. always   4. sometimes

     2. almost always   5. seldom or never

     3. frequently

18. After I binge eat I turn to one of several strict methods to try to keep from gaining weight (vigorous exercise, strict dieting, fasting, self-induced vomiting, laxatives, or diuretics).

     1. never or I don't binge eat   4. a lot of the time

     2. rarely   +5. most or all of the time

     3. occasionally

19. X I have tried to lose weight by fasting or going on strict diets.

     1. not in the past year   4. 4–5 times in the past year

     2. once in the past year   5. more than 5 times in the past year

     3. 2–3 times in the past year

20. X I exercise vigorously and for long periods of time in order to burn calories.

     1. average or less than average   4. much more than average

     2. a little more than average   5. a great deal more than average

     3. more than average

21. When engaged in an eating binge, I tend to eat foods that are high in carbohydrates (sweets and starches).

    +1. always   4. sometimes

     2. almost always   5. seldom, I don't binge

     3. frequently

22. Compared to most people, my ability to control my eating behavior seems to be:

     1. greater than others' ability   4. much less

     2. about the same   + 5. I have absolutely no control

     3. less

23. I would presently label myself a 'compulsive eater' (one who engages in episodes of uncontrolled eating).

+1. absolutely
2. yes
3. yes, probably
4. yes, possibly
5. no, probably not

24. I hate the way my body looks after I eat too much.

1. seldom or never
2. sometimes
3. frequently
4. almost always
+5. always

25. When I am trying to keep from gaining weight, I feel that I have to resort to vigorous exercise, strict dieting, fasting, self-induced vomiting, laxatives, or diuretics.

1. never
2. rarely
3. occasionally
4. a lot of the time
+5. most or all of the time

26. Do you believe that it is easier for you to vomit than it is for most people?

+1. yes, it's no problem at all for me
2. yes, it's easier
3. yes, it's a little easier
4. about the same
5. no, it's less easy

27. X I use diuretics (water pills) to help control my weight.

1. never
2. seldom
3. sometimes
4. frequently
5. very frequently

28. I feel that food controls my life.

+1. always
2. almost always
3. frequently
4. sometimes
5. seldom or never

29. X I try to control my weight by eating little or no food for a day or longer.

1. never
2. seldom
3. sometimes
4. frequently
5. very frequently

30. When consuming a large quantity of food, at what rate of speed do you usually eat?

+1. more rapidly than most people have ever eaten in their lives
2. a lot more rapidly than most people
3. a little more rapidly than most people
4. about the same rate as most people
5. more slowly than most people (or not applicable)

31. X I use laxatives or suppositories to help control my weight.
1. never   4. frequently
2. seldom   5. very frequently
3. sometimes

32. Right after I binge eat I feel:
+1. so fat and bloated I can't stand it
2. extremely fat
3. fat
4. a little fat
5. OK about how my body looks or I never binge eat

33. Compared to other people of my sex, my ability to always feel in control of how much I eat is:
1. about the same or greater   4. much less
2. a little less   +5. a great deal less
3. less

34. In the last 3 months, on the average how often did you binge eat (eat uncontrollably to the point of stuffing yourself)?
1. once a month or less (or never)
2. 2–3 times a month
3. once a week
4. twice a week
+5. more than twice a week

35. Most people I know would be surprised at how fat I look after I eat a lot of food.
+1. yes, definitely   4. yes, possibly
2. yes   5. no, probably not or I never eat a lot
3. yes, probably   of food

36. X I use diuretics (water pills) to help control my weight.
1. 3 times a week or more   4. once a month
2. once or twice a week   5. never
3. 2–3 times a month

Scoring: X denotes questions whose answers are not added to determine the total BULIT-R score; + denotes the most strongly symptomatic response, which receives a score of five points

Appendix 4-B: Questionnaire for Eating Disorder Diagnoses (Q-EDD)

Please complete the following questions as honestly as possible. The questions refer to *current behaviors and beliefs*, meaning those that have occurred in the past 3 months.

Sex: (Please circle)   Male   Female

Age: _____

School/Occupational Status: (Please circle)

Junior High or younger (*specify* grade: _____)

High School Freshman

High School Sophomore

High School Junior

High School Senior

College Freshman

College Sophomore

College Junior

College Senior

Not in School/Employed (specify: _____)

Race/Ethnicity: Caucasian/White

(Please circle)   African-American/Black

Hispanic /Latino/Mexican-American

American Indian

Asian-American/Pacific Islander

Other: _____ (specify)

Present height: _____ feet _____ inches

Present weight: _____ pounds

My body-frame is: small   medium   large (Please circle)

I would like to weigh   _____ pounds.

1. Do you experience recurrent episodes of binge eating, meaning eating in a discrete period of time (e.g., within any 2-hour period) an amount of food that is definitely larger than most people would eat during a similar time period?

    YES   NO

    If YES: Continue to answer the following questions.

    If NO: Skip to Question #4 (on the next page)

2. Do you have a sense of lack of control during the binge-eating episodes (i.e., the feeling that you cannot stop eating or control what or how much you are eating)?

    YES   NO

3. Circle the answers within the *two* sets of [**bold brackets**] below that best fit for you:

   On the average, I have had [**1, 2, 3, 4, 5, 6 or more**] binge-eating episodes a *WEEK* for at least

   [**1 month, 2 months, 3 months, 4 months, 5 months, 6–12 months, more than one year**]

4. Please circle the appropriate responses below concerning things you may do *currently to prevent weight gain*. If you circle yes to any question, please indicate how often on the average you do this and how long you have been doing this.

   a) **Do you make yourself vomit?**   YES   NO

      How often do you do this?

      Daily   Twice/Week   Once/Week   Once/Month

      How long have you been doing this?

      1 month   2 months   3 months   4 months   5–11 months   More than a year

   b) **Do you take laxatives?**   YES   NO

      How often do you do this?

      Daily   Twice/Week   Once/Week   Once/Month

      How long have you been doing this?

      1 month   2 months   3 months   4 months   5–11 months   More than a year

   c) **Do you take diuretics (water pills)?**   YES   NO

      How often do you do this?

      Daily   Twice/Week   Once/Week   Once/Month

      How long have you been doing this?

      1 month   2 months   3 months   4 months   5–11 months   More than a year

   d) **Do you fast (skip food for 24 hours)?**   YES   NO

      How often do you do this?

      Daily   Twice/Week   Once/Week   Once/Month

      How long have you been doing this?

      1 month   2 months   3 months   4 months   5–11 months   More than a year

   e) **Do you chew food but spit it out?**   YES   NO

      How often do you do this?

      Daily   Twice/Week   Once/Week   Once/Month

      How long have you been doing this?

      1 month   2 months   3 months   4 months   5–11 months   More than a year

   f) **Do you give yourself an enema?**   YES   NO

      How often do you do this?

      Daily   Twice/Week   Once/Week   Once/Month

      How long have you been doing this?

      1 month   2 months   3 months   4 months   5–11 months   More than a year

g) Do you take appetite control pills? YES NO
How often do you do this?
Daily Twice/Week Once/Week Once/Month
How long have you been doing this?
1 month 2 months 3 months 4 months 5–11 months More than a year

h) Do you diet strictly? YES NO
How often do you do this?
Daily Twice/Week Once/Week Once/Month
How long have you been doing this?
1 month 2 months 3 months 4 months 5–11 months More than a year

i) Do you exercise a lot? YES NO
How often do you do this?
Daily Twice/Week Once/Week Once/Month
How long have you been doing this?
1 month 2 months 3 months 4 months 5–11 months More than a year

5. If you answered YES to "exercise a lot," please answer questions #5a, 5b, 5c, and 5d. If you answered NO to "exercise a lot," skip to question #6.

5a. Fill in the blanks below:
   I _____ (types of exercise, e.g., jog, swim) for an average of _____ hours at a time.

5b. My exercise sometimes significantly interferes with important activities.
   YES   NO

5c. I exercise despite injury and/or medical complications.
   YES   NO

5d. Is your primary reason for exercising to counteract the effects of binges or to prevent weight gain?
   YES   NO

For the following questions, circle the response that best reflects your answer:

6. Does your weight and/or body shape influence how you feel about yourself?

1	2	3	4	5
Not at all	A Little	A moderate amount	Very Much	Extremely or Completely

7. How afraid are you of becoming fat?

1	2	3	4	5
Not at all	A Little	A moderate amount	Very Much	Extremely or Completely

8. How afraid are you of gaining weight?

1	2	3	4	5
Not at all	A Little	A moderate amount	Very Much	Extremely or Completely

9. Do you consider yourself to be:

1	2	3	4	5	6
Grossly Obese	Moderately Obese	Overweight	Normal Weight	Low Weight	Severely Underweight

10. Certain parts of my body (e.g., my abdomen, buttocks, thighs) are too fat.

   YES   NO

11. I feel fat all over.

   YES   NO

12. I believe that how little I weigh is a serious problem.

   YES   NO

13. I have missed at least 3 consecutive menstrual cycles (not including those missed during a pregnancy).

   YES   NO

Source: Mintz, L. B., O'Halloran, M. S., Mulholland, A. M., and Schneider, P. A.

Appendix 4-C: Multidimensional Body-Self Relations Questionnaire (MBSRQ)

INSTRUCTIONS — PLEASE READ CAREFULLY

The following pages contain a series of statements about how people might think, feel, or behave. You are asked to indicate *the extent to which each statement pertains to you personally.* Your answers to the items in the questionnaire are anonymous, so please do not write your name on any of the materials. In order to complete the questionnaire, read each statement carefully and decide how much it pertains to you personally. Using a scale like the one below, indicate your answer by entering it to the left of the number of the statement.

1	2	3	4	5
Definitely Disagree	Mostly Disagree	Neither Agree Nor Disagree	Mostly Agree	Definitely Agree

EXAMPLE:

_____ I am usually in a good mood.

In the blank space, enter a 1 if you *definitely disagree* with the statement; a **2** if you *mostly disagree*; a 3 if you *neither agree nor disagree*; a 4 if you *mostly agree*; or enter a **5** if you *definitely* agree with the statement. There are no right or wrong answers. Just give the answer that is most accurate for you. Remember, your responses are anonymous, so please be *completely honest* and answer all items.

1	2	3	4	5
Definitely Disagree	Mostly Disagree	Neither Agree Nor Disagree	Mostly Agree	Definitely Agree

_____ 1. Before going out in public, I always notice how I look.

_____ 2. I am careful to buy clothes that will make me look my best.

_____ 3. I would pass most physical-fitness tests.

_____ 4. It is important that I have superior physical strength.

_____ 5. My body is sexually appealing.

_____ 6. I am not involved in a regular exercise program.

_____ 7. I am in control of my health.

_____ 8. I know a lot about things that affect my physical health.

_____ 9. I have deliberately developed a healthy life style.

_____ 10. I constantly worry about being or becoming fat.

_____ 11. I like my looks just the way they are.

_____ 12. I check my appearance in a mirror whenever I can.

_____ 13. Before going out, I usually spend a lot of time getting ready.

_____ 14. My physical endurance is good.

_____ 15. Participating in sports is unimportant to me.

_____ 16. I do not actively do things to keep physically fit.

_____ 17. My health is a matter of unexpected ups and downs.

_____ 18. Good health is one of the most important things in my life.

_____ 19. I don't do anything that I know might threaten my health.

_____ 20. I am very conscious of even small changes in my weight.

_____ 21. Most people would consider me good-looking.

_____ 22. It is important that I always look good.

_____ 23. I use very few grooming products.

_____ 24. I easily learn physical skills.

_____ 25. Being physically fit is not a strong priority in my life.

_____ 26. I do things to increase my physical strength.

_____ 27. I am seldom physically ill.

_____ 28. I take my health for granted.

_____ 29. I often read books and magazines that pertain to health.

_____ 30. I like the way I look without my clothes on.

_____ 31. I am self-conscious if my grooming isn't right.

_____ 32. I usually wear whatever is handy without caring how it looks.

_____ 33. I do poorly in physical sports or games.

_____ 34. I seldom think about my athletic skills.

_____ 35. I work to improve my physical stamina.

_____ 36. From day to day, I never know how my body will feel.

_____ 37. If I am sick, I don't pay much attention to my symptoms.

_____ 38. I make no special effort to eat a balanced and nutritious diet.

_____ 39. I like the way my clothes fit me.

_____ 40. I don't care what people think about my appearance.

_____ 41. I take special care with my hair grooming.

_____ 42. I dislike my physique.

_____ 43. I don't care to improve my abilities in physical activities.

_____ 44. I try to be physically active.

_____ 45. I often feel vulnerable to sickness.

_____ 46. I pay close attention to my body for any signs of illness.

_____ 47. If I'm coming down with a cold or flu, I just ignore it and go on as usual.

_____ 48. I am physically unattractive.

_____ 49. I never think about my appearance.

_____ 50. I am always trying to improve my physical appearance.

_____ 51. I am very well coordinated.

_____ 52. I know a lot about physical fitness.

_____ 53. I play a sport regularly throughout the year.

_____ 54. I am a physically healthy person.

_____ 55. I am very aware of small changes in my physical health.

_____ 56. At the first sign of illness, I seek medical advice.

_____ 57. I am on a weight-loss diet.

For the remainder of the items use the response scale given with the item, and enter your answer in the space beside the item.

____ 58. I have tried to lose weight by fasting or going on crash diets.
      1. Never
      2. Rarely
      3. Sometimes
      4. Often
      5. Very Often

____ 59. I think I am:
      1. Very Underweight
      2. Somewhat Underweight
      3. Normal Weight
      4. Somewhat Overweight
      5. Very Overweight

____ 60. From looking at me, most other people would think I am:
      1. Very Underweight
      2. Somewhat Underweight
      3. Normal Weight
      4. Somewhat Overweight
      5. Very Overweight

61–69. Use this 1 to 5 scale to indicate *how satisfied you are* with each of the following areas or aspects of your body:

1	2	3	4	5
Very Dissatisfied	Mostly Dissatisfied	Neither Satisfied Nor Dissatisfied	Mostly Satisfied	Very Satisfied

____ 61. Face (facial features, complexion)
____ 62. Hair (color, thickness, texture)
____ 63. Lower torso (buttocks, hips, thighs, legs)
____ 64. Mid torso (waist, stomach)
____ 65. Upper torso (chest or breasts, shoulders, arms)
____ 66. Muscle tone
____ 67. Weight
____ 68. Height
____ 69. Overall appearance

Part II

The Characteristics of Stress

5

Definition of Stress

Teddy L. Jones

CONTENTS

5.1   Learning Objectives

After completing this chapter you should be able to:

- Define stress as the term is commonly used by laypersons and by professionals studying stress in humans;
- Identify both positive and negative aspects of stress in humans;
- Comprehend at least one framework for analyzing approaches to help people to deal more effectively with stress.

5.2   Research Background

5.2.1   Definition of Stress — A Source of Confusion

Looking for a villain? STRESS. Yes, stress is a source of negative conditions experienced by people of all ages from a variety of cultures The popular view points to stress as a basis for or factor in headaches, premenstrual tension, back pain, childhood tantrums, eating disorders, marital discord, substance abuse, high blood pressure, some types of cancer, heart disease, road rage, and poor work performance. The term itself has become part of the common vocabulary in the United States and much of Western culture. Yet, the meanings attributed to this term vary widely, according to whether it is being used in popular or scientific literature. Conceptual definitions of stress tend to be viewed in two major ways: as a cause or as a result. Stress resulting from either of those conceptual positions has been defined and measured using either psychological or physical methods reflecting the researcher's position on the subject.

Why does such confusion exist about something that we all experience? One possible reason is that stress is a borrowed term. Stress has a precise meaning in physics, and it was in borrowing that term from physics to use as an analogy for what he had observed as the "syndrome of just being sick" that Hans Selye first used "stress" as a concept. Knapp[1] expounds on the lack of precision in stress researchers' use of the term by stating that Selye, in later works, acknowledged that his initial unfamiliarity with English prompted him to fail to make the distinction between "stress" (the cause of wear and tear) and "strain" (the effect — or the wear and tear itself). Selye called them both stress initially and then later chose the word "stressor" to refer to the cause. Knapp's suggestion is to resolve the confusion by following Selye's approach and using "stressors" instead of "strains" to refer to causes of stress, and devoting research efforts to finding methods of measuring stress and stressors. This chapter therefore uses Selye's conceptual definition of stress as "…the nonspecific response of the body to any demand made upon it"[2] and defines stressor as that which produces stress. It is important to bear in mind the decades of work by Selye and others have produced much elaboration on the specifics of stress and its effects. When Selye first began, in the 1940s, he studied stress as a biological phenomenon. His initial subjects were not human.[3] Over time, human studies have detailed stress from the biophysical perspective. Additionally, psychologists and other researchers have explored the psychological aspects of stress. Among them one of the most influential, Richard Lazarus, stated in his introduction to an anthology on stress that it is "…any event in which environmental demands, internal demands, or both tax or exceed the adaptive resources of an individual, social system, or tissue system."[4] To integrate these approaches, a professional should choose the perspective that stress in humans is a whole-person response, a nonspecific one, that is evidenced in every aspect of the being.

5.2.2 What Is Happening When Stress Is Present?

Based on the complex history of research on stress, it is difficult to provide a clear, comprehensive explanation of what is happening to a person when stress is present, for the reason that different perspectives on the study of stress result in differing approaches in describing it. As Cohen and Kessler[5] explain, one view, the biological, focuses on pathophysiological reactions; another perspective, the psychological, concerns itself with a psychologic appraisal of events and response capabilities; and yet another view is more epidemiological, in that it is concerned with identifying types of variables (of environmental exposures) that increase risks of adverse outcomes. In an attempt to integrate these approaches, a schematic representation of the relationships among stressors and the stress response in humans is provided in Figure 5.1. The stressor is the source of arousal to the organism. It may be environmental (extreme cold, for example), physical (e.g., extended athletic competition), or psychosocial (e.g., sick family member).

Regardless of the stressor, certain automatic responses occur, as first noted by Selye. After decades of research, vast amounts are known about the particular bio-

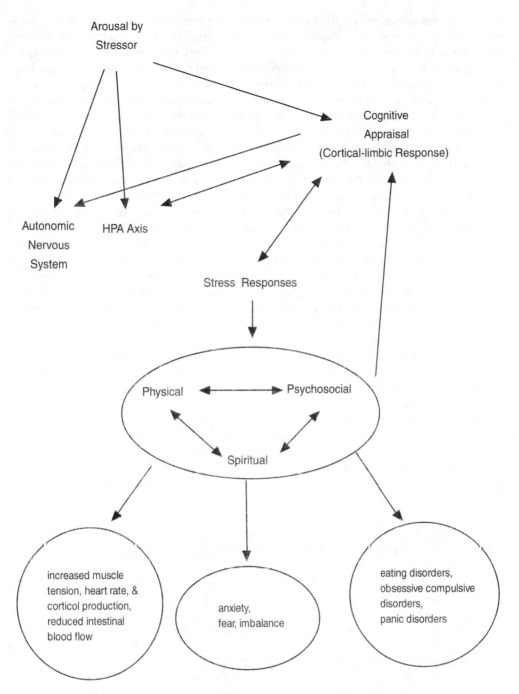

FIGURE 5.1
Relationships of stressors and stress responses in humans.

chemical pathways triggered by certain types of stressors and in stress-inducing situations of varying durations in organisms with varying genetic makeups with and without pre-existing diseases. Although much of the research is extremely specific and therefore not widely applicable, one major set of responses does appear to be present across all research categories, those responses that are set in motion at the hypothalamus, pituitary, adrenal axis (HPA Axis). This set of interrelated endocrine glands initiates the signals provoking the cascade of responses that constitute the stress response, originally called the General Adaptation Syndrome by Selye. These responses are recognized as those which allowed primitive humans (and other living organisms) to survive in hostile environments, as they prepared for fight or flight.

Tsigos and Chrousos[6] offer an excellent discussion of the biochemistry of the HPA axis. A key neuroendocrine effector of the stress response is corticotropin-releasing hormone (CRH), which is produced in the hypothalamus along with arginine vaso-pressin (AVP). Acting together, they prompt the pituitary to produce ACTH (adrenal corticotrophic hormone). In non-stressful conditions, baseline levels of these hormones are produced, with variations that are cyclical throughout the day (diurnal) and can be interrupted by stress. ACTH acts upon the adrenal glands to affect the production of glucocorticoids and adrenal androgens, and it also affects the control of aldosterone in the adrenal glands. These adrenal glucocorticoids are the main effectors of stress at the cellular level of the whole organism, as receptors for glucocorticoids are present throughout the body. Thus, stimulation of glucocorticoid production above baseline levels affects virtually every system in the body. These systems transmit inhibitory messages to the hypothalamus and the pituitary. When these messages are effective, the result is a limitation of the exposure of tissues to the potentially destructive results of longer-term glucocorticoid exposure. These destructive effects become pronounced when chronic stress alters the inhibitory mechanism and include tissue catabolism (breakdown), lipogenesis (inappropriate fat conversion), reproductive suppression, and immune system suppression.

Both the sympathetic and parasympathetic aspects of the autonomic nervous system also respond to stress. The result is that epinephrine, norepinephrine, and acetylcholine production are altered. Receptors throughout the body respond to these neurotransmitter substances, including the vascular smooth muscle, fat, kidney, and intestine, among others. An array of other neurochemicals have been identified as the messengers for these three chemicals, which act to produce the readiness for fight or flight.

One other set of chemical interactions produces central nervous system responses to stressors. These act within the cortical and limbic aspects of the brain and are thought to mediate the emotional aspects (appraisals) of stress. To complicate this already complex set of interactions, each affects and can prompt others. Thus, a primarily emotional stressor can trigger the same cascade of chemical reactions and resulting behavioral responses that exposure to extreme cold (primarily a physical stressor) might. In Figure 5.1, note that the elements of the stress response interact with one another and that, at the organic response level, the entire organism — body, mind, and spirit — is affected. The responses range from reduced intestinal blood flow, muscle tension, heart rate (autonomic response), and cortisol production (HPA axis) to anxiety or fear (cortical-limbic response). If the stressor is acute and of short duration, the organism moves from the initial alarm phase to a stage of resistance, and then returns to a stage of readiness. It has adapted. If the initial resistance phase is ineffective, exhaustion and death can occur.

Chronic exposure to stressors can result in either maladaptation or adaptation. In maladaptive responses, the effects can be destructive, as mentioned earlier, and can affect growth; reproduction; thyroid function; fat, muscle and bone metabolism; gastrointestinal function; and the immune system and inflammatory response. In addition, when the maladaptation is expressed via functions triggered by the corticolimbic system, psychoemotional disorders can ensue. Some of the ones in which stress has been implicated include obsessive-compulsive disorders, eating disorders, and panic disorders.

Research continues on a variety of fronts, toward the goal of understanding this very complex set of reactions. For example, Dorn and Chrousos have studied stress in adolescents.[7] Tsigos and Chrousos[8] have explored the connection of the HPA axis to psychiatric and autoimmune disorders. Gullette et al.[9] have looked at emotional stress and reduced cardiac blood flow. Family stressors and their effects on adolescents have served as the focus for Forehand et al.[10] Woods et al.[11] have researched stress and premenstrual syndrome. Stress and eating disorders have been studied by Fryer, Weller and Kroese,[12] Gold et al.,[13] and Kaye et al.,[14] among many others. The relationship of stress to depression has received much research attention, as in the study by Connor and Leonard.[15] Due to the vast number of studies focused on immune function and stress, meta-analytic research, which attempts to synthesize common themes, has become important, as evidenced in the work by Herbert and Cohen.[16]

5.2.3   Approaches to the Study of Stress

An abundance of research from the biological perspective exists to describe in minute detail the variety of biochemical responses that are elements of the stress syndrome. It is beyond the scope of this chapter to attempt to explain in detail those complex biochemical pathways. (More information on these biochemical pathways can be found in Chapter 7.) However, it is important to note that there is a growing recognition that stress is implicated in a variety of dysfunctions. One study which, though conducted from the biological perspective also recognized a possible emotional stimulus, looked at the so-called "white coat effect." It is often noted that blood pressure measured for the same subject in a clinical setting is higher than in a non-clinical setting. One theory suggests that this difference is prompted by the situation itself, where white coats indicate the presence of health-care providers. The study confirmed a highly positive correlation between a mental stress activity (having one's blood pressure checked in a clinical setting) and the "white coat" setting itself. Thus, Lantelme et al.[17] concluded that the white coat effect is the result of the stress of the situation.

Another research approach uses a more psychological perspective and includes measurement of either individual perceptions and/or standard measures of psychological stress and coping, rather than biological measures such a blood pressure reading. Marlowe[18] recorded headaches, stressful events, appraisal processes, and coping responses in 114 headache patients over a 28-day period. He concluded that stressful events may be causally related to headaches, and that the ways in which headache patients respond to these stressful events may have implications for the number and intensity of those headaches. Gilbert, Bazak, and Harel[19] also studied headache patients from the psychological viewpoint. They concluded that women should receive special psychological interventions including counseling on developing coping skills, in addition to medical intervention. This conclusion stemmed from their finding that in a sample of 65 women and 26 men, women had more severe psychological symptoms than men in six subscales measuring psychological symptoms.

The epidemiological approach is evident in a review of research by King,[20] who looked at the question of whether school uniforms should be mandated in elementary schools. He found no evidence for the claim that stress from competition would be lowered by requiring uniforms. A similar research perspective guided Fiscella and Franks[21] in considering psychological distress as a contributor to racial and socioeconomic disparities in mortality. They concluded that psychological distress as a mediator of the effects of race or class on health was not supported by the data from a large national sample in the U.S.

5.2.4   Related Concepts

Over time, several concepts have gained broad acceptance in the field of stress research. These ideas, like the notion of stress itself, have entered the popular vocabulary and are

TABLE 5.1

General Adaptation Syndrome

Stage	Mechanism of Response	Potential Result
Alarm	Autonomic nervous system Hypothalamic-pituitary-adrenal axis, cortico-limbic system	Mobilize resistance ("flight or fight") or death if stressor is overwhelming
Resistance	Physical, psychological, spiritual adaptive responses	Adaptation or move to exhaustion if chronic stress depletes adaptive energy
Exhaustion	Reserve of adaptive energy	Uses reserve OR/until death ensues

familiar to many. Eustress, distress, adaptation, coping, and anxiety are all terms relevant to understanding stress, and for that reason, these concepts merit discussion.

The idea of a stress-free existence may be attractive to each of us at some time. Just think — no worries, no discomfort, no excitement, no threats. Selye recognized that not all stress is bad. In fact, without any stress, an organism can lose its abilities to respond. For those humans conditioned to action and accomplishment, lack of stress can itself become stressful. To explain the idea that each organism has an ideal level of stress, Selye used the term eustress. For damaging stress, he used the term distress.[22] Inherent in these concepts is that the ideal or eustress level varies by individual, depending on individual characteristics. For that same reason, what characterizes distress varies individually, as well.

Adaptation is a term used to explain the more global reaction of an organism to its environment. It is the automatic adjustment made in response to stressors. In Selye's work[23] there are three phases of what he called the General Adaptation Syndrome. (see Table 5.1). First is the alarm reaction, which occurs upon initial exposure to a stressor. As mentioned earlier, the organism can die if the initial stressor is so powerful that it overcomes the normal levels of defense. One example of this is what can occur with massive burns wherein general adaptation begins with resistance. This occurs if the organism is able to respond with the series of biochemical reactions described earlier and if the response is sufficient to deal with the stressor. For example, if the stressor is a large animal advancing threateningly, the biochemical reactions that occur make running away a successful response. When the person returns to a calmer state and the animal is no longer a threat, adaptation has occurred. If continued exposure to stressors is present, it is possible for adaptive energy, which is thought to be finite for each individual organism, to become depleted. If this occurs, the organism undergoes a phase of exhaustion. The alarm response recurs but is ineffective and death ensues. Thus, adaptation describes one aspect of the stress syndrome, a condition in which the organism is successfully defending itself against the stressor. It is doing so at the expense of adaptive energy.

Coping can be thought of as one aspect of humans' efforts to adapt. Because human beings are equipped with thought and feelings and the ability to make choices, they tend to make appraisals of the demands (stressors) affecting them. Coping refers to "an individual's efforts to master demands (conditions of harm, threat, or challenge) that are appraised (or perceived) as exceeding or taxing his or her resources."[24] The choices one makes about how to cope vary, based on knowledge, skills, and emotions. Choices tend to reflect both personality and prior experience. Coping responses can be learned, in contrast to the simpler automatic aspects of adapting. Thus, many researchers believe that learning coping responses is one way in which humans can improve their overall ability to adapt to stress.

One final term which is often a part of discussions about stress is anxiety. Stress and anxiety are not synonymous. However, anxiety can be a factor in the initial arousal prompted by a stressor. In contrast to fear, an emotion aroused when a threat is actual or imminent, anxiety is prompted by anticipation. Particularly, anxiety is an emotion "...arising when harm is anticipated, when the harm (or the coping required by it) is ambiguous, and when that harm tends to be symbolic rather than concrete (as in fright) and concerns a central feature of the person's identity or self."[25] Awareness that one's popularity is slipping, a concern over parental approval of a college major, or worry about body size are examples of perceived threats to the ideal self. The emotion generated by these appraisals is anxiety. The appraisals or perceptions are stressors which, because they are somewhat symbolic and are not necessarily observable, are often very difficult to alter as sources of stress in the individual. Feeling anxious frequently suggests that one is experiencing stress without coping satisfactorily. But stress also can occur accompanied by fright or fear when the stressor is an actual direct or potential harm rather than a symbolic one.

5.2.5 A Framework for Approaches to Managing Stress

It is appropriate to construct a framework for developing approaches to managing stress effectively. A Stress Management Strategies Worksheet, which will help you identify an appropriate strategy for managing stress, can be found in Appendix 5-A. This framework consists of four strategic approaches to the stress problem: (a) leave the stressor; (b) change the appraisal of the stressor; (c) improve the organism's readiness to deal with stress; and (d) combined approaches with elements of two or more of the other strategies.

Leaving the stressor sounds very simple. Just go. Removing the stressor from one's context can be very effective, particularly if the removal can be for a period of time long enough or to a distance great enough to eliminate the threat. Examples of this method might range from running away from a mugger or dropping a class to taking a route to work with less traffic. Other examples include walking out of the room where your child is having a tantrum, coming indoors from a very cold and wet storm, or leaving a job where there is extreme deadline pressure every day.

Changing the appraisal of the stressor must be accomplished by several means. In any use of this strategy, the purpose is to help the individual see a perceived threat as being of less importance or effect, or to help the person cope with an ability that is equal to the demand. The coping mechanisms of denial or ignoring are two ways to lessen the effects of appraisal of threat. Those methods have some short-term benefits and may be satisfactory when the stressor is neither long term, recurring, nor particularly damaging. Denial of the chest pain of a myocardial infarction is an example of one inappropriate use of that defense.

Crisis intervention is a process in which a person being affected by a stressor learns to reappraise the stressor. Through a structured process, the individual is taught to focus on immediate demands and on the ability and strength to deal effectively with the situation. Longer-term counseling or group support activities can help one to learn different appraisals of stress-inducing situations. Kirkland[26] studied coping strategies among female African-American nursing students. Strategies most frequently and most successfully used in the sample were taking action to remove or circumvent the stressor; seeking social support for assistance, information or advice; and seeking social support for emotional reasons. King et al.[27] studied social support using three groups for comparison, healthy, mildly asthmatic and severely asthmatic, during academic exams. Social support was found to protect against immune system decrements during times of stress, such as school exams for asthmatic adolescents.

Improving readiness to react to stressors can be accomplished in several ways. Improved diet, adequate rest, and regular exercise improve overall health and therefore readiness. Health risk assessments and substance abuse and safety education are examples of educational techniques addressing this strategy. Various forms of meditation and relaxation training designed to elicit the relaxation response can enhance one's ability to respond effectively to stressors. When one has a habitual stress-prone style, such as the so-called Type A personality, stress is a common occurrence. Numerous illnesses such as cardiovascular diseases have been correlated with this personality type. Yet, a study in Sweden demonstrated that an intervention aimed at reducing hostility and time pressure was effective in changing the stress-producing behaviors that are characteristic of Type A.[28] Another study linked step aerobics performance to a reduction in tension, depression, fatigue, and anger and an increase in vigor.[29] Cancer patients demonstrated reduced stress in experiments on learning relaxation and meditation techniques in McNeil's research.[30] These studies suggest that while the stressors are not necessarily removed, individuals' abilities to respond can be enhanced by techniques aimed at improving the organism's overall health and readiness to respond.

The fourth strategy, combining two or more of the other strategies, has the potential to be most useful when a professional has the opportunity to do a personal assessment of the person experiencing distress. Based on the assessment of the individual, his or her state of general health, daily habits, the typical stressors experienced and the way in which adaptation and coping are being expressed, a plan reflecting the efforts most likely to be acceptable to and effective for that person can be developed. For example, some individuals are not likely to be willing to join a support group as a first step if part of their pattern is to have relatively few social contacts. While the social support may be a very important long-term goal, it would likely not be the first technique used with these people. Rather, individual instruction in meditation might be a good initial effort, along with some counseling. This might need to be combined with consultation with a dietitian to correct poor dietary patterns which have resulted in obesity. Each combination of techniques would be designed to fit the needs of a particular individual.

5.3   Application of Research Question

In the framework of this chapter, Definition of Stress, a relevant application from one area of the research on this rather global topic is the use of a technique to identify and quantify a person's perception of stress. One method designed for that purpose is the "Perceived Stress Scale" by Cohen, Kamarck, and Mermelstein.[31] This tool is included in Appendix 5-B and can be easily self-administered. Because it asks the respondent to reflect on the past month, it can be used repeatedly. For example, one could use the scale before and after learning or practicing some stress-reduction activities. This could be an indication of the effectiveness of the efforts to reduce stress. The scale has 14 items, each of which is marked on a 5-point scale from 0 to 4, indicating the extent to which the person has experienced certain feelings in the last month. Scoring is determined by summing the answers for all 14 items, with 7 of the items being scored in the reverse. In reported research, the $\times$ and SD values for two separate groups of female college students sampled were 23.57 $\pm$ 7.55 and 24.71 $\pm$ 6.29. The $\times$ and SD values in a community sample were slightly higher, 25.6. $\pm$ 8.24. Both coefficient alpha and test-retest reliability were high.

References

1. Knapp, T., Stress versus strain: a methodological critique, *Nursing Research*, 37, 181, 1988.
2. Selye, H., *Stress without Distress*, J. B. Lippincott, Philadelphia, 1974, 27.
3. Selye, H., *Stress*, Acta, Montreal, 1950.
4. Monat, S., and Lazarus, R. *Stress and Coping: An Anthology*, 3rd ed., Columbia University Press, New York, 1991, 3.
5. Cohen, S., and Kessler, R. C., Strategies for measuring stress in studies of psychiatric and physical disorders, in *Measuring Stress – A Guide for Health and Social Scientists*, Cohen, S., Kessler, R. C., and Gordon, L. G., Eds., Oxford University Press, New York, 3.
6. Tsigos, C. and Chrousos, G. P., Physiology of the hypothalamic-pituitary-adrenal axis in health and dysregulation in psychiatric and autoimmune disorders, *Endocrinology and Metabolism Clinics of North America*, 23, 451, 1994.
7. Dorn, L. D. and Chrousos, G. P., The endocrinology of stress and stress system disorders in adolescence, *Endocrinology and Metabolism Clinics of North America*, 22, 685, 1993.
8. Tsigos, C., and Chrousos, G. P., Physiology of the hypothalamic-pituitary-adrenal axis in health and dysregulation in psychiatric and autoimmune disorders, *Endocrinology and Metabolism Clinics of North America*, 23, 451, 1994.
9. Gullette, E. C. D., Blumenthal, J. A., Babyak, M., Mittleman, M. A., and McClure, M. Do everyday emotional stresses provoke myocardial ischemia?, *Consultant*, 37, 2360, 1997.
10. Forehand, R., Biggar, H., Kotchick, B.A., Cumulative risk across family stressors: short and long term effects for adolescents, *Journal of Abnormal Child Psychology*, 26, 119, 1998.
11. Woods, N. F., Lentz, M. J., Mitchell, E. S., Shaver, J., and Heitkemper, M., Luteal phase ovarian steroids, stress arousal, premenses, perceived stress, and premenstrual symptoms, *Research in Nursing and Health*, 21, 129, 1998.
12. Fryer, S., Waller, G., and Kroese, B. S., Stress, coping, and disturbed eating attitudes in teenage girls, *International Journal of Eating Disorders*, 22, 427, 1997.
13. Gold, P. W., Gwirtsman, H., Avgerinos, P., et al., Abnormal hypothalamic-pituitary-adrenal function in anorexia nervosa: pathophysiologic mechanisms in underweight and weight-corrected patients, *New England Journal of Medicine*, 314, 1335, 1986.
14. Kaye, W. H., Gwirtsman, H. E., George, D.T., et al., Elevated cerebrospinal fluid levels of immunoreactive corticotropin-releasing hormone in anorexia nervosa: relation to state of nutrition, adrenal function, and intensity of depression, *Journal of Clinical Endocrinology and Metabolism*, 64, 203, 1987.
15. Connor, T. J. and Leonard, B. E., Depression, stress and immunological activation: the role of cytokines in depressive disorders, *Life Sciences*, 62, 583, 1998.
16. Herbert, T. B. and Cohen, S., Stress and immunity in humans: a meta-analytic review, *Annals of Behavioral Medicine*, 55, 364, 1993.
17. Lantelme, P., Milon, H., Gharib, C., Gayet, C., and Fortrat, J. O., White coat effect and reactivity to stress: cardiovascular and autonomic nervous system responses, *Hypertension*, 31, 1021, 1998.
18. Marlowe, N., Stressful events, appraisal, coping and recurrent headache, *Journal of Clinical Psychology*, 54, 247, 1998.
19. Cilbar, O., Bazak, Y., and Harel, Y., Gender, primary headache, and psychological distress, *Headache*, 38, 31, 1998.
20. King, K., Should school uniforms be mandated in elementary schools? *Journal of School Health*, 68, 32, 1998.
21. Fiscella, K. and Franks, P., Does psychological distress contribute to racial and socioeconomic disparities in mortality? *Social Science and Medicine*, 45, 1805, 1997.
22. Selye, H., *Stress without Distress*, J. B. Lippincott, Philadelphia, 1974, 138.
23. Selye, H., *Stress without Distress*, J. B. Lippincott, Philadelphia, 1974, 38.
24. Monat, S., and Lazarus, R., *Stress and Coping: An Anthology*, 3rd ed., Columbia University Press, New York, 1991, 5.
25. Lazarus, R., *Patterns of Adjustment*, 3rd ed., New York, McGraw Hill, 1976, 73.

26. Kirkland, M. L., Stressors and coping strategies among successful female African American baccalaureate nursing students, *Journal of Nursing Education*, 37, 5, 1998.
27. Kang, D. H., Coe, C. L., Karaszewski, J., and McCarthy, D. O., Relationship of social support to stress responses and immune function in healthy and asthmatic adolescents, *Research in Nursing and Health*, 21, 117, 1998.
28. Karlsberg, L., Kakau, I., and Unden, A., Type A behavior intervention in primary health care reduces hostility and time pressure: a study in Sweden, *Social Science and Medicine*, 46, 397, 1998.
29. Kennedy, M. and Newton, M., Effect of exercise intensity on mood in step aerobics, *Journal of Sports Medicine and Physical Fitness*, 37, 200, 1997.
30. McNeil, C., Stress reduction: three trials test its impact on breast cancer progression, *Journal of the National Cancer Institute*, 90, 12, 1998.
31. Cohen, S., Kamarck, T., and Mermelstein, R., A global measure of perceived stress, *Journal of Health and Social Behavior*, 24, 394, 1983.

Appendix 5-A: Stress Management Strategies Worksheet

Stressor: Strategies:
                                         Leave the stressor
                                         Change the appraisal of the stressor
                                         Improve the organism to deal with the stressor
                                         Combine strategies

Directions:
Mark a + or – below each stress management strategy as you analyze it in regard to a particular stressor in your life. Total the + marks and subtract the – marks beneath each strategy. If only one strategy has 2 or more + marks remaining, choose it as your strategy. If more than one have 2 or more + marks, consider combining strategies.

How to Analyze the Strategies:
Consider the following characteristics of each strategy <u>for you at this time</u>:

1. Feasibility - Do you have the knowledge or skill to use this strategy? yes = + no = –
2. Resources - Do you have the financial or other material resources to use this strategy? yes = + no = –
3. Support - Would at least one person important to you support the use of this strategy? yes = + no = –
4. Barriers - Are there significant barriers to prevent your using the strategy? List each barrier. Each barrier = –
5. Courage/motivation - Do you have the courage and/or motivation to choose this strategy? yes = + no = –

Tally Sheet
Leave the stressor
1.____ 2.____ 3.____ 4.____ 5.____ Total +'s____ Total –'s____ Remaining +'s____

Change the appraisal of the stressor
1.____ 2.____ 3.____ 4.____ 5.____ Total +'s____ Total –'s____ Remaining +'s____

Improve the organism to deal with the stressor
1.____ 2.____ 3.____ 4.____ 5.____ Total +'s____ Total –'s____ Remaining +'s____

Combine strategies
1.____ 2.____ 3.____ 4.____ 5.____ Total +'s____ Total –'s____ Remaining +'s____

Insights gained from this exercise:

Appendix 5-B: Perceived Stress Scale

The questions in this scale ask you about your feelings and thoughts during the last month. In each case, you will be asked to indicate *how often* you felt or thought a certain way. Although some of the questions are similar, there are differences between them and you should treat each one as a separate question. The best approach is to answer each question fairly quickly. That is, don't try to count up the number of times you felt a particular way, but rather indicate the alternative that seems like a reasonable estimate. *For each question choose from the following alternatives:*

0. Never
1. Almost never
2. Sometimes
3. Fairly often
4. Very often

1. In the very last month, how often have you been upset because of something that happened unexpectedly? _____
2. In the last month, how often have you felt that you were unable to control the important things in your life? _____
3. In the last month, how often have you felt nervous and "stressed"? _____
4. ªIn the last month, how often have you dealt successfully with irritating life hassles? _____
5. ªIn the last month, how often have you felt that you were effectively coping with important changes that were occurring in your life? _____
6. ªIn in the last month, how often have you felt confident about your ability to handle your personal problems? _____
7. ªIn the last month, how often have you felt that things were going your way? _____
8. In the last month, how often have you found that you could not cope with all the things that you had to do? _____
9. ªIn the last month, how often have you been able to control irritations in your life? _____
10. ªIn the last month, how often have you felt that you were on top of things? _____
11. In the last month, how often have you been angered because of things that happened that were outside of your control? _____
12. In the last month, how often have you found yourself thinking about things that you have to accomplish? _____
13. ªIn the last month, how often have you been able to control the way you spend your time? _____
14. In the last month, how often have you felt difficulties were piling up so high that you could not overcome them? _____

ª Scored in the reverse direction.

6

The Psychology of Stress and Coping

Cathy Thompson and Stephen Cook

CONTENTS

6.1   Learning Objectives

After completing this chapter you should be able to:

- Understand the relationships among stress, coping, and psychological distress;
- Understand gender differences in stress experience and coping;
- Identify methods for helping individuals to evaluate their current coping behaviors.

6.2   Research Background

The most cursory inspection of our popular culture reveals that contemporary American has become very interested, indeed almost obsessed, with stress and how to cope with it. Self-help books, advice columns, popular magazines, and talk shows provide endless suggestions about how to deal with interpersonal problems that may arise in a romantic relationship or in the workplace, as well as other problems that may cause depression or anxiety. There is much we still do not know, and many people have recognized the importance of looking closely at the relationships between coping and psychological distress,[1-3] and coping and physical distress.[4]

0-8493-2027-5/01/$0.00+$.50
© 2001 by CRC Press, Inc.

6.2.1 Stress and Coping Defined

It is important to establish definitions of *stress* and *coping*. Aldwin[5] defines stress as "that quality of experience, produced through a person-environment transaction, that, through overarousal or underarousal, results in psychological or physiological distress." Stoyva and Carlson[6] define psychological stress as "a situation in which the challenges or threats facing the individual exceeds his or her estimated coping resources." After reviewing the history of the term "stress" and the implications of various definitions, Lazarus and Folkman[7] state, "Psychological stress is a particular relationship between the person and the environment that is appraised by the person as taxing or exceeding his or her resources and endangering his or her well-being." Put more simply, *stress* is our reaction in response to a demand. This demand or event that overwhelms us or disturbs our equilibrium is known as a *stressor*.

A stressor can be physical in nature, such as a broken arm, or emotional, such as the breakup of a romantic relationship. As indicated by the previous definitions, stressors are typically considered to be aspects of the environment, but stressors can also be internal, such as the demands associated with having the flu. It is important to remember that stress can be an adaptive response to stressors or demands to help us deal more effectively with problems we encounter. Just as experiencing the demands associated with lifting weights helps our muscles to become stronger, experiencing stressors in various situations can help us grow stronger psychologically.[8] Most people function best under moderate levels of stress.[9] However, under conditions of persistent high stress, people can develop a variety of damaging physical and psychological symptoms.[10]

Early research explored the relationship between stressful events and individual distress but found that the stressful event accounted for only 10% of the changes in distress.[11] Obviously there are other factors which must be considered when examining the roots of human emotional and physical distress, and some researchers have hypothesized that the coping behaviors of an individual may play a role in determining the amount of distress he or she experiences.

Webster's Dictionary[12] defines "cope" as a verb: "To strive; to struggle or contend with something." Parkes[13] points out that coping is a "multidimensional" construct which "involves both behavioral and cognitive strategies which may be directed towards altering, re-evaluating or avoiding stressful circumstances, or alleviating their adverse effects." Lazarus and Folkman[7] define coping as "constantly changing cognitive and behavioral efforts to manage specific external and/or internal demands that are appraised as taxing or exceeding the resources of the person." Lazarus and Folkman note that coping is limited to stressors that are consciously perceived as especially stressful. Not everyone agrees with Lazarus and Folkman's conceptualization of coping as involving constantly changing behaviors, however, and some evidence suggests that coping behaviors are more stable than Lazarus and Folkman theorize.[13,14] This issue, along with the concept of appraisal, will be discussed further in this chapter. Holahan et al.[11] define coping as "a stabilizing factor that can help individuals maintain psychosocial adaptation during stressful periods; it encompasses cognitive and behavioral efforts to reduce or eliminate stressful conditions and associated emotional discomfort." Using information from these various definitions, coping can be defined more simply as what an individual consciously does to deal with the effects of a stressor or personal problem. The coping response can include behavioral, cognitive, or even affective strategies to handle a stressor.[15]

Lazarus and Folkman's[7] transactional model of stress and coping views the stressor and a person's response to that stressor as affecting each other. An individual first experiences a stressor and then must evaluate that stressor and determine the meaning it holds for him or her. That step is called appraisal. Appraisal is the way a person cognitively evaluates the significance of an experience, and determines which coping responses could be used most effectively. Lazarus and Folkman have identified three kinds of cognitive appraisal: primary, secondary, and reappraisal. Primary appraisal involves judging an encounter as irrelevant, positive, or as involving harm, loss, threat, or challenge. Secondary appraisal involves a judgment about the availability and likely efficacy of coping behaviors. Reappraisal refers to "a changed appraisal based on new information from the environment and/or the person." The appraisals of an individual change as he or she moves through a stressful situation and applies various coping strategies. Similarly, coping is seen as a process that changes over time in response to both the changing demands of the stressful situation and the individual's subjective appraisal of that situation. Other researchers[17,18] have proposed similar theories of coping. Common to these theories is the importance placed on both appraisals and coping strategies used by individuals as they cope with a stressor.

Holahan et al.[11] also emphasize the importance of considering dispositional and contextual variables in the study of coping. They describe dispositional variables as those having to do with a consistent, stable use of coping strategies across various situations. Contextual or situational variables are described as those concerned with how particular characteristics of a stressful event influence the various coping strategies. Holahan et al.[11] propose an integrative conceptual framework, which emphasizes how enduring personal factors, as well as more changeable situational factors, shape coping efforts.

Holahan et al.[11] also distinguish between two relatively stable factors in the coping process: (a) the environmental system, which is composed of ongoing life stressors (e.g., chronic physical illness) and social coping resources (e.g., support from family members); and (b) the personal system which includes an individual's sociodemographic characteristics and personal coping resources (e.g., self-confidence). The authors conceptualize these relatively stable variables as influencing the life crises and transitions individuals face. These events often reflect significant changes in life circumstances.

The combined influences of the environmental system, personal system, and life crises and transitions shape health and well-being both directly and indirectly through the process of cognitive appraisal and specific coping responses. For instance, if a person has relatively few ongoing life stressors, receives strong support from family members, and has a high sense of self-efficacy for dealing with personal problems, he or she will be able to cope more effectively with a life crisis (such as the death of a loved one) and will in turn exhibit relatively fewer symptoms of distress during his or her response to this crisis. It is important to note that the causal paths in the framework are bi-directional, indicating that reciprocal feedback can occur at each stage. For example, if someone copes effectively with a life crisis such as the death of a loved one, this will in turn give that person a higher sense of self-efficacy for dealing with personal problems. The researchers point out that this framework "emphasizes the central mediating role of cognitive appraisal and coping responses in the stress process."

Some people suggest that most existing theories of coping are not fully applicable to the stressors women face and their subsequent coping strategies. Banyard and Graham-Bermann[19] take issue with current theories of coping which fail adequately to consider the unique perspective of women. They point out that theories which portray women as using less "healthy" coping behaviors often do not consider the ways in which a woman's social experience differs from a man's, and how a careful consideration of those differences may reveal that coping strategies previously labeled "bad" (e.g., emotion-focused coping) are actually quite adaptive. The authors propose an alternative model of coping theory, which acknowledges that women experience stress differently than men do, rather than considering stress as a homogeneous concept. Additionally, this alternative model would "understand that coping occurs in a context shaped by social forces based on gender, race, class, age, and sexual orientation." The proposed theory of coping would redefine the meaning of coping to include those actions "used to maximize the survival of others (such as children, family, and friends)." Descriptions of coping strategies would also be revised to remove the pejorative meanings often associated with different types of coping. The implication is that different responses might be needed for women and men who are attempting to cope with eating disorders.

6.2.2   Assessment of Coping

The theoretical position one accepts with regard to the definition of coping influences how one identifies and measures coping behaviors. The assessment of coping has a rocky history, and a multitude of measures exist (for reviews of coping assessment, see Aldwin,[5] Parker and Endler,[20] and Schwarzer and Schwarzer[21]). Most of these are not without their problems, and when looking at the research on coping it is important to have a basic understanding of the methods used to measure coping (see Appendix 6-A for a coping measure entitled *Problem-Focused Styles of Coping*).

In a review of coping assessment, Parker and Endler[20] list 14 coping measures, each of which assesses coping along different dimensions. For example, the original Ways of Coping (WOC) scale[22] distinguishes between problem-focused coping and emotion-focused coping. Problem-focused coping is aimed at active problem-solving or doing something to change the source of the stress. Emotion-focused coping is aimed at reducing or managing the distress associated with the stress. Parker and Endler point out that other coping instruments assess a variety of activities, including seeking social support, venting of emotions, aggression, distraction, self-destruction, endurance, superstitious thinking, resignation, self-isolation, wishful thinking, being confrontative, being humorous, and relaxing.

The researchers conclude that the proliferation of coping scales makes it difficult to generalize empirical findings from one population to another. They also criticize the psychometric properties of many of the scales, and point to such weaknesses as low internal reliabilities, a lack of construct validity, a lack of empirical validation, and an unsubstantiated factor structure. Certainly there is much overlap among the many coping behaviors assessed by different instruments, although it appears that three basic dimensions are being measured:[20,22,24] (1) task-oriented coping, which refers to strategies used to solve a problem or minimize its effects; (2) emotion-oriented coping, which refers to strategies used to manage the emotions related to the problem, including seeking social support; and (3) avoidance-oriented coping, which refers to strategies used to avoid a stressful situation.

6.2.3   Stress, Coping, and Psychological Distress

Questions about the nature of coping have relevance for the study of the development of psychopathology and the treatment of mental illness. Holahan et al.[11] point out that "coping is a stabilizing factor that can help individuals maintain psychosocial adaptation during stressful periods…" Thus it naturally follows that when coping behaviors become inadequate, an individual may no longer be able to function adaptively. This concept is reflected repeatedly in the *Diagnostic and Statistical Manual of Mental Disorders*, Fourth Edition (DSM-IV),[25] which specifies that the symptoms for many disorders must "cause clinically significant distress or impairment in social, occupational, or other important areas of functioning." When adaptive functioning has been disrupted, the primary clinical goal is often re-establishing effective coping.

Endler and Parker[17] examined the relationships between state and trait anxiety, depression, and coping styles in 55 male and 155 female college undergraduates and found that participants who reported higher levels of depressive symptoms also reported using more emotion-focused coping behaviors than those who reported lower levels of depressive symptoms. Task-oriented coping was positively related to lower levels of depressive symptoms. There was no significant relationship between depressive symptoms and avoidance-oriented coping. Although such correlational data cannot provide information regarding a causal link between coping and distress, there is ample evidence indicating that the coping strategies and behaviors employed by an individual are related to the presence or absence of psychological distress.

Higgins and Endler[2] explored the relationship of stressful life events and coping to physical and psychological distress. The researchers assessed three styles of coping (emotion-oriented, task-oriented, and avoidance-oriented) and administered measures of recent life stressors, physical symptoms, and psychological symptoms. The sample consisted of 101 male and 104 female undergraduate college students. Results indicated that emotion-oriented coping was a significant, positive predictor of distress for both males and females while task-oriented coping was negatively related to distress only for males. Women reported using more emotion-oriented coping than men did, and they reported more distress. While this study further highlights possible gender differences in coping and the experience of distress, it also emphasizes the importance of exploring the relationships between stressors, coping, and distress.

Neckowitz and Morrison[26] investigated the coping strategies reportedly used by bulimic women when coping with a stressor involving someone known intimately and someone not known intimately. Results indicated that bulimic women differed from a comparison group, in that they felt more threatened and made greater use of avoidant coping behaviors. The problem of using avoidance as a coping strategy is highlighted by this excerpt from Neckowitz and Morrison:

> Undue reliance on escape-avoidance as a coping option can be hazardous…Over the long term, this can interfere with the processes of information seeking, anticipation, and planning that are often necessary for developing an effective response to a threat or challenge. With the development of potential steps of positive action disrupted, the sense of instrumentality, interpersonal effectiveness, and agentic self-esteem would predictably be diminished, and chronic feelings of pessimism and apathy may develop…In turn, this would understandably contribute to continued reliance on avoidant coping styles rather than active responses to stressors.[26]

It seems logical, then, that one focus of treatment of an eating disorder among women would be to assess the effectiveness of each individual's current coping behaviors and assist her in finding more adaptive coping behaviors.

In their exploration of coping behaviors in eating-disordered women, Troop, Holbrey, Trowler, and Treasure[27] also found that women diagnosed with eating disorders relied more on avoidant coping behaviors than did women in a normal comparison group. However, no difference between the two groups was apparent in their use of problem-focused coping strategies, and no relationship existed between coping behaviors and the severity of the eating disorder. In women with anorexia nervosa or bulimia nervosa, avoidant coping behaviors were positively related to symptoms of depression. The researchers suggested that when treating an eating disorder patient, it may prove helpful to include a focus on methods to improve the efficacy of coping efforts.

In sum, it appears that at least a moderate correlation exists between coping behaviors and distress for a variety of people with a variety of problems. Emotion-focused coping appears to be consistently related to the presence of psychological distress.[2,3,17,28,29] The relationships between task-oriented coping, avoidance-oriented coping, and distress are less clear. Some researchers have found a positive correlation between task-oriented coping and psychological well-being,[17,28,30] while others have found gender differences that would indicate this relationship exists only for men.[2] Evidence suggests that avoidance-oriented coping may be negatively correlated with psychological well-being[1], but evidence also suggests no relationship between avoidance-oriented coping and well-being.[31] However, there seems to be an indication that people with eating disorders rely more on avoidance coping than people who have not been diagnosed with eating disorders although, curiously, nothing indicates that people with eating disorders use more task-oriented coping strategies.

Some researchers have found little evidence of a significant relationship between coping and distress. Zautra, Sheets, and Sandler[32] explored the ability of coping behaviors to predict individual differences in adjustment to life stressors in a sample of recently divorced mothers and found that coping dispositions assessed at one point in time failed to account for changes in distress over a period of 5 months. The researchers concluded that "the evidence strongly suggests that trait-based measures do not discriminate those who adjust well to life stress from those who do not." It cannot be said with certainty that the way in which a person copes causes or alleviates psychological symptoms such as depression or anxiety; indeed, it is possible that psychological symptoms may influence the way an individual copes. Although there appears to be a significant amount of evidence supporting the hypothesis that coping is correlated with psychological distress, certainly more research is needed to sort out the relationship between coping and the presence or absence of psychological distress.

6.2.4   Dispositional vs. Situational Approaches to the Study of Coping

The dispositional approach to the study of coping assumes that individuals are predisposed to use habitual coping strategies across different types of stressful situations or at different points in time. Scientists using this approach attempt to identify basic coping styles that are relatively stable within the person. Several schools of thought provide a basis for describing person-based variables, including psychoanalysis with its emphasis on defense mechanisms,[33] and personality theorists who view coping styles as basic personality traits.[34] This approach uses coping scores from the same individual compiled over different measurement occasions, or scores collected on a single occasion to represent a stable index of the individual's coping styles, and compares that person's response with those of others. This method allows one to assess individual differences in the use of coping strategies. If one accepts the hypothesis that the basis for coping lies within the individual, it makes sense to attempt to identify and quantify individual characteristics that determine (or significantly influence) the choice and implementation of coping behaviors. However, attempts to identify person-related predictors of coping have been somewhat less than successful. Amirkhan[14] points out that over the last 20 years, researchers have found "only sporadic correlations between personality test scores and modes of coping, and this rather chaotic pattern of findings continues to characterize the literature today."

In a review of the literature, Parkes[13] states that relatively few dimensions of personality have been found to be related to coping: locus of control, hardiness, Type A behavior, neuroticism, and dispositional optimism. Researchers subscribing to theories of coping which hold that coping is a dispositional construct have attempted to relate coping to stable personality characteristics and have had moderate success. Should coping be related to stable personality characteristics, it naturally follows that individuals should be fairly consistent in their situational coping behaviors. There is some evidence to suggest that this is the case, but there is also research indicating very little individual consistency in coping.

The situational approach assumes that individuals have a repertoire of coping options available to them from which they can choose, depending on the characteristics of the situation (e.g., the stressor's intensity, duration, and controllability) and appraisal factors. This approach is often associated with Lazarus and Folkman[7] who, as discussed previously, have advocated a transactional view of stress and coping. A person's response to stress is seen as a continually developing process rather than a discrete behavior dependent on stable personality characteristics. According to this view, a person's response to stressful events may vary, depending on situational factors and other person variables, such as how the individual appraises both the stressor and his or her own coping resources. Lazarus and Folkman's contextual model relies heavily on this concept. Situational research paradigms based on this theory often study behaviors and cognitions of the same person or the same group of persons across different types of situations to determine how characteristics of those situations influence individual coping.

Appraisal is a key concept of coping theories that emphasize situational characteristics. Many environmental events have the potential to be stressful, but will only become so as a function of the meaning attributed to those events by the individual.[7] As stated previously, the transactional approach to coping holds that person variables, such as appraisal, can influence responses to stressful events. However, Cassidy and Burnside[35] point out that attempts to produce a model of cognitive appraisal have met with little success. They identify several variables as contributing to psychological vulnerability including achievement motivation, attributional style, problem-solving style, emotional reactivity, hopelessness, perceived control, and perceived social support. The researchers characterize these variables as contributing to the ways people think about and give meaning to their experience in the process of appraisal. The researchers tested the relationship between these variables and a variety of measures of life stress, work stress, depression, anxiety, hostility, positive affect, life satisfaction, and job commitment, and their data support an explanatory role for seven variables associated with cognitive vulnerability and appraisal. The researchers suggest that these variables could be used in an integrative model of a cognitive appraisal of stress and could prove valuable in guiding psychotherapeutic interventions.

Transactional theorists, such as Lazarus and Folkman,[7] argue that coping behavior depends on successive processes of cognitive appraisal and reappraisal, with resulting adjustments made in coping. As a stressful episode develops over time, there is a continuous interaction between appraisal, coping, and emotion, each fluctuating and evolving as the transaction unfolds. Given this constant evolution, a person's coping activities may change depending on the characteristics of the situation and an appraisal of both the stressor and his or her own coping resources. Thus it follows that there would be little consistency in an individual's coping behavior across situations. However, theorists such as Amirkhan[36] point out that it seems unlikely people are born anew in every crisis they encounter; they must carry person-bound factors with them from stressor to stressor, factors that also influence the choice of a coping strategy. Whether these are personality dispositions, motivational or affective tendencies, or even accumulated coping resources, they should produce some consistency in response across stressful situations. The evidence regarding consistency and flexibility in coping is ambivalent, with empirical support for both dispositional and situational theories of coping.

6.2.5   Gender Differences in Coping

A significant area in coping research has focused on gender differences in coping and subsequent changes in distress. It seems particularly relevant to explore gender differences as they apply to eating disorders, since anorexia nervosa and bulimia nervosa are diagnosed more often in women than men.[37] Therefore, it is helpful to explore how women in particular cope with personal problems. Aldwin[5] cites evidence indicating that gender differences in seeking social support begin to emerge between the ages of 6 and 9 years, with girls seeking more support than boys. However, Amirkhan[14] points out that results regarding gender differences and coping are equivocal. Some studies find that women use more emotion-focused strategies than men, yet others find that women use more problem-focused strategies.

McDaniel and Richards[38] explored gender differences in how college students cope with sad moods. A small group of college students who reported experiencing depressive feelings during the last year and did not seek professional assistance to cope with those feelings were interviewed about the nature of their problems, the coping behaviors they used, and the consistency and effectiveness of coping. The results indicate that women reported more sad moods than men, both retrospectively and currently. Further, men reported using more coping techniques than women and tended to use relaxation, self-reward, and situational changes more frequently. The researchers concluded that "women profit more from more 'emotion-focused' techniques...whereas men profit from more 'problem-focused' procedures..."

Nolen-Hoeksema[39] argues that one explanation for the consistent finding that approximately twice as many adult women are depressed as adult men may be found in sex differences in response to depression that stem from gender stereotypes. Women appear more likely to engage in ruminative responses when depressed, thereby amplifying their symptoms and extending depressive episodes. Men appear more likely to distract themselves from depressed moods, thereby dampening their symptoms. Being active and controlling one's moods are part of the masculine stereotype; being inactive and emotional are part of the feminine stereotype.[39] Ruminating can be conceptualized as an emotion-focused coping strategy. Ruminations are defined as thoughts and behaviors that focus an individual's attention inward on his or her depressed state, and the research indicates that such a response serves to exacerbate and extend a depressive episode.

Endler and Parker[17] explored the relationship between state and trait anxiety, depression, and coping styles in a sample of undergraduate students. Generally, women reported more emotion-oriented and avoidance-oriented strategies than men, but no gender differences were found for the use of task-oriented coping behaviors. Participants who reported more emotion-oriented coping and less task-oriented coping reported higher levels of depressive symptoms.

Leong et al.[29] tested the hypothesis that students' styles of coping influence their adjustments to college. College freshmen completed a measure of college adjustment and coping. No significant gender differences were noted with regard to college adjustment; however, females reported significantly higher levels of emotional venting and seeking social support. No gender differences were found in task-oriented coping.

Ptacek, Smith, and Zanas[40] explored the relationship between gender, appraisal, and coping. College undergraduates recorded daily information about the most stressful event of the day for 21 consecutive days. The researchers found evidence to support a socialization hypothesis of coping, which suggests that men and women are socialized to cope with stressful events in different ways. Sex-role stereotypes and gender-role expectations serve to socialize men to deal instrumentally with stress, while women are socialized to express emotion, use emotion-focused coping behaviors, and seek the support of others.

Porter and Stone[41] also tested the hypothesis that there are differences in the way men and women experience daily problems, as well as in the coping behaviors they employ, using longitudinal daily data. Married couples completed daily questionnaire booklets that included a mood assessment, a daily event checklist and appraisal section, questions about symptomatology, and a coping measure. Results indicated that men and women reported differences in the content of stressors they experienced, but not in the manner in which they appraised those situations or in the coping behaviors they used to deal with them. Women reported more problems focused on the self, more parenting problems, and more problems involving other people. Men reported more work-related problems and more miscellaneous problems than women. The researchers point out that these results are consistent with what would be expected based on traditional roles and point out that studies that have found little difference in the types of problems experienced by men and women often use college populations in which men and women occupy similar roles. Women and men generally appraised their problems as equally severe, chronic, and controllable, although women appraised problems focused on the self as more chronic than did men. There were no gender differences noted in coping across problem-content categories, and the researchers suggested that their results do not support the socialization hypothesis, which implies that men use more problem-focused coping and women use more emotion-focused coping.

Hamilton and Fagot[42] compared different college undergraduate coping strategies to test the theory that men use instrumental coping strategies more frequently than women, and that women employ more emotion-focused behaviors. With the exception of women reporting more overall stress, no gender differences emerged for frequency of stressful events or proportion of problem-solving behavior. The researchers suggest that the results of studies which find a difference in coping behaviors between men and women (i.e., women use emotional expressiveness to a greater degree, while men exhibit higher levels of active problem-solving) may be due, in part, to differential recall of female-specific events using retrospective methods. Moreover, stressors that involve interpersonal conflict may not be addressed as effectively with instrumentality and are perhaps solved more easily by self-soothing strategies, such as asking advice from friends. The ability to use both instrumental and expressive modes of coping seems important for both men and women in daily living, and both modes are differentially applied to stressful events.[42]

In sum, Hamilton and Fagot[42] found no evidence to support the hypothesis that men and women differ in the actual coping behaviors they use, but they raise some interesting questions about the possibility of differential recall of stressors and the resulting effect on coping assessment. Perhaps men and women do not differ significantly with respect to actual coping behaviors, but do differ with respect to the stressors they recall and reference when describing their coping strategies. One possibility is that men may think primarily of the way they cope with problems at work, whereas women may think primarily of ways in which they cope with interpersonal problems. This hypothesis may also explain some of the inconsistencies found in the literature assessing coping behaviors within participants, across participants, and between genders. This hypothesis also has particular relevance for assessing the coping styles of women with eating disorders. For instance, do women find coping with eating disorders much more difficult than men, because problems with eating are not similar to interpersonal problems, with which women feel more comfortable coping?

The hypothesis that men and women mentally reference different situations when attempting to describe general coping styles may be at least partially supported by gender-role theory. Boyle and Paludi[43] define gender norms as "prescribed behaviors that combine to make up a [gender] role." These norms are dictated by society. Boyle and Paludi state that the primary gender role for women in this society is motherhood, with the role of wife coming in a close second. Both of these socially prescribed roles involve intense interpersonal relationships with one's children and husband. In order to carry out these roles successfully a woman must develop certain interpersonal skills, such as openness and empathy, which are not seen as central to gender norms for men. Rather than revolving around parenting and marriage, men's gender roles involve other themes significantly less dependent on relationships with others. Boyle and Paludi describe five elements central to acceptable gender roles for males in this society. This first is called an "antifeminine element" in which "men are admonished never to act in any way that may be interpreted as feminine." A second element dictates that men should strive to "prove their masculinity by being better than others at work and sports." This is referred to as the "success element." The "aggressive element" decrees that men should be prepared to fight for what they consider right and shun "feminine" means of settling conflict. The "sexual element" emphasizes the importance of sexual conquest and initiating sex. Finally, the "self-reliant" element of male gender norms admonishes men to "be cool, unflappable, in control, and tough."

Thus, it would appear that socially prescribed gender norms dictate different priorities for men and women, with the primary role of a woman being defined by her relationship with someone else (i.e., child, husband). Although their published study found no significant difference in the frequency of stressful events reported by men and women, Hamilton and Fagot[42] state that in previous pilot studies, women reported experiencing significantly more stressful interpersonal events, such as unfriendly people, prejudicial acts, and conflicts with roommates, instructors, and romantic partners. Since the basis for female gender norms appears to lie in an interpersonal domain, it would logically follow that problems in this area would be considered more important and more familiar to women than problems in other areas, such as school or work. On the other hand, consideration of the elements of male gender norms which emphasize success and self-reliance would suggest that men have a greater investment in coping adaptively with academic and occupational problems.

Thus, it seems logical to hypothesize that men and women may prioritize stressful situations differently, based on the threats they pose to their respective gender roles. When asked to describe how they cope with problems in general or any specific problem they have recently experienced, they may reference different problems based on this prioritization. Although many studies have produced evidence to indicate that women report more psychological distress than men,[2,38,42] research regarding gender differences in coping remains equivocal. It has long been believed that women use emotion-focused coping to a greater extent than men, and there is some support for this belief.[2,17,29,44] Support for the belief that men use more problem-focused coping[40,44] also exists. Other researchers have found little evidence of gender differences.[41,42]

6.3   Application of Research Question

Now we can apply what we know about stress and coping to the task of assisting someone with an eating disorder. Disordered eating could be partially conceptualized as a maladaptive way of coping. It follows that one way of helping someone caught in the dangerous cycle of an eating disorder is to help that individual evaluate the effectiveness of current coping behaviors and assist the person in developing more effective coping techniques. Indeed, some psychotherapy treatment approaches to eating disorders employ specific techniques to modify coping strategies in response to high-risk situations.[37] Following are some guidelines and suggestions for assisting a person exhibiting an eating disorder.

Since initial research has indicated more avoidant coping among women with eating disorders than among those without, this suggests a possible area of intervention. Namely, it might be helpful to help women with eating disorders modify their coping responses, so that they rely less on avoidant responses to stressors in their lives. The initial research also indicates that women with eating disorders do not differ from women not diagnosed with eating disorders in the amounts of task-oriented coping used in response to stressful situations. This suggests that women with eating disorders have the ability to use task-oriented, and perhaps more adaptive, coping strategies but again, problems arise due to the number of avoidant coping strategies they employ.

Perhaps teaching women with eating disorders how to purposely escape being avoidant could prove a useful intervention. However, research in this area so far cannot produce definitive conclusions concerning whether such intervention might truly be effective. To begin with, it is important to have a good understanding of how people cope in a variety of situations, as well as how they appraise the stressors in their lives. An understanding of the cognitive processes involved in coping is important in planning interventions for reducing maladaptive responses to stress.[45,46] Lightsey[47] offers several recommendations for counselors based on his review of literature concerning the psychological resources of positive thoughts, hardiness, generalized self-efficacy, and optimism. Specifically, he recommends that clinicians "help the client to develop active problem-solving skills" and "teach a variety of coping skills, because some contexts require skills other than active problem solving."

One way to explore how people cope with different problems is to ask them, very specifically, how they typically deal with common problems in a variety of domains. It should not be assumed that disordered eating is how a particular individual may cope with *all* of the problems in her life; there is likely to be at least one stressor with which the individual deals effectively. Ask her how she copes with problems in her family (e.g., What do you do when your parents fight? What do you do when you fight with your brother or your sister? How did you react when your parents split up?), at school (e.g., How do you react when you get a disappointing grade on a test or an assignment? How do you approach a difficult math problem?), and with her friends (What kinds of things do you like to do with your friends? How do you cope when you have a disagreement with a friend?). It is important to explore all areas of the individual's life thoroughly, even those aspects that do not appear to be directly related to the eating disorder, with the goal of delineating areas of effective coping, as well as areas that appear to be plagued by problematic coping strategies.

The next step is to ask the individual how well the coping strategies used for any particular problem appear to be working. Is she accomplishing her goal? How would she like things to be different? Once she has identified areas in need of change, the task then becomes one of finding more effective coping strategies. One way to accomplish this is to discuss areas in which she appears to be coping well. Even effective coping with a relatively small and specific problem may be generalized to encompass a larger, more complex problem. For example, suppose the individual states that while she makes good grades in math and actually enjoys solving complex algebra problems, she feels overwhelmed by the demands of school, a regular babysitting job, and participation in athletics. It may be possible to help her reduce her avoidant responses to these situations and draw on her more basic and logical problem-solving techniques.

However, it is important not to assume that there is one "best" style of coping. It is often tempting to consider problem-focused coping as effective with all problems, but that is not the case. For example, it may prove more adaptive to use an avoidant or emotion-focused coping strategy when faced with a situation about which nothing can be done (e.g., a terminally ill friend), and a more problem-focused coping strategy when the problem does have a potential solution (e.g., a flat tire). More research is needed in this area to determine the adaptivity of particular coping strategies.

Once situations have been identified in which a person's coping responses do not seem adaptive and are actually increasing distress, one can work with her in developing alternative coping behaviors. Has she ever faced a similar problem in the past? How did she cope with that problem? Would those same coping behaviors work in this situation? How would she like things to be different, and how can she accomplish that objective? Educating the individual about basic problem-solving strategies[48] can also be helpful.

References

1. Deisinger, J. A., Cassisi, J. E., and Whitaker, S. L., Relationships between coping style and PAI profiles in a community sample, *Journal of Clinical Psychology*, 52, 303, 1996.
2. Higgins, J. E. and Endler, N. S., Coping, life stress, and psychological and somatic distress, *European Journal of Personality*, 9, 253, 1995.
3. Kuiper, N. A., Olinger, L. J., and Air, P. A., Stressful events, dysfunctional attitudes, coping styles, and depression, *Personality and Individual Differences*, 10, 229, 1989.
4. Olff, M., Brosschot, J. F., and Godaert, G., Coping styles and health, *Personality and Individual Differences*, 15, 81, 1993.
5. Aldwin, C. M., *Stress, Coping, and Development*, Guilford Press, New York, 1994, 22.
6. Stoyva, J. M. and Carlson, J. G., A coping/rest model of relaxation and stress management, in *Handbook of Stress: Theoretical and Clinical Aspects*, 2nd ed., Goldberger, L. and Breznitz, S., Eds., Free Press, New York, 1993, 724.
7. Lazarus, R. S. and Folkman, S., *Stress, Appraisal, and Coping*, Springer, New York, 1984, 19.
8. Hann, N., The assessment of coping, defense, and stress, in *Handbook of Stress: Theoretical and Clinical Aspects*, 2nd ed., Goldberger, L. and Breznitz, S., Eds., Free Press, New York, 1993.
9. Yerkes, R. M. and Dodson, J. D., The relation of strength of stimulus to rapidity of habit-formation, *Journal of Comparative Neurology and Psychology*, 18, 459, 1908.
10. Seleye, H., History of the stress concept, in *Handbook of Stress: Theoretical and Clinical Aspects*, 2nd ed., Goldberger, L. and Breznitz, S., Eds., Free Press, New York, 1993.
11. Holahan, C. J., Moos, R. H., and Schaefer, J. A., Coping, stress resistance, and growth; conceptualizing adaptive functioning, in *Handbook of Coping: Theory, Research, Applications*, Zeidner, M. and Endler, N. S., Eds., John Wiley & Sons, New York, 1996, 24.
12. Nichols, K., et al., *Webster's Dictionary*, Nickel Press, New York, 1991.
13. Parkes, K. R., Personality and coping as moderators of work stress processes: models, methods, and measures, *Work and Stress*, 8, 110, 1994.
14. Amirkhan, J. H., Seeking person-related predictors of coping: exploratory analyses, *European Journal of Personality*, 8, 13, 1994.
15. Carver, C. S. and Scheier, M. F., Situational coping and coping dispositions in a stressful transaction, *Journal of Personality and Social Psychology*, 66, 184, 1994.
16. Heppner, P. P., Cook, S. W., Wright, D. M., and Johnson, W. C., Jr., Progress in resolving problems: a problem-focused style of coping, *Journal of Counseling Psychology*, 42, 279, 1995.
17. Endler, N. S. and Parker, J. D. A., State and trait anxiety, depression and coping styles, *Australian Journal of Psychology*, 42, 207, 1990.
18. Endler, N. S. and Parker, J. D. A., Assessment of multidimensional coping: task, emotion, and avoidance strategies, *Psychological Assessment*, 6, 50, 1994.
19. Banyard, V. L. and Graham-Bermann, S. A., Can women cope? A gender analysis of theories of coping with stress, *Psychology of Women Quarterly*, 17, 303, 1993.
20. Parker, J. D. and Endler, N. S., Coping with coping assessment: a critical review, *European Journal of Personality*, 6, 321, 1992.

21. Schwarzer, R. and Schwarzer, C., A critical survey of coping instruments, Zeidner, M. and Endler, N. S., Eds., *Handbook of Coping: Theory, Research, Applications*, John Wiley & Sons, New York, 1996, 107.

22. Folkman, S. and Lazarus, R. S., An analysis of coping in a middle-aged community sample, *Journal of Health and Social Behavior*, 21, 219, 1980.

23. Amirkhan, J. H., A factor analytically derived measure of coping: the coping strategies indicator, *Journal of Personality and Social Psychology*, 59, 1066, 1990.

24. Cook, S. W. and Heppner, P. P., A psychometric study of three coping measures, *Educational and Psychological Measurement*, 57, 906, 1997.

25. American Psychiatric Association, *Diagnostic and Statistical Manual of Mental Disorders*, 4th ed., Washington, D.C., 1994, 327.

26. Neckowitz, P. and Morrison, T. L., Interactional coping strategies of normal-weight bulimic women in intimate and nonintimate stressful situations, *Psychological Reports*, 69, 1167, 1991.

27. Troop, N. A., Holbrey, A., Trowler, R., and Treasure, J. L., Ways of coping in women with eating disorders, *The Journal of Nervous and Mental Disease*, 182, 535, 1994.

28. Heppner, P. P., Cook, S. W., Strozier, A. L., and Heppner, M. J., An investigation of coping styles and gender differences with farmers in career transition, *Journal of Counseling Psychology*, 38, 167, 1991.

29. Leong, F. T., Bonz, M. H., and Zachar, P., Coping styles as predictors of college adjustment among freshmen, *Counselling Psychology Quarterly*, 10, 211, 1997.

30. Vollrath, M., Alnaes, R., and Torgersen, S., Differential effects of coping in mental disorders: a prospective study in psychiatric outpatients, *Journal of Clinical Psychology*, 52, 125, 1996.

31. Petrosky, M. J. and Birkimer, J. C., The relationship among locus of control, coping styles, and psychological symptom reporting, *Journal of Clinical Psychology*, 47, 336, 1991.

32. Zautra, A. J., Sheets, V. L., and Sandler, I. N., An examination of the construct validity of coping dispositions for a sample of recently divorced mothers, *Psychological Assessment*, 8, 256, 1996.

33. Kelly, W. L., *Psychology of the Unconscious: Mesmer, Janet, Freud, Jung, and Current Issues*, Prometheus Books, New York, 1991.

34. Shevrin, H., Bond, J. A., Brakel, L. A. W., Hertel, R. K., and Williams, W. J., *Conscious and Unconscious Processes: Psychodynamic, Cognitive, and Neurophysiological Convergences*, Guilford Press, New York, 1996.

35. Cassidy, T. and Burnside, E., Cognitive appraisal, vulnerability and coping: an integrative analysis of appraisal and coping mechanisms, *Counseling Psychology Quarterly*, 9, 261, 1996.

36. Amirkhan, J. H., Extroversion: a "hidden" personality factor in coping? *Journal of Personality*, 63, 189, 1995.

37. Wilson, G. T. and Pike, K. M., Eating disorders, in *Clinical Handbook of Psychological Disorders: A Step-by-Step Treatment Manual*, Barlow, D. H., Ed., Guilford Press, New York, 1993.

38. McDaniel, D. M. and Richards, C. S., Coping with dysphoria: gender differences in college students, *Journal of Clinical Psychology*, 46, 896, 1990.

39. Nolen-Hoeksema, S., *Sex Differences in Depression*, Stanford University Press, Stanford, CA, 1990.

40. Ptacek, J. T., Smith, R. E., and Zanas, J., Gender, appraisal, and coping: a longitudinal analysis, *Journal of Personality*, 60, 747, 1992.

41. Porter, L. S. and Stone, A. A., Are there really gender differences in coping?: A reconsideration of previous data and results from a daily study, *Journal of Social and Clinical Psychology*, 14, 184, 1995.

42. Hamilton, S. and Fagot, B. I., Chronic stress and coping styles: a comparison of male and female undergraduates, *Journal of Personality and Social Psychology*, 55, 819, 1988.

43. Boyle, J. A. and Paludi, M. A., *Sex and Gender: The Human Experience*, 3rd ed., Brown & Benchmark Publishers, Madison, WI, 1995.

44. Ptacek, J. T., Smith, R. E., and Dodge, K. L., Gender differences in coping with stress: when stressor and appraisals do not differ, *Personality and Social Psychology Bulletin*, 20, 421, 1994.

45. Horowitz, M. J., Znoj, H. J., and Stinson, C. J., Defensive control processes: use of theory in research, formulation, and therapy of stress response syndromes, in Zeidner M. and Endler, N. S., Eds., *Handbook of Coping: Theory, Research, Applications*, John Wiley & Sons, New York, 1996, 532.

46. Horowitz, M. J., *Formulation as a Basis for Planning Psychotherapy Treatment*, American Psychiatric Press, Inc., Washington, D.C., 1997.

47. Lightsey, O. R., What leads to wellness? The role of psychological resources in well-being, *The Counseling Psychologist*, 24, 589, 1996.

48. D'Zurilla, T. J. and Nezu, A. M., Clinical stress management, in *Clinical Decision Making in Behavior Therapy: A Problem-Solving Perspective*, Nezu, A. M. and Nezu, C. M., Eds., Research Press, Champaign, IL, 1989, 371–400.

Appendix 6-A: Problem-Focused Styles of Coping (PF-SOC)

The Problem-Focused Styles of Coping (PF-SOC: Heppner, Cook, Wright, and Johnson, 1995) is an 18-item questionnaire that measures the degree to which adults use cognitive, behavioral, and affective strategies to resolve the variety of personal problems in their lives. The PF-SOC provides scores for the following coping styles:

Reflective Style: This is a primarily cognitive coping style that describes the tendency to plan, reflect, and examine causes when dealing with personal problems. This coping style generally conveys efforts to approach or engage in the resolution of problems.

Reactive Style: This a coping style that includes primarily emotional and cognitive responses that deplete the individual or distort attempts to solve problems. People who score high on this factor tend to respond impulsively or be confused in response to personal problems, which tends to inhibit effective problem resolution.

Suppressive Style: This coping style describes a tendency to avoid or deny when responding to personal problems. This style portrays escapism, confusion, and a lack of persistence when coping which inhibit successful problem resolution.

As conveyed in the definitions, the three coping scales describe both a particular style of dealing with problems and the degree to which coping responses are leading to the successful resolution of problems. The Reflective Style describes generally successful efforts to resolve problems, while the Reactive and Suppressive Styles describe generally a lack of progress toward resolving problems. Initial information about the reliability and validity of the PF-SOC can be found in Heppner et al. (1995). This questionnaire has been used primarily with college student samples. Following are the ranges of mean scores and standard deviations in three samples of women college students from two universities in the Midwest and Southwestern United States ($\underline{N}$ = 93 to 380; Heppner et al, 1995): Reflective Style: $\underline{M}$ = 20.0 to 22.9, $\underline{SD}$ − 4.9 to 5.6; Reactive Style: $\underline{M}$ = 12.0 to 14.4, $\underline{SD}$ = 3.6 to 4.0; and Suppressive Style: $\underline{M}$ = 12.3 to 13.1, $\underline{SD}$ == 3.6 to 4.2

To score the PF-SOC, enter the responses in the corresponding blanks below and sum the responses for each scale.

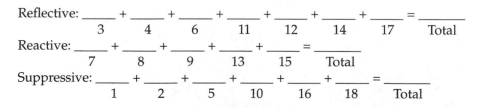

The authors would appreciate any information concerning the results you obtain using the PF-SOC. Please send such information to P. Paul Heppner, Ph.D., 16 Hill Hall, Department of Educational and Counseling Psychology, University of Missouri-Columbia, Columbia, MO 65211, or e-mail: HeppnerP@missouri.edu. If you would like additional information about this measure, please contact P. Paul Heppner, Ph.D.

The Problem-Focused Styles of Coping (PF-SOC)

Directions

This inventory contains statements about how people think, feel, and behave as they attempt to resolve personal difficulties and problems in their day-to-day lives. These are personal problems that come up from time to time, such as feeling depressed, getting along with friends, choosing a career, or deciding whether to get married or divorced. In considering how you deal with such problems, think about successful and unsuccessful outcomes, and what hinders or helps you in solving these problems. Please respond to the items as honestly as possible so as to accurately portray how frequently you do what is described in each item. Do not respond to the items as you think you should; rather respond in a way that most accurately reflects how you actually think, feel, and behave when you solve personal problems.

Please read each statement on the following page and indicate how often each item describes the way you typically respond to problems. In doing so, use the following alternatives:

1. ALMOST NEVER
2. OCCASIONALLY
3. ABOUT HALF OF THE TIME
4. OFTEN
5. ALMOST ALL OF THE TIME

Some people may find that a number of these items are typical of their responses all of the time, other items are occasionally used, while others are almost never typical of their responses. For example, consider this statement:

I think about past failures to help me solve my problems.

If you do this often, you would indicate number 4 on the questionnaire.
Now, please respond to the items on the following page.

_____ 1. I am not really sure what I think or believe about my problems.

_____ 2. I don't sustain my actions long enough to really solve my problems.

_____ 3. I think about ways that I solved similar problems in the past.

_____ 4. I identify the causes of my emotions which helps me identify and solve my problems.

_____ 5. I feel so frustrated I just give up doing any work on my problems at all.

_____ 6. I consider the short-term and long-term consequences of each possible solution to my problems.

_____ 7. I get preoccupied thinking about my problems and overemphasize some parts of them.

_____ 8. I continue to feel uneasy about my problems, which tells me I need to do some more work.

_____ 9. My old feelings get in the way of solving current problems.

_____ 10. I spend my time doing unrelated chores and activities instead of acting on my problems.

_____ 11. I think ahead, which enables me to anticipate and prepare for problems before they arise.

_____ 12. I think my problems through in a systematic way.

_____ 13. I misread another person's motives and feelings without checking with the person to see if my conclusions are correct.

_____ 14. I get in touch with my feelings to identify and work on problems.

_____ 15. I act too quickly, which makes my problems worse.

_____ 16. I have a difficult time concentrating on my problems (i.e., my mind wanders).

_____ 17. I have alternate plans for solving my problems in case my first attempt does not work.

_____ 18. I avoid even thinking about my problems.

Source: From Heppner, P. P., Cook, S. W., Wright, D. M., and Johnson, W. C., Jr., Progress in resolving problems: a problem-focused style of coping, *Journal of Counseling Psychology*, 42, 279, 1995. With permission.

7

Physiology of Stress

Jacalyn J. Robert-McComb

CONTENTS

7.1 Learning Objectives

After reading this chapter, the reader should understand:

- The relationship between stress and eating disorders;
- The physiological reactions associated with stress the response, specifically hormone secretions and targeted organs;
- The physiological consequences of chronic stress;
- The physiological reactions associated with stress management;
- Physiological measurements of stress;
- Plausible stress management techniques.

7.2   Research Background

7.2.1   The Relationship between Stress and Eating Disorders

Even though the relationship among stress, coping strategies, and eating disorders is not clearly understood, it seems that stressors are associated with disturbed eating attitudes. Furthermore, stressful life events precede the onset of anorexia nervosa and bulimia nervosa in most cases.[1,2] Disordered eating is often an unhealthy attempt at coping with stress.[3] The interpersonal stress theory states that binge eating is triggered by a stressful antecedent.[4] Support for this theory comes from observations that binge eating often occurs in frustrating and problematic situations associated with negative feelings such as anxiety.[5,6] Although individuals may use eating disorders as a method of coping, they soon are caught in a negative cycle, increasingly using ineffective behaviors in attempts to cope with stress.

However, in some laboratory paradigms, the eating habits of bulimic women following stressors have not been significantly different from the habits of the control subjects. Levine and Marcus[7] observed the eating behaviors of women with bulimic symptoms following exposure to an interpersonal stressor. They found that even though the consumption of carbohydrates increased following a stressor, the eating behaviors of these women were not significantly different from the eating behaviors of nonbulimic women. Their conclusion was that women with bulimic symptoms are not substantially more vulnerable to eating in response to stress than women without bulimic symptomatology. However, this outcome may result from the difficulty in evaluating the effects of stress on eating behaviors in a laboratory setting.

Other studies have suggested that stress is a consequence rather than a cause of eating disorders.[8] Sharpe, Ryst, and Steiner[9] found that even though eating disorder subjects reported more stressful life events than did noneating disorder subjects, the differences were driven by the disorder-specific events.

In summary, stress is almost certainly involved at some point in the continuum of the pathology of eating disorders. Distress may occur prior to, during, or following the attitudes and behaviors associated with anorexia, bulimia, eating-disorder-not-otherwise-specified or binge-eating disorder. Finally, attempts to use preventive interventions with populations at high risk for developing eating disorders should consider stress as both a risk factor and target for intervention.

7.2.2   Physiological Reactions Associated with the Stress Response

7.2.2.1   The Human Nervous System

To lay the groundwork for an understanding of the stress response, let us first briefly discuss the human nervous system[10,11] with an overview that has been simplified to meet the objectives of this chapter.

The basic anatomical unit of the human nervous system is the neuron (see Figure 7.1). Impulses from neuron to neuron are chemical. Impulse transmission from neuron to neuron occurs via the release of a neurotransmitter substance, either acetylcholine or norepinephrine.

The human nervous system consists of the central nervous system (CNS) and the peripheral nervous system (PNS). The brain and the spinal cord form the CNS, and the peripheral nervous system consists of all neurons in the body exclusive of the CNS (see Figure 7.2).

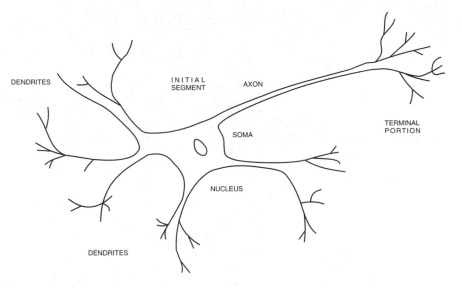

FIGURE 7.1
A neuron is the functional unit of the nervous system.

The peripheral nervous system is divided into the autonomic and somatic nervous systems. The autonomic system is concerned with the regulation of the internal environment of the body or with the maintenance of homeostasis. The autonomic system controls heart rate, blood pressure, hormonal balance, respiration, metabolism and reproduction; in essence, it supplies motor fibers to smooth and cardiac muscles and glands. The autonomic nervous system is further divided into two distinct branches or systems, sympathetic and parasympathetic. The autonomic system will be discussed in more detail later in the chapter, since it is central to understanding the stress response.

The somatic pathway is involved in impulse conduction that relays sensory and motor information between the CNS (brain and spinal cord) and receptors in the body. The pathway for conduction of nervous impulses from the periphery to the CNS is direct (see Figure 7.3). Whereas, in the sympathetic autonomic nervous system, the cell body of the first neuron is located in the brain or spinal cord, the neuron then synapses with one or more nerve fibers outside the central nervous system (ganglia) before the nerve fibers pass into various tissues and organs (see Figure 7.3).

7.2.2.1.1 Central Nervous System

Parts of the Brain
The three major parts of the brain are the cerebrum, the cerebellum, and the brainstem. The cerebrum is responsible for rational and moral thought including memory, interpretation of sensation, and decision making. The cerebellum is mainly involved in the control of muscular activity. The brainstem is composed of the medulla oblongata, pons, midbrain, and diencephalon. The medulla oblongata is involved in the control of breathing, blood circulation, and heart rate. The pons is a neural pathway for the brain. The midbrain is a small region of the brainstem located between the pons and the diencephalon. The diencephalon includes the thalamus and hypothalamus. The thalamus transmits information to various parts of the brain and the hypothalamus regulates hunger, thirst, and temperature. The hypothalamus functions along with the thalamus to determine pleasure and pain and establish emotional state. The hypothalamus is also important in releasing neurohormones responsible for the control of endocrine function in the body.

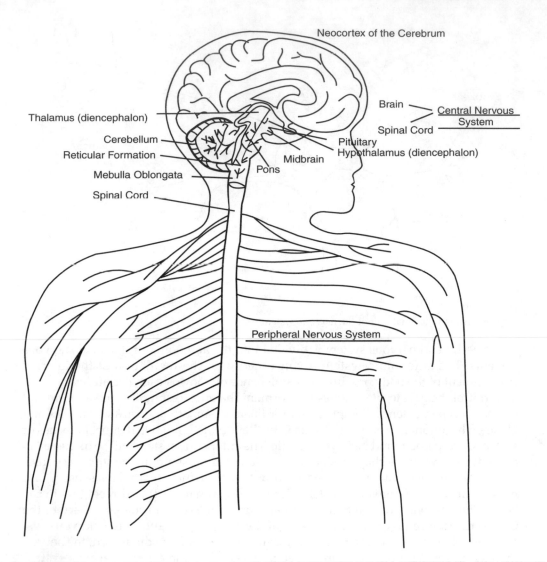

FIGURE 7.2
The brain and the spinal cord.

Functional Organization of the Brain

From a functional point of view, the emotional or affective brain can be considered to be divided into three different but interrelated levels (see Figure 7.4). There is a hierarchical organization of the brain, meaning that the functions of lower levels are influenced by the higher levels, and that higher level functions can override lower level functions.

The neocortical level represents the highest organization of the brain. The neocortex, primarily the frontal lobe and to a lesser degree the temporal lobe, decodes and interprets sensory signals received from the limbic system, and processes the information and exerts control by being excitatory or inhibitory. The neocortex presides over imagination, logic, decision making, problem solving, planning, organization, and memory.

The limbic system represents the major component of the second level of the brain, and is the brain's control center. It is composed of numerous neural structures, three of which are central to the stress response: the hypothalamus, thalamus, and pituitary gland. These three glands work together to maintain a level of homeostasis in the body.

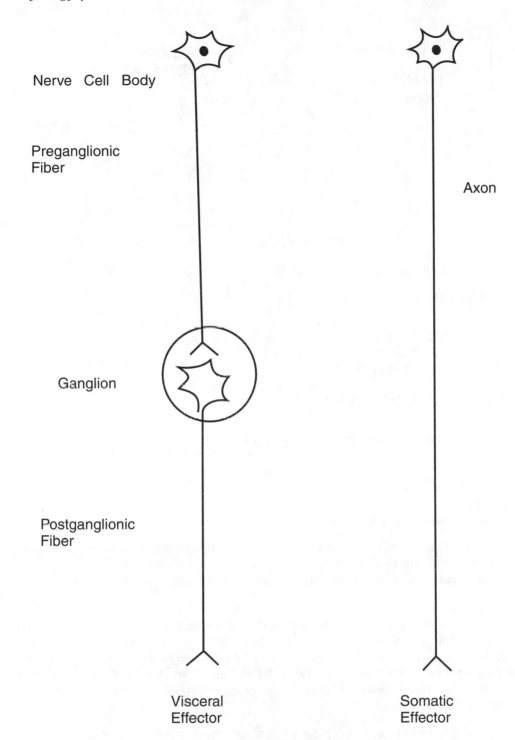

FIGURE 7.3
The differences between the somatic and autonomic neural pathways to effector organs.

The brainstem and reticular formation form the lowest functional level of the human brain, referred to as the vegetative level. This level is concerned with respiration, heart rate, etc. The reticular formation is a diffuse network that extends from the spinal cord to the lower brain centers and is concerned with sensory and motor impulses. The

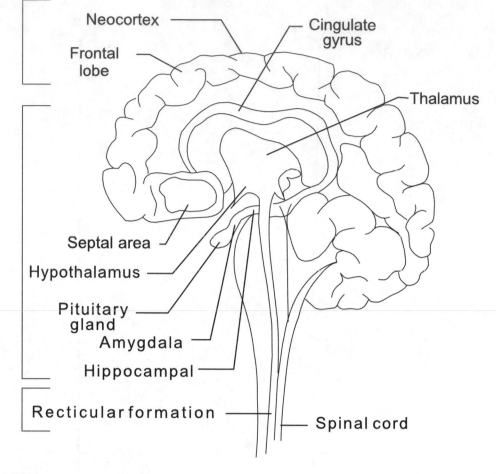

FIGURE 7.4
Hierarchical organization of the brain.

reticular activating system is selective, and only certain stimuli will arouse other portions of the brain through this selective pathway. Along with the spinal cord, this pathway uses neurons to send information to and from parts of the body and the brain.

Spinal Cord
The lowest part of the brain stem, the medulla oblongata, is continuous below the spinal cord. The spinal cord is composed of tracts of nerve fibers that allow two–way conduction of nerve impulses. The sensory (afferent) fibers carry neural signals from sensory receptors, such as those located in the muscles and joints, to the upper level of the CNS. Motor (efferent) fibers from the brain and spinal cord travel down to the end organs (muscles, glands).

7.2.2.1.2   Autonomic System of the Peripheral Nervous System
Sympathetic Branch
The sympathetic nerves originate in the spinal cord between the thoracic and lumbar segments and innervate various organs and tissues (see Figure 7.5).

Parasympathetic Branch
The parasympathetic nerves have fibers located in several cranial nerves, a few sacral nerves, and primarily the vagus nerve (see Figure 7.6). These nerve fibers similarly

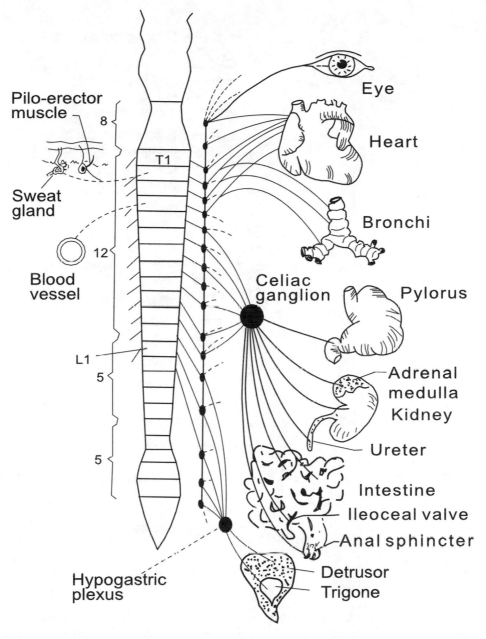

FIGURE 7.5
Sympathetic nervous system.

innervate various tissues and organs, as does the sympathetic autonomic nervous system. However, in the parasympathetic system, the preganglion fibers pass uninterrupted to the organ or tissue innervated.

All preganglion neurons of both the sympathetic and parasympathetic nervous systems release the same neurotransmitter, acetylcholine, which will excite both the sympathetic and parasympathetic postganglion neurons. However, postganglion fibers of the sympathetic nervous system also release norepinephrine (also known as noradrenalin) as a neurotransmitter. In general, postganglion fibers of the sympathetic nervous system release norepinephrine as a neurotransmitter, and postganglion fibers of the parasympathetic nervous system release acetylcholine as a neurotransmitter.

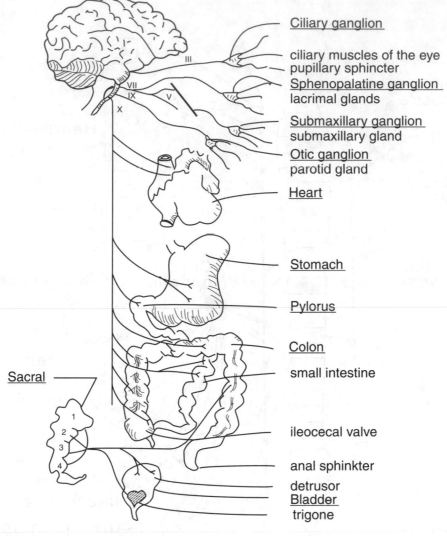

FIGURE 7.6
Parasympathetic nervous system.

7.2.2.1.3 *The Stress Response*

The stress response evoked results from an individual's cognitive interpretation of the event rather than the actual event; it is a process of arousal and involves pathways. Pathways control the glands that produce the hormone or chemical messenger, the circulation of the hormone to the target organ or gland, and the release of the chemical responsible for preparing the body for the stressful encounter. Three main physiological pathways or axes are activated upon elicitation of the stress response, the neural, the neural endocrine axis, and the endocrine pathways.[11] All of the pathways are interrelated; however, these pathways will be discussed separately and will begin with the initial physiological response to a stressor and culminate with the body's most pronounced physiological response.

7.2.2.1.4 *Neural Pathways*

Signals from either an internal (a cognitive state or internal physical sensation) or external (through sensory receptors of the peripheral nervous system) source are sent

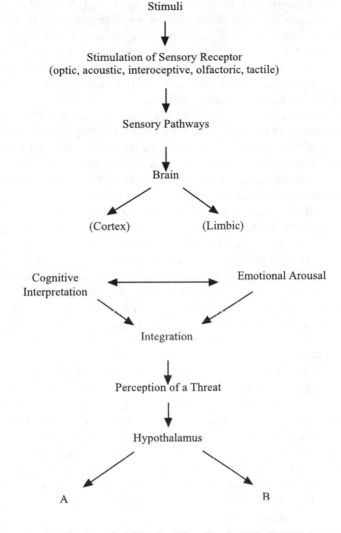

FIGURE 7.7
Initial activation of the stress response.

via sensory neural pathways toward the brain. The information is both rationally and emotionally integrated. The hypothalamus functions along with the thalamus to determine emotional state and activate autonomic nervous system activity (see Figure 7.7).

If a stimulus is perceived as threatening, the stress response is elicited. During the stress response, an increased sympathetic discharge occurs. The degree of sympathetic activation depends on the perceived severity of the threat. A serious threat will result in increased end-organ response caused by the recruitment of sympathetic end-organ activity (see Figure 7.5). During the stress response, myocardial contractility, heart rate, and blood pressure will increase. Sympathetic stimulation causes the vasculature of the body to constrict. Blood is shunted away from the periphery. In some instances, spinchter tone increases, peristaltic movement in the gastrointestinal tract is inhibited, and blood flow to the digestive organs decreases.

Sympathetic activation may also dilate the bronchi and constrict blood vessels in the respiratory system, even though the effect is mild. Sympathetic activation also has an effect on the glands of the body, causing increased perspiration along with increased skin conductivity. Constriction occurs in the secretory capacity of the nasal, salivary, lacrimal, and many gastrointestinal glands. The pupil of the eye dilates during sympathetic activation, and the subject exhibits increased mental alertness, muscular strength, and increased basal metabolic response (increase in blood levels of glucose resulting from hepatic glucose release and glycogenolysis in muscle). Conversely, activity in the ducts of the gall bladder, liver, urethra, and bladder is inhibited. All of these physiological responses are preparing the body for the increased demands it may be called upon to meet in order to overcome the perceived threatening situation. The neural transmission during the stress response is very rapid because the pathways involved are neural. However, the effects do not last long due to the rapid disintegration and re-uptake of the neurotransmitter substance. Also, the stores of the neurotransmitter substance can become exhausted under intense and constant stimulation.

Even though there is increased sympathetic discharge during the stress response, the parasympathetic nervous system also exerts an influence. Most organs of the body are innervated by both the sympathetic and parasympathetic nervous systems, and some parasympathetic end-organ stress reactions may occur. The primary role of the parasympathetic nervous system is to relax the body and return it to a restful state. Parasympathetic end-organ stress reactions include decreased blood pressure, heart, and respiration rates, and increased vagal tone. Parasympathetic response coupled with sympathetic arousal following a stressor (i.e., shunting of blood from the periphery, a decrease in venous return) may also cause a condition known as syncope or, more commonly, fainting.

The effects of autonomic neural activation on end-organs during the stress response are immediate but not long lasting. In order to maintain levels of stress arousal for a longer time, an additional psychophysiological axis must be activated. Sympathetic arousal stimulates the particular organs that are needed for the "fight or flight" response.

7.2.2.1.5 Neuroendocrine Pathways

Cannon was the first to describe the "fight or flight response" response.[12] During this response the body is prepared for heightened muscular activity so that it may either fight or flee the perceived danger. The stress response occurs as a result of both neural and endocrine activity and is neuroendocrine in nature. The flight or fight response has its origin in the dorsomedial–amygdalar complex. Neural impulses continue to flow through the hypothalamus, thoracic spinal cord, and eventually innervate the adrenal medulla (see Figure 7.8).

Adrenal medullary stimulation results in the release of adrenalin and noradrenalin into the systemic circulation. The effects of this pathway are similar if not identical to direct sympathetic arousal. The difference between these two pathways is that the measurable effects are delayed (20 to 30 s). Furthermore, the duration of the stimulation is increased tenfold. This pathway has been termed the intermediate phase of

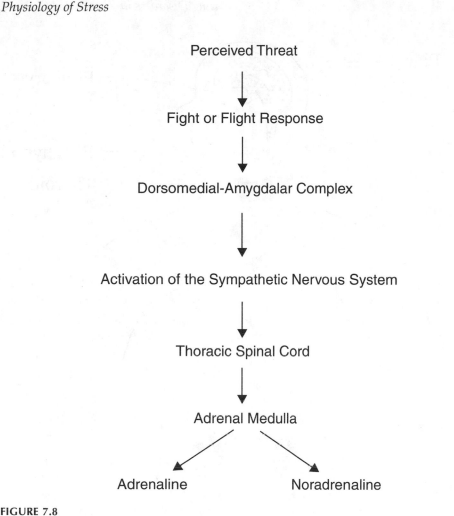

FIGURE 7.8
Intermediate activation of the stress response.

activation in the stress response. Some of the physiological effects of adrenal medullary axis stimulation are as follows (a) increased arterial blood pressure and cardiac output; (b) increased plasma levels of free fatty acids, triglycerides, and cholesterol; (c) increased muscular tension; and (d) decreased amount of blood flow to the kidneys and periphery of the skin.

7.2.2.1.6   *Endocrine Pathways*

Several endocrine glands are involved in physiological response to stress. Figure 7.9 illustrates the main endocrine glands that are involved in the stress response. A longer time is required both for endocrine hormonal release and for the hormones to be transported through the circulation. The three main endocrine pathways that have been implicated in the stress response are termed the adrenal cortical axis, the somatotropic axis, and the thyroid axis. The most chronic and prolonged somatic response to stress is the result of these endocrine pathways.

The Adrenal Cortical Axis

The septal-hippocampal complex appears to be the highest point of origin for the adrenal cortical axis (see Figure 7.10). Neural impulses then descend into the median eminence of the hypothalamus. The neurosecretory cells in the median eminence of

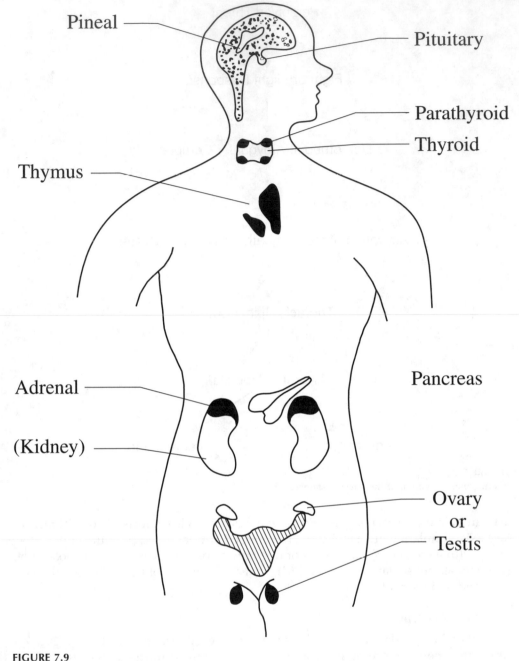

FIGURE 7.9
Major endocrine glands of the body.

the hypothalamus release corticotropin releasing factor (CRF) into the hypothalamic hypophyseal portal system. The CRF descends into the infundibular stalk to the anterior pituitary cells. The anterior pituitary is sensitive to CRF and responds by releasing adrenocorticotropic hormone (ACTH) into the systemic circulation. ACTH then stimulates the adrenal cortex to release glucocorticoids (cortisol and corticosterone) and mineralocorticoids (aldosterone and deoxycorticosterone) into the systemic circulation. Some of the physiological effects of glucocorticoids and mineralocorticoids are listed on Table 7.1.

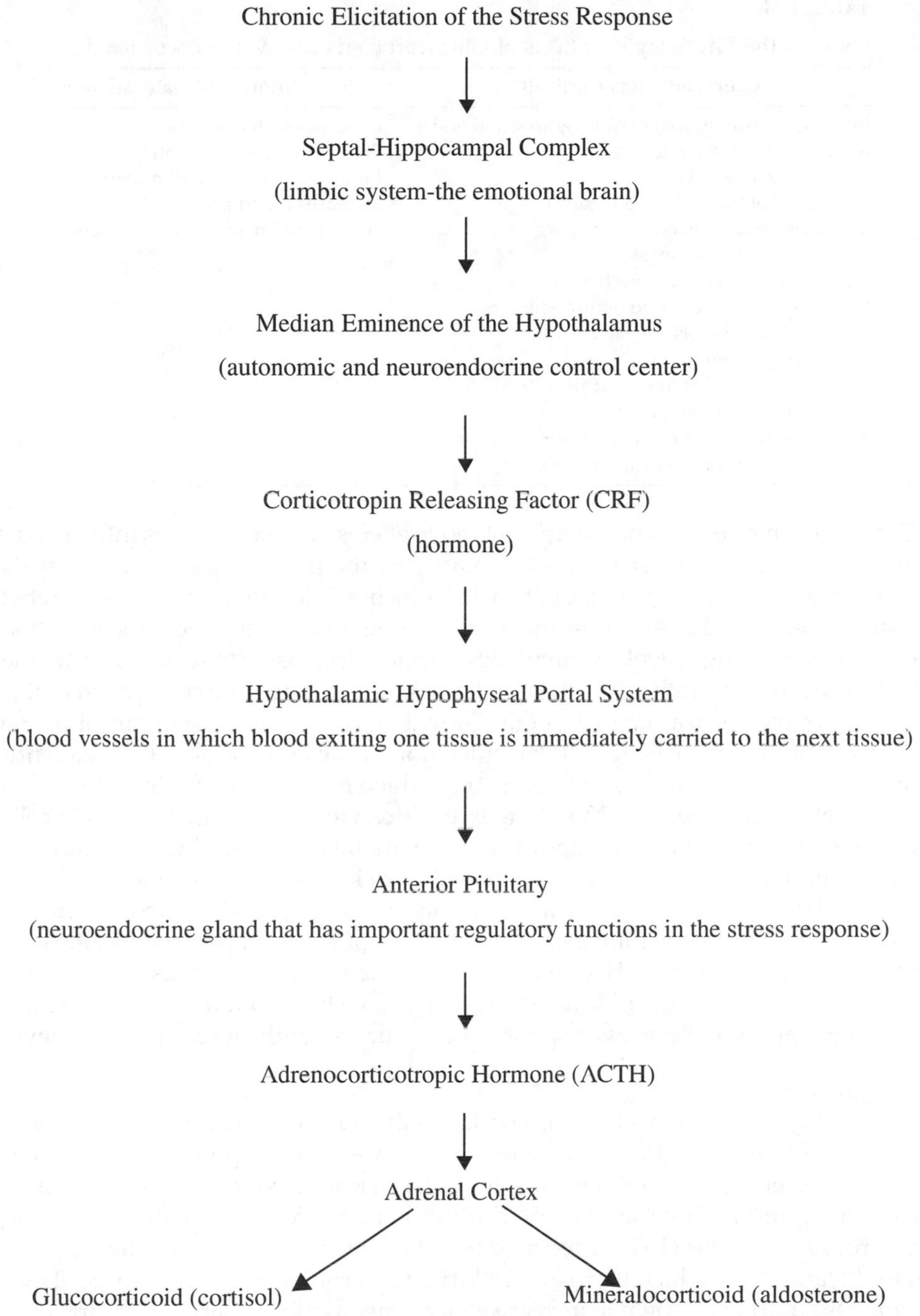

Chronic Elicitation of the Stress Response

↓

Septal-Hippocampal Complex

(limbic system-the emotional brain)

↓

Median Eminence of the Hypothalamus

(autonomic and neuroendocrine control center)

↓

Corticotropin Releasing Factor (CRF)

(hormone)

↓

Hypothalamic Hypophyseal Portal System

(blood vessels in which blood exiting one tissue is immediately carried to the next tissue)

↓

Anterior Pituitary

(neuroendocrine gland that has important regulatory functions in the stress response)

↓

Adrenocorticotropic Hormone (ACTH)

↓

Adrenal Cortex

Glucocorticoid (cortisol)   Mineralocorticoid (aldosterone)

FIGURE 7.10
The adrenal cortical axis.

The Somatotropic Axis
The somatotropic axis has the same basic pathway, beginning from the septal-hippocampal complex through the hypothalamic hypophyseal portal system as the adrenal cortical axis, with the exception that the somatotropin releasing factor stimulates the pituitary to release growth hormone (somatotropin) into the systemic circulation (see Figure 7.11).

TABLE 7.1

Some of the Physiological Effects of Glucocorticoids and Mineralocorticoids

Glucocorticoids (cortisol)	Mineralocorticoids (aldosterone)
Increases serum glucose levels (gluconeogenesis)	Increases water retention
Increases free fatty-acid release into systemic circulation	Promotes sodium retention
Increases ketone body production	Enhances potassium elimination
Increases arterial blood pressure	Increases blood pressure because of increased water retention
Exacerbates herpes simplex	
Suppresses the immune system	
Increases susceptibility to nonthrombotic myocardial necrosis	
Mobilizes proteins	
Elevates the level of amino acids in the blood, especially from muscle tissue	
Enhances amino acid transport into the liver, which contributes to gluconeogenesis	

   Growth hormone (GH) has many metabolic effects, and secretion is influenced not only by the stress response but also primarily by the prevailing circulating levels of metabolites such as amino acids, fatty acids, glucose, and other hormones secreted in the stress response. For example, the hormone epinephrine enhances the secretion of the GH, whereas high levels of circulating cortisol decrease GH secretion. The role of GH during stress is to stimulate the uptake of amino acids by the cells and to mobilize energy resources such as fat in the body. Growth hormone enhances amino acid transfer across the cell, increasing cellular utilization of these substrates. Consequently, a reduction in cellular glucose uptake ensues, which may then result in a rise in blood sugar levels. This increase in blood sugar levels can in turn stimulate the beta cells of the pancreatic islets of Langerhans to secrete extra insulin. It has been suggested that overstimulation of GH can produce a diabetic-like insulin-resistant effect and act as a potential diabetogenic agent. Growth hormone also has an effect on many of the electrolytes in the body. GH influences the retention of sodium, potassium, phosphate, and calcium in the body. GH secretion in response to stress is not as frequent as the cortisol response. However, elevated GH levels have been found in the blood following the elicitation of the stress response in conjunction with elevated cortisol levels.

The Thyroid Axis
The pathway of the thyroid axis is similar to the adrenal cortical and somatotropic axes. The difference begins at the median eminence of the hypothalamus where thyrotopin-releasing factor (TRF) is sent through the portal system to the anterior pituitary (see Figure 7.12). From the anterior pituitary, thyroid-stimulating hormone or thyrotrophic hormone (TTH) is released into the systemic circulation. The target is the thyroid gland, from which thyroxine and triiodothyronine are then released. Thyroid hormones have been shown to increase general metabolism, heart rate, heart contractility, peripheral vascular resistance, and the sensitivity of some tissues to catecholamines. Figure 7.13 depicts the relationships among the immediate, intermediate, and long-term effects of the body's physiological reactions to a stressor.

7.2.3   Physiological Consequences of Chronic Stress

The process by which external stressors cause changes in internal bodily functions is only partially understood. However, it seems that illness occurs because of the chronic

Chronic Elicitation of the Stress Response

↓

Septal-Hippocampal Complex

(limbic system-the emotional brain)

↓

Median Eminence of the Hypothalamus

(autonomic and neuroendocrine control center)

↓

Somatotropin Releasing Factor

(hormone)

↓

Hypothalamic Hypophyseal Portal System

(blood vessels in which blood exiting one tissue is immediately carried to the next tissue)

↓

Anterior Pituitary

(neuroendocrine gland that has important regulatory functions in the stress response)

↓

Somatotropin Hormone (Growth Hormone)

FIGURE 7.11
The somatotropic axis.

and excessive elicitation of stress hormones and the body's continual physiological attempts to overcome the perceived threat. Hans Seyle[13] theorized a three-component model to explain the stress response. The chronic and continual secretion of the hormones associated with stress may ultimately lead to illness (see Table 7.2). In his model, the first phase is called *alarm reaction*. The alarm reaction is characterized by the release of adrenal medullary and cortical hormones into the bloodstream. This phase parallels the fight or flight response proposed by Cannon. The second phase of GAS is termed the *stage of resistance*. Cortisol secretion is heightened and the body functions at elevated metabolic levels. The last phase is the *stage of exhaustion*. Endocrine activity is

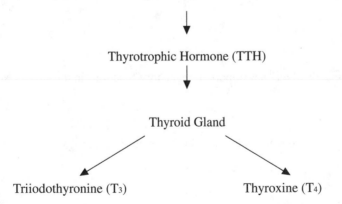

Chronic Elicitation of the Stress Response

↓

Septal-Hippocampal Complex

(limbic system-the emotional brain)

↓

Median Eminence of the Hypothalamus

(autonomic and neuroendocrine control center)

↓

Thyrotopin Releasing Factor (TRF)

(hormone)

↓

Hypothalamic Hypophyseal Portal System

(blood vessels in which blood exiting one tissue is immediately carried to the next tissue)

↓

Anterior Pituitary

(neuroendocrine gland that has important regulatory functions in the stress response)

↓

Thyrotrophic Hormone (TTH)

↓

Thyroid Gland

Triiodothyronine (T_3)   Thyroxine (T_4)

FIGURE 7.12
The thyroid axis.

increased, and high circulatory levels of cortisol begin to produce pronounced effects on the circulatory, digestive, immune, and other systems of the body. In this final stage of exhaustion cardiovascular, gastrointestinal, immune, respiratory, and musculoskeletal disorders occur.

A brief overview of possible disease conditions seen in the stage of exhaustion related to chronic stress follows. The cardiovascular system is thought by many researchers to be the primary target end-organ for the stress response.[14] Cardiovascular disorders most often associated with the stress response are essential hypertension, arrhythmias,

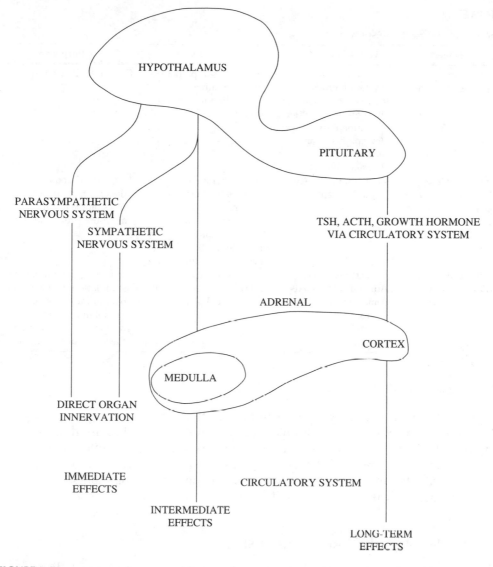

FIGURE 7.13
Relationships among stress pathways.

migraine headaches, and Raynauds' phenomenon (vasoconstriction in the hands, fingers, feet, or toes). The two gastrointestinal disorders most often linked to the stress response are peptic ulcers and ulcerative colitis. A combination of emotional factors (anger and rage) and genetic factors appear to be involved in the pathogenesis of gastrointestinal disorders associated with stress. Anxiety or stress may also cause or exacerbate bronchial asthma. The inability to breathe following contraction of the bronchiole airways is anxiety producing, thus provoking a bronchial asthma attack. Chronic stress may also contribute to low back pain. The back muscles play an obvious role in the fight or flight response. During the stress response, blood flow increases to the muscles needed for fight or flight, back muscles contract, and if there is no associated action and contraction continues, metabolites increase, blood flow ultimately decreases, and pain may result.

Common stress-related disorders of the skin include eczema, acne, urticaria, and psoriasis. The mechanisms of involvement are not clearly understood, and the

TABLE 7.2

Stages of the Stress Response

Stages	Pathways or Axes	Effects	Purpose
Immediate (quickest response)	Autonomic Nervous System Pathway:[a] Results in the release of the neurotransmitter, norepinephrine (sympathetic) or acetylcholine (parasympathetic)	End-organ sympathetic or parasympathetic stimulation for a short duration (2–3 sec)	Overall body arousal
Intermediate (20 to 30 second delay for onset of measurable effects)	Neuroendocrine Axis:[b] "Fight or flight"	The adrenal medulla secretes the hormones epinephrine (adrenaline) and norepinephrine (noradrenalin), prolonging the effects of sympathetic stimulation	Heightened body arousal; the effects on the physiological symptoms are more pronounced
Prolonged effects Minutes, hours, days, or weeks	Endocrine Axises Adrenal cortical axis Somatropic axis Thyroid axis General adaptation syndrome[c]	Numerous hormones are released, depending on the targeted gland.	Requires greater intensity stimulation; however, the overall metabolic effect is to mobilize energy resources in preparation for the stressful encounter

[a] See Figure 7.7.
[b] See Figure 7.8.
[c] See Figures 7.10 to 7.13.

relationship between stress and skin disorders rests on clinical case reports. It has also been stated that excessive and chronic stress can exert a generalized immunosuppressive effect. However, the effects of stress on immunity are very complex, and the relationship between stress and disease is multifactorial and interactive. Most scientists who investigate stress and immunity do so in the context of a common-sense belief in the existence of a causal relationship between stress and disease.

7.2.4 Physiological Measurements of Stress

The physiological measurement of the stress response is a complex task. In this section physiological end-organ responses as well as chemical measurements will be discussed. It must be noted that because of the multifactorial nature of the stress response, several measurements are needed, psychological as well as physiological. Numerous psychological tools to evaluate the stress response can be found in the literature; however, it is beyond the scope of this chapter to discuss psychological assessments and their importance.

Physiological end-organ measurements commonly seen in the literature include heart rate, breathing rate, and blood pressure. It is important to obtain baseline measurements of these variables for each individual, since variations exist among individuals from day to day. Published norms are presented in Table 7.3. Elevation from normal in any one or any combination of these variables is an indication of sympathetic arousal and/or heightened adrenal medullary activity.

Plasma levels of catecholamines can be measured in blood samples by several techniques. Radioimmune assay methods are frequently used. It must be remembered that blood levels of these hormones vary from laboratory to laboratory and depend

TABLE 7.3

Average Values for Heart Rate, Blood Pressure, and Respiratory Rate in Adults

Heart Rate	Blood Pressure	Respiratory Rate
60–80 bpm	Normal	Normal
74 bpm (women)	Systolic (mm Hg) <130	12 breaths per min
72 bpm (men)	Diastolic (mm Hg) <85	.5 L per breath

TABLE 7.4

Catecholamine and 17-Hydroxycorticosteroid (17-OHS) Hormone Levels in Adults

Condition	Epinephrine	Norepinephrine	17-OHS
Plasma Levels (ng/ml)			
Normal	0.05	0.20	
Severe Stress	0.27	4.10	
Average 24-h			
Urinary Levels (µg)			
Normal	2 to 51	25 to 50	
Stress	>51	>51	
Plasma (µg/100ml)			
Normal			
8:00 A.M.			5.5 to 26.3
4:00 P.M.			2.0 to 18.0
Stress			>26
Urine (µg/24-h sample)			
Normal			
8:00 A.M.			20 to 100
Stress			>100

on test conditions, time of sampling, and the state of the individual being tested.[15] Twenty-four hour urine samples of catecholamines are also measured in many laboratories. Typical values for total urinary catecholamines can range from 0 to 100 µg/24 sample.[16] Under psychological stress, urine catecholamine excretions can approach 300 µg per day.[17] Table 7.4 depicts average values of the hormones epinephrine and norepinephrine in adults in normal and distressed states.[17–19]

Corticosteroid levels, although fairly accurately assessed, also depend on the psychological and physiological state of the subject, the test conditions, the methods used, the adequacy of the sample collection, and the means of the assay. Cortisol (adrenal cortical hormone) is secreted at an average rate of 20 mg/day.[20] Blood concentrations of cortisol fluctuate diurnally and average 12 µg percent.[20] A group of urinary metabolites of cortisol, the 17-hydroxycorticosteroids (17-OHCS), can be used to estimate the daily cortisol excretion rates. Table 7.4 lists 17-OHCS values observed in normal and distressed states.[15,21]

Clinical biofeedback is also used to measure physiological responses to stress. However, biofeedback is used more as an educational tool to teach individuals how to listen to their bodies' physiological responses to stress and control the response through learned relaxation techniques.[22,23] There are many types of biofeedback equipment.[24] Electromyographic feedback monitors electrical impulses produced by the muscles. The electroencephalographic biofeedback detects and monitors brain waves. Cardiovascular biofeedback is often used to augment an individual's ability to control heart

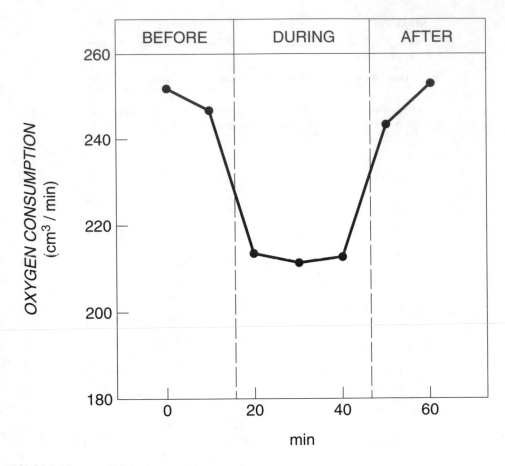

FIGURE 7.14
Changes in oxygen consumption during the practice of the relaxation response.

rate. Thermal biofeedback measures the flow of blood to a specific area by the heat emitted. Electrodermal biofeedback measures the electrical conduction of the skin. For more information on clinical biofeedback training, contact the Biofeedback Certification Institute of America at http://www.biof.com/neurofeedback.html.

7.2.5 Physiological Reactions Associated with Relaxation

Studies have shown that the regular practice of relaxation techniques is associated with a decrease in oxygen uptake, carbon dioxide production, heart rate, blood lactate, and systolic blood pressure while at rest.[25] A group of researchers at Harvard Medical School carried out a number of experiments investigating the physiological response of eliciting what has come to be known as the "relaxation response." The regular practice of the relaxation response also produces a significant decrease in VO_2, rate of perceived exertion, systolic blood pressure, rate-pressure product, and frequency of breathing during submaximal exercise.[26,27] In one experiment, individuals who had been meditating anywhere from 1 month to over 9 years (20 minutes in the morning and 20 minutes in the evening) participated in data collection in which oxygen consumption was measured before, during, and after the meditation period. The experiments showed that during meditation, there was a marked decrease in the body's oxygen consumption.[28] (see Figure 7.14). This change in oxygen consumption

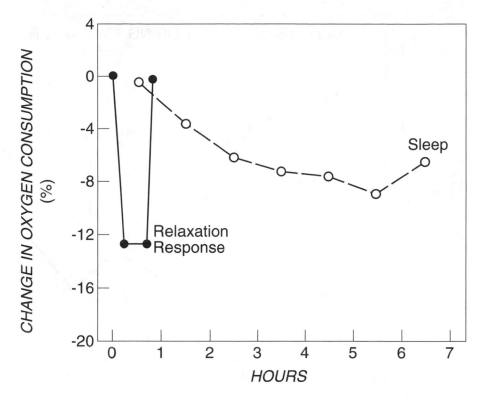

FIGURE 7.15
Comparison between the level of oxygen consumption during the practice of the relaxation response and sleep.

during meditation is markedly different from the change in oxygen consumption during sleep (see Figure 7.15). Meditation is therefore not a substitute for sleep or vice versa. Blood lactate levels also fall rapidly during the first 10 minutes of meditation and remain at extremely low levels during meditation[29] (see Figure 7.16). These results during meditation, along with the additional findings of decreased heart rate and respiration rates, signify decreased activity of the sympathetic nervous system during the elicitation of the relaxation response.

7.3 Application of Research Question

The focus of this chapter has been on the physiological consequences of distress. Stress is inevitable, yet distress is negotiable. How do we manage or negotiate the stress in our lives before it becomes distress? In 1975, Herbert Benson, M.D. wrote a book entitled *The Relaxation Response*[30] which discusses various techniques employed to achieve a relaxation response. These techniques come from many sources and cultures, some of which are Yoga, Zen Buddhism, Transcendental Meditation, and Christian Mysticism. Whatever the source, the experience is unique and deeply personal. However, there appear to be four basic elements underlying the elicitation of the relaxation response.

The first element is a *quiet environment* (internally and externally). It is best to choose an environment that has a calming effect, one that fosters a state of deep

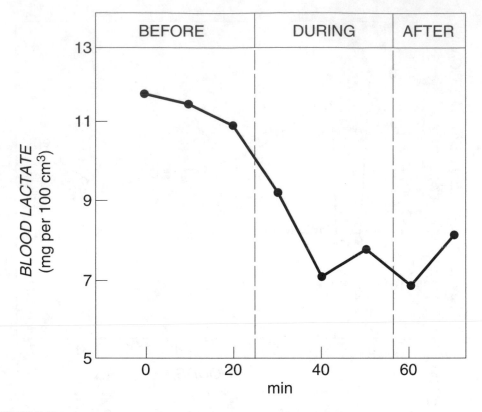

FIGURE 7.16
Changes in blood lactate during the practice of the relaxation response.

relaxation and has as few distractions as possible. The environment should be comforting and may be a place of worship, a backyard, or a bedroom. The second element is an *object to dwell upon*, to help clear the mind of distracting thoughts. One of the major difficulties in eliciting the relaxation response is mind wandering. Having an object to gaze upon or a word or phrase to repeat helps shift the mind away from external distracting thoughts. The third element, a *passive attitude*, is perhaps the most essential factor in eliciting the relaxation response. Diligent effort should be made to eliminate the intrusion of thoughts and distractions. If distracting thoughts interfere, they should be disregarded. That means redirecting attention to the object to be focused upon or the phrase to be repeated. The fourth element is a *comfortable position* that can be maintained for at least 20 minutes and allow the practitioner to remain awake. A sitting position is recommended for that reason, but a prone position may work better for some individuals.

More than one method can work in achieving the relaxation response; however, these four components should be included in whichever method is used. It is not even important to understand how or why this method works; however, it is imperative to perform the steps. The technique chosen to elicit a deep state of relaxation should be practiced daily for at least twenty minutes, if possible. However, it is imperative to set a practical time limit that can be easily be met. A method by which daily relaxation practice can be easily logged has been included in Appendix 7-A. Below is a sample exercise; however, the best method is one that is unique to the individual. Sample relaxation techniques, including a progressive muscle relaxation, a yoga stretch, and a breathing exercise[31,32] are included in Appendices 7-B through 7-D. Remember, for these techniques to be effective, they must be practiced on a regular basis.

SAMPLE BODY SCAN EXERCISE

Sit or lie quietly in a comfortable position. Close your eyes. Breathe deeply; as you inhale, feel your chest expand and abdomen rise slightly. As you exhale, feel the chest fall with a sigh of release. Become aware of your breathing. Begin focusing on parts of your body; scan your body with your breathing. Beginning with your toes, direct your attention and breathe into your toes. Continue breathing fully and deeply as you scan your body in an organized format, giving each part of your body attention with the direction of your breath. First your right toe, then your right heel, the top of your foot, your tibia, your calf muscle, your hamstrings, your thighs; linger at each body part with your breathing, and direct attention to that body part; then repeat with the other leg. Become aware of how each part of your body feels; be sensitive to it, and honor each part of your body with your breath.

Next, go to the pelvic region. Feel any sensations or lack of sensations here; shift your breath's attention to this part of your body. Feel your abdomen; feel it rise and fall with your breathing; feel your rib cage expand as you breathe in and fall as you breathe out deeply, rhythmically. Next, direct your breath's attention to the fingers on the right hand. Do any fingers hurt? Take your breath there. Continue scanning your right arm, being attentive to the feelings or lack of feelings in your arm. Become aware of your body; honor your body with your attention. Repeat the same with your left arm.

When your mind starts to wander, and it will, gently bring it back into your breathing and the scan of your body. Don't try too hard; you must maintain a passive attitude. The practice is enough to bring about relaxation if performed regularly and thoughtfully. Direct your breath's attention to your shoulder region; feel the tension. Breathe deeply, as if blowing out the tension with each breath. Scan your neck; feel the sensations in your neck as you inhale and exhale; linger here. Next, let your breath's attention go to your face. Are your lips pursed tightly or relaxed? Are your teeth clenched or relaxed? How about your jaw? Soften these parts of your body by bringing your breath's attention to the parts of your face and neck that are tight and tense. Breathe, simply breathe, honoring any sensation or lack of sensation you feel in this region; just be conscious of each body part. Concentrate on your eyes. Are they tired or do they need rest? Honor this.

Next, focus on the top of your head. Breathe deeply through your mouth and nose; then let your breath resonate from deep down, and let your diaphragm expand on each inhalation and contract fully on each exhalation. Just lie there breathing deeply for a few minutes. When you are ready, gently open your eyes and affirm yourself for taking this time to nourish your sense of relaxation.

In closing, do not worry about whether you are successful in achieving a deep level of relaxation. Maintain a passive attitude, and let relaxation occur at its own pace. When distracting thoughts occur, try to ignore them and gently bring your concentration back to your breathing, directing your attention to your body scan. To see the benefits of the relaxation response, you must practice it almost daily. It is your special time to honor yourself with relaxation and ultimately better health.

References

1. Schmidt, U.H., Tiller, J.M., Andrews, B., Blanchard, M., and Treasure, J., Is there a specific trauma precipitating onset of anorexia nervosa?, *Psychological Medicine*, 27(3), 523, 1997.
2. Fryer, S., Waller, G., Kroese, B. S., Stress, coping, and disturbed eating attitudes in teenage girls, *International Journal of Eating Disorders*, 22(4), 427, 1997.

3. Soukup, V. M., Beiler, M. E., and Terrell, F., Stress, coping style, and problem-solving ability among eating-disordered inpatients. _Journal of Clinical Psychology_, 46(3), 592, 1990.

4. Laessle, R. G., Beumont, P. J., Butow, P., Lennerts, W., O'Conner, M., Pirke, K. M., Touyz, S. W., and Waadt, S., A comparison of nutritional management with stress management in the treatment of bulimia nervosa, _British Journal of Psychiatry_, 159, 250, 1991.

5. Abraham, S. F., and Beumont, P. J., How patients describe bulimia or binge-eating. _Psychological Medicine_, 12(3), 625, 1982.

6. Catteanach, Malley, and Rodin, Psychologic and physiologic reactivity to stressors in eating disordered individuals. _Psychosomatic Medicine,_ 50(6), 591, 1988.

7. Levine, M. D. and Marcus, M. D., Eating behavior following stress in women with and without bulimic symptoms, _Annals of Behavioral Medicine,_ 19(2), 132, 1997.

8. Rosen, J. C., Compas, B.E., and Tracy, B., The relationship among stress, psychological symptoms, and eating disorder symptoms: a prospective analysis. _International Journal of Eating Disorders_, 14(2), 153, 1993.

9. Sharpe, T. A., Ryst, E., and Steiner, H., Reports of stress: a comparison between eating disordered and non-eating disordered adolescents, _Child Psychiatry and Human Development_, 28(2), 117, 1997.

10. Asterita, M. F., _The Physiology of Stress_, Human Sciences Press, New York, 1985, chap. 3 and 6.

11. Everly, G. S., and Rosenfeld, R., _The Nature and the Treatment of the Stress Response_, Plenum Press, New York, 1983, chap. 2, 3, and 4.

12. Cannon, W. B. and Paz, D. Emotional stimulation of adrenal gland secretion. _American Journal of Physiology,_ 28(1), 64, 1911.

13. Seyle, H., The general adaptation syndrome and the gastrointestinal disease of adaptation, _American Journal of Proctology,_ 2, 167, 1951.

14. Matthews, K.A., Owens, J.F., Kuller, L.W., Sutton-Tyrrell, K., Lassilia, H.C., and Wolfson, S.K., Stress-induced pulse pressure change predicts women's carotid atherosclerosis, _Stroke,_ 29(8), 1525, 1998.

15. Tietz, N. M., _Fundamentals of Clinical Chemistry,_ W.B. Saunders, Philadelphia, 1976.

16. Asterita, M., _The Physiology of Stress_, Human Sciences Press, New York, 1985, chap. 2 and 3.

17. Williams, R.H., _Textbook of Endocrinology,_ W. B. Saunders, Philadelphia, 1981.

18. Goodman, L.S. and Gilman, A., _The Pharmacological Basis of Therapeutics_, Macmillan, New York, 1980.

19. Engelman, K. and Portnoy, B. A., Sensitive double-isotope derivative assay for norepinephrine and epinephrine: normal resting human plasma levels, _Circulation Research_, 26(1), 53, 1970.

20. Guyton, A.C., _Textbook of Medical Physiology,_ W. B. Saunders, Philadelphia, 1981.

21. Tepperman, J., _Metabolic and Endocrine Physiology_, Yearbook Medical Publishers, Inc., Chicago, 1980.

22. Miller, N.E., What biofeedback does (and does not) do, _Psychology Today_, 23, 22, 1989.

23. Fisher-Williams, M., _A textbook of Biological Feedback_, Human Sciences Press, New York, 1986.

24. Seaward, B., _Managing Stress,_ Jones and Bartlett Publishers, Boston, 1994.

25. Beary, J.F. and Benson, H. A simple psychophysiologic technique which elicits the hypometabolic changes of the relaxation response, _Psychosomatic Medicine,_ 36(5), 115, 1974.

26. Benson, H., Dryer, T., and Hartley, L. H., Decreased VO_2 consumption during exercise with elicitation of the relaxation response, _Journal of Human Stress_, 4(2), 38, 1978.

27. Gervino, E. V., and Veazey, A. E., The physiological effects of Benson's relaxation response during submaximal aerobic exercise, _Journal of Cardiac Rehabilitation_, 4, 254, 1984.

28. Wallace, R.K., Benson, H., and Wilson, A wakeful hypometabolic physiologic state, _American Journal of Physiology,_ 221(3), 795, 1971.

29. Wallace, R.K., Physiological effects of transcendental meditation, _Science_, 167(926), 1751, 1970.

30. Benson, H., _The Relaxation Response,_ William Morrow and Company, Inc., New York, 1975, chap. 4.

31. Bernstein, D. A. and Borkovec, T. D., _Progressive Relaxation Training: A Manual for Helping Professions_, Research Press, Champaign, IL, 1973.

32. Luby, S., _Hatha Yoga for Total Health_, Prentice-Hall, Englewood Cliffs, NJ, 1977.

Appendix 7-A: Log Sheet to Record Relaxation Periods

On a scale of 1 to 10, with 10 being the highest, rate your level of stress before and after the practice of the relaxation response. Many techniques can be used. Briefly describe the technique you used. You may want to journal any insights you gained about yourself from this practice. Also by recording the time, you may notice that mornings or evenings work best for you.

| | 1 | 2 | 3 | 4 | 5 | 6 | 7 | 8 | 9 | 10 | |

low stress (1–2); low-moderate stress (3–4); moderate stress (5–6); high-moderate stress; (7–8) high stress (9–10)

Week 1	Time	Stress Level Before	Technique Used	Stress Level After	Insights
M					
T					
W					
TH					
F					
S					
SU					
Week 2					
M					
T					
W					
TH					
F					
S					
SU					

Appendix 7-B: Breathing Meditation

Why Breathing Meditation?

- The techniques are easy to learn.
- Most breathing exercises can be done anywhere.
- Respiration is directly linked with the autonomic nervous system that controls (speeds up) sympathetic activation and (slows down) parasympathetic activation.

Points to Remember

- Breathing through the nose is preferred rather than breathing though the nose and mouth. The nasal passages warm and filter the air coming in.
- Breathing cycles should be natural and gentle.
- Avoid hyperventilation or artificially deep successive breathing patterns.
- Training in relaxation should never be substituted for medical treatment if needed.

Abdominal Breathing

The Practice

- Find a quiet environment.
- Lie down in a comfortable position.
- Observe the natural rhythm of your breath.
- After a couple of minutes extend your breath, making it a little longer than usual while maintaining the natural rhythm.
- Put one hand just below your rib cage on the solar plexus.
- Focus your attention on this area.
- As you breathe out, notice your hand sinking; the diaphragm is assuming it's natural dome shape, pushing the air out of the lungs.
- Maintain the natural rhythm of your breathing, gently extending your breathing cycle.
- As you inhale, feel your hand rise as the diaphragm flattens out to make room for the expansion of air in your lungs.
- Let your mind follow the path of your breath.
- Be mindful of the sensations of breathing, cool air coming in, warm air going out.
- When distracting thoughts occur, acknowledge them and turn your attention back to your breathing.
- Be mindful of the slowing of your breathing pattern; in a restful state your body doesn't require the oxygen content it did before you began your relaxation period.
- Continue in this deep state of relaxation just a few minutes longer.

Appendix 7-C: Progressive Muscular Relaxation

Why Progressive Muscular Relaxation?
Relaxation follows tensing the muscles.
You will be asked to concentrate on the feelings that accompany the tensing and relaxing of the muscles; you may not have been aware of moments of tension in your body before.

Points to Remember
The contraction of the muscles is carried out all at once, not gradually. Tension is maintained in the muscles for 5–7 seconds.
Relaxation of the muscle follows contraction. The relaxation period is 30–40 seconds. It is important to notice the feelings that accompany the tensing and relaxing of your muscles.
Training in relaxation should never be substituted for medical treatment if needed.

Bernstein and Borkovec's Progressive Muscular Relaxation

The Practice
Sit in a reclining chair or in a chair with a high back and arms.
There are 16 areas of concentration that will be tensed and relaxed.
The procedure is the same for each muscle group.

Procedure
Tense each area of concentration separately, however, follow this same outline.
Tense the concentrated area as tightly as possible, feel the tension, hold the tension for 5–7 seconds, then relax. Notice the sensations you feel in this area when you relax. Feel the relaxation flowing through the surrounding areas in your body. Compare the way this area of your body feels when it is tensed to when it is relaxed. Sequentially tense and relax the following areas of concentrations. You can alter or summarize the areas of selected concentration to fit your needs both physically (individuals with high blood pressure may need to concentrate only on the relaxation phase of the cycle) and mentally (time constraints, etc.).

Areas of Concentration
1. Make a fist with the dominant hand without involving the upper arm.
2. Using the same arm, push your elbow down on the arm of the chair.
3–4. Do the same sequence with the nondominant hand.
5. Raise your eyebrows.
6. Wrinkle your nose and squeeze your eyes shut.
7. Pull back the corners of your mouth and clench your teeth.
8. Pull the chin down and press the head against the back of the chair.
9. Bring the shoulders back.
10. Tighten the abdominal muscles.
11. Contract the thigh and hamstring muscles at the same time.
12. Point the dominant foot down.
13. Pull the dominant foot up.
14. The nondominant leg repeats the same sequence, beginning with the contraction of the thigh and hamstring.

Appendix 7-D: Yoga Sun Salutation Stretch

1. Stand straight-palms together, take a *complete breath* and bring calmness to your mind.
2. *Inhale* and raise both arms over your head, slightly leaning back.
3. *Exhale* and reach out in front and lower your hands to the floor.
4. Bend your knee while sliding your right foot as far back as you can, look up and *inhale*.
5. Slide your left foot back to meet your right foot, retain your breath.
6. *Exhale* as you bring your knees to the floor, bend your elbows and slowly lower your chest to the floor.
7. Keep the lower part of your body on the floor, *inhale* as you look up.
8. Curl your toes under, raise your hips until your arms and legs are straight, *exhale*.
9. Shift your weight to your left foot, bring your right foot forward in line with your hands, *inhale*, look up, and straighten the left knee.
10. Bring your left foot beside the right and *exhale* as you place both hands on the floor beside your feet, ribs and chest towards the thighs.
11. *Inhale,* as you reach out, concaving the spine and bringing your arms up.
12. *Exhale,* as you return to the original starting position. Do not rush. Repeat the round starting with the other foot. Breathe deeply and fully. Do as many times as necessary for a nice warm-up; four times is recommended.

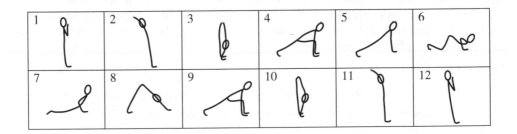

8

Stress Inventories Used in Clinical and Non-Clinical Settings

Robert W. Grant

CONTENTS

8.1 Learning Objectives

After completing this chapter the reader should be able to:

- Identify the desirable psychometric characteristics of stress assessment instruments;
- Understand the underlying stress theory that justifies the use of a particular instrument as a stress assessment device;
- Identify two or three assessment devices that reflect each of three theoretical approaches to understanding stress;
- Compose a brief but comprehensive battery of stress assessment devices to be used in a non-clinical or clinical setting.

8.2   Research Background

The psychological assessment of stress is a complex undertaking, both theoretically and practically. As has been described previously, stress is a multi-dimensional construct, elements of which have been found to reside in the environmental events of life, in the biological reactions to such events, in the strains of interpersonal relationships, and in the multiple psychological symptoms and coping responses made in reaction to the challenges and annoyances we face daily. Stress can be viewed as a truly holistic concept that unites the psyche, the soma, and the social and physical environments. The assessment of stress is as multifaceted as its empirical study.

Due to the complex and, at times, seemingly contradictory nature of theories of stress, a multitude of instruments have been developed or employed in its measurement. Reviewing all of the relevant test instruments would be a monumental task beyond the scope of this chapter. Instead, the intention here will be to familiarize the reader with some of the more popular and practical test instruments that are readily available. Taken together, these assessment devices offer the reader a flexible and effective battery from which to choose for screening individuals who may be at risk for developing, or who may presently be experiencing, an eating disorder. The psychological stress assessment instruments presented here will necessarily reflect the multidimensional nature of this construct.

In selecting stress inventories for use in clinical and non-clinical settings, several criteria should be employed. First, tests should be used only if they have met psychometric standards appropriate for their purposes. In most cases, adequate reliability in terms of internal consistency of items and test-retest stability over time should be demonstrated. Such statistics help insure that a test or scale measures a single variable (or set of specific variables), and that the measurement of that variable will not be affected by temporary or chance conditions that may be operating at a particular time. Test instruments should also have demonstrated evidence of validity; that is, some evidence must be available to support the contention that the test measures what it was designed to measure, and not some related or unrelated variable. Scores obtained with a particular test should correlate significantly and, at least moderately, with other tests known to measure the same or similar constructs. On the other hand, such scores should not correlate with instruments measuring opposite, irrelevant, or common confounding variables such as social desirability or a "yes" response set. Other types of test validity considered might be the predictive accuracy of a test (ability to predict which subjects will later develop physical or psychological pathologies as a result of stress) and discriminant validity (ability to differentiate between subjects falling into various populations, e.g., to differentiate between depressed patients and normal subjects). In addition, reliability and validity data, as well as the norms presented for a test, must have been based on an adequate sampling of the population, both in terms of numbers and characteristics of subjects. This helps insure that, in interpreting an individual's test score, the result is compared to the population to which that person belongs so that inferences of probability can be accurately drawn from the score.

Secondly, tests should be selected based on compatibility with existing theories of stress. The instruments presented here have, in most cases, either been developed by stress theorists and researchers for use in empirical theory validation, or are existing, well-studied tests that have been adopted as stress measures, because the variables they tap represent reasonable definitions of stress. Some of the tests presented, have not been widely used in stress research, but are well-developed instruments that clearly measure constructs related to stress theory. In general, tests that represent measures of stimulus or event-oriented aspects of stress theory, response-oriented theories, and interactional approaches to stress should be selected. In the stimulus or event-oriented category, instruments measuring major life events and minor daily stressors or "hassles" are included. Within the response-oriented category are questionnaires related to physical health factors and psychological symptoms that are likely to represent reactions to stress. Stress measurement devices based on an interactional model of stress include those which assess adaptive coping and other cognitive-perceptual mechanisms, as well as tests measuring aspects of social and interpersonal relations.

It is always helpful, whenever possible, to use stress assessment instruments which are easily obtained and cost effective. Instruments should be appropriate for use with the specific population that is being assessed. Most important in this regard is whether the assessment device is designed for use with adults, adolescents, or children, and whether the persons to be assessed are from a clinical or non-clinical group.

8.2.1   Stimulus-Event Measures

Stimulus-oriented measures of stress are designed from the perspective that stress is an inherent potential within environmental events or occurrences which impact the individual, usually in negative ways. This view of stress is analogous with an engineering conceptualization in which each individual is seen as having an innate capacity to tolerate or cope with environmental pressures.[1] When the environment produces stress in excess of the individual's ability to withstand it, the individual experiences a deterioration in physical or psychological functioning, much as a support beam might buckle and break under an excessive load. Stimulus-oriented stress assessment devices thus focus primarily on the measurement of accumulated external environmental demands such as major life events and daily irritants or "hassles". A variety of studies have shown stimulus-oriented stress measures to be fairly sensitive predictors of stress-related sequelae such as medical and psychological illness.[2–4]

8.2.1.1   *Social Readjustment Rating Scale (SRRS)*

Authors:	Thomas H. Holmes and Richard H. Rahe
Number of Items:	43
Age Range:	Adults
Time:	5 to 10 min
Purpose:	To assess the severity of stress experienced by an individual related to major life events that have occurred within a recent, specified time period.
Availability:	See Reference 5, the social readjustment rating scale by Holmes and Rahe.

Description: The SRRS[5] is a questionnaire designed to assess the occurrence and magnitude of stressful life events experienced by an individual within a recent, specified period of time, and which are likely to increase the person's risk of developing a physical or psychological illness. Stress, for the purposes of the SRRS, is defined in terms of the total amount of life change and readjustment required by the life events the individual has experienced.

The SRRS consists of 43 common events covering both positive and negative life changes. Examples include death of spouse, high mortgage, outstanding personal achievement, and vacation. Each item has an associated scale of impact value, or life change unit (LCU) value. These values were determined by having subjects rate the magnitude of life changes or readjustments that they believed would be experienced if the event actually occurred to them. These ratings were then averaged across subjects, resulting in an average LCU for each item. The SRRS is scored by summing the LCUs or scale of impact values for each item endorsed as having been experienced by the individual. This total score can then be used to evaluate the overall level of event-related stress the person has undergone and to assess the risk for future development of physical or psychological illness.

Scores below 100 are considered very low. Scores between 100 and 199 are labeled low. Scores between 200 and 299 are considered moderate, and those 300 and above are high. Both retrospective and prospective studies by Holmes and Rahe[5] have found that scores in the high range are associated with an 80 percent probability of developing a major illness within the following two years, while moderate and low scores reflect a 50 percent and 30 percent probability of illness, respectively.

More detailed information about the specific areas of life in which stress occurs may be very important in designing and planning interventions. Such information can be gleaned from the SRRS by analyzing scores on various subfactors that have been defined through factor analysis. Masuda and Holmes[6] defined three such factors: personal and social change, loss of loved one, and change in marital status. Based on a sample of 353 adults, Skinner and Lie[7] described six factor-analytically derived subfactors which include: (1) personal and social activities, (2) work changes, (3) marital problems, (4) residence changes, (5) family issues, and (6) school changes.

Psychometrics: Internal consistency reliability for the SRRS has been estimated to be between .72 and .80.[7] This reflects adequate but not superior internal consistency. Test-retest reliability estimates of the SRRS have varied considerably from study to study, but this appears mainly to be due to the length of time between testing. With a one-week test-retest, correlations have ranged between .87 and .90.[8,9] When the test-retest interval is extended to 6 to 12 months, the correlations range between .64 and .74.[9–11] Although sometimes criticized, longer retest interval reliabilities are actually very good, especially considering that the SRRS scores are event-related, and individuals would be expected to experience many different stressors in an intervening 6- to 12-month period.

Multiple studies have found that individuals from groups having various types of physical and psychological problems report a higher incidence of stressful life events than individuals from normal control groups. Such results have been seen with the SRRS in studies of child-abusing parents,[12,13] psychiatric inpatients,[14] and pediatric cancer patients.[15] Holmes and Masuda[16] have summarized several studies showing a positive correlation between SRRS scores and myocardial infarction, fractures, and other health changes. Other investigations have found significant correlations between SRRS scores and surgery for duodenal ulcers,[17] and inpatient treatment for substance abuse.[18] Well-controlled prospective studies have even shown that subjects with higher SRRS scores are more likely to develop cold symptoms than those with low scores, when directly exposed to rhinovirus in a controlled environment.[19,20] Prospective studies have also shown that SRRS scores predict later serious illness and level of health care services utilization.[21]

The content validity of the SRRS appears to be good. The items were developed from the Life Chart of Adolf Meyers[22] which is composed of biological, psychological and social events that relate to the development of illness. There appears to be good concordance among various sociodemographic groups with regard to the perception and ranking of life events comprising the scale.[6] Married individuals between the ages of 25 and 55, however, seem to show the greatest concordance in the perception of and ranking of SRRS items and, therefore, this test may be particularly well suited for that population.

The numbers of subjects and range of populations on which normative and validity data for the SRRS have been collected is very strong. Tennen, Affleck and Herzberger[23] have catalogued over 13 populations studied with the SRRS.

Uses: The SRRS may be used in stress-related research, clinical evaluation and preventive efforts. In individuals who are already known to have eating disorders, the SRRS can be used to identify precipitating stressors and to target life-areas for special interventions, such as grief and loss counseling, relationship skills enhancement, family therapy, general stress management techniques, or assertiveness training. Similar targeting for preventative intervention can also be useful, for individuals who may be assessed as being at risk for future development of an eating disorder.

8.2.1.2   *Life Event Scale – Children (LES-C)*

Author:	R. Dean Coddington
Number of Items:	35
Age Range:	6 to 11
Time:	5 min
Purpose:	To assess the severity of stress experienced by children related to the occurrence of major life events.
Availability:	See Reference 24, *Life Event Scale – Children* by R.D. Coddington.

Description: The LES-C[24] is a children's-age-level, event-related stress inventory similar to the SRRS. It is a 35-item questionnaire comprised of stressful life events, to be completed by the child's parent. The LES-C is printed on a single page, with life change unit weightings alongside each item. To the right of the items are four columns labeled summer, fall, winter, and spring. The instructions tell the parents to write the item weighting into the appropriate column if their child experienced the event in the previous 12 months. A total score is obtained by adding the numbers in each column. The 6-, 9-, and 12-month scores are adjusted for the passage of time. The resultant score is then compared to the 75th percentile score for normative population. Scores above the 75th percentile are considered to represent high levels of stress and a high risk for the development of emotional, behavioral, or medical problems.

Psychometrics: Internal consistency estimates are not given. Interrater reliability for the life change unit ratings of items by professional adults was high (.92).[25] Test-retest reliability was .89 when the retest was given immediately, and .69 and .67 at three- and six-month intervals, respectively.[26] Support for the validity of the LES-C comes primarily in the form of predictive and discriminative studies. Heisel and colleagues[27] found children hospitalized for medical reasons to have high LES-C scores. Children who had behavior problems in the classroom were found by Coddington[26] to have significantly higher LES-C scores than children who did not have behavior problems. High LES-C scores were also found to be as predictive of poor grades as low aptitude scores. The LES-C normative data were based on a sample of 3600 normal elementary school children.[24]

Uses: The uses of the LES-C are basically similar to those for the SRRS. The LES-C has a wide range of applications, including research on stress, screening for risk and prevention, assessment of intervention effectiveness, progress, and outcome. This scale can be used by educators, social workers, psychologists, psychiatrists, and pediatricians, as well as other paraprofessionals. It can provide rapid insight into the stressors in a child's life and can assist in determining a more productive focus for an interview.

8.2.2 Response-Oriented Measures

Response-oriented measures of stress are designed from the perspective that stress is evident in an organism's physical and psychological reactions to the events it experiences. This view was most notably elucidated originally by Walter Cannon[28] and later by Hans Selye[29] in his famous description of the General Adaptation Syndrome (GAS). Psychological aspects of stress response are generally thought of in terms of emotional or behavioral symptoms and excessive, disorganized, or maladaptive reactions to events. Physical stress responses are usually viewed in terms of physical symptoms of disease or distress, as well as in terms of more fundamental physiological measurements, such as heart rate and cortisol levels. Although they have natural and obvious relationships to stress theory and the measurement of stress, most of the assessment devices in the category of response-oriented measurements were developed as clinical and clinical research instruments in the areas of psychopathology and general health assessment. Generally, the psychological response-oriented instruments that have been used to assess stress are psychological symptom inventories and questionnaires addressing mood and affect. Response-oriented measures of physical reactions to stress are primarily health inventories that assess physical symptoms and/or the respondents' perceptions of their levels of well-being in general areas of health. These response-oriented instruments have been used extensively in stress research and have been found to be sensitive to stressful events, stress related to physical illness, the effects of interventions aimed at reducing stress, and the occurrence of physical illness related to stress.[30]

8.2.2.1 Beck Depression Inventory (BDI)

Author:	Aaron Beck
Number of Items:	21
Age Range:	13 to Adult
Time:	5 to 10 min
Purpose:	To measure the presence and degree of depression.
Availability:	The Psychological Corporation Order Service Center P.O. Box 839954 San Antonio, TX 78283-3954

Description: The BDI[31] is a 21-item self-report measure of depression. The items of the BDI were constructed to address specific symptoms and characteristics that are specific to depressed patients. The items are presented in a multiple-choice format, with each item having four choices, each of which is assigned a weight of zero, one, two or three points. The choices are rank ordered and weighted to reflect the range of severity of the symptom assessed by the item. Respondents are asked to select the answers which best reflect how they have felt over the previous week, including on the day they complete the inventories. If more than one choice applies equally to the respondent, he or she is requested to circle each appropriate statement. The score is obtained by summing the highest-ranked choice circled for each item. The following guidelines are given for interpreting individual scores: 0 to 9, normal; 10 to 15, mild depression; 16 to 19, mild to moderate depression; 20 to 29, moderate to severe depression; 30 to 63, severe depression.

Psychometrics: Internal consistency reliability for the BDI has been found to range from .86 to .93.[32] All item-total correlations were significant at the .001 level. Test-retest reliability has been estimated at greater than .90. Changes in the BDI scores over time have been shown to correspond highly with changes in clinicians' ratings of depression among psychiatric patients.[32] The BDI has also demonstrated concurrent validity through highly significant correlations with standard measures of depression, such as the Depression Adjective Checklist and the MMPI Depression Scale. These correlations were .66 and .75 respectively. The subjects utilized in constructing the BDI were two groups of psychiatric outpatients totaling 409 individuals.[32] The first group was comprised of 226 patients and the second of 183 patients.

Uses: The BDI is useful for clinical screening of depressive states, as well as in research where depression is a variable under study. Its ease of administration and simple scoring method make it an excellent tool for assessing change at multiple points in time. The BDI has been used extensively in a variety of settings, including both inpatient and outpatient psychiatric settings, counseling centers, schools, and industrial settings. In the same way, it has become a standard in a variety of research applications. The BDI can be administered and scored by clerical or paraprofessional staff. Interpretation for clinical purposes should be done by a professional with appropriate background and training. For purposes of categorization for research, where specific cutoff scores are utilized, less training is required. Because norms for the BDI were not established on a "normal" population, it may have shortcomings related to interpretation of the meanings of scores when applied to nonclinical populations.

8.2.2.2 Reynolds Child Depression Scale (RCDS) and Reynolds Adolescent Depression Scale (RADS)

Author:	William M. Reynolds
Number of Items:	30
Age Range:	8 to 12 for RCDS, 12 to 18 for RADS
Time:	10 min
Purpose:	To provide a measure of self-reported symptoms of depression in children and adolescents by way of group or individual assessment.
Availability:	Psychological Assessment Resources, Inc. P.O. Box 998 Odessa, FL 33556

Description: The RCDS and RADS[33,34] are reviewed together because they were devised by the same person and are very similar in construction. The RCDS and RADS are self-report inventories comprised of 30 Likert-type items, which are rated on a 4-point scale as occurring almost never, sometimes, a lot of the time, or all the time. Items are rated according to how often the respondent has experienced the symptom or feeling over the previous 2 weeks. Item content reflects DSM-III and DSM-III-R[35] criteria for major depression and dysthymic disorder, and evaluates the affective, cognitive, behavioral, and physical components of depression. Both the RCDS and RADS come with answer sheets that can be scored manually and scoring keys. Mail-in scoring and computerized scoring software are also available from the publisher. These scales may be administered in groups or individually. Items can be read and answered by the respondents, or items presented orally in cases where reading is problematic. The RCDS and RADS are quick and easy to administer and score. The manual provides percentile ranks and cutoff scores for interpretation of the results. Six items are considered critical and individuals endorsing four or more of these items, regardless of their total scores, should be given more thorough assessments.

Psychometrics: Internal consistency reliability for the Reynolds depression scales is quite good. Coefficient alphas for the RCDS are reported to range from .88 to .90[36], while internal consistency coefficients for the RADS have been between .92 and .96[34]. Test-retest reliability is also very good. Correlation of scores on the RCDS over a 3$^1/_2$ to 4$^1/_2$-week interval was found to be .85, with reliabilities for various demographic groups ranging from .72 to .92. Stability for the RADS for a 6-week interval was found to be .84.

Content validity of the RCDS and RADS is demonstrated by the similarity of items to DSM-III and DSM-III-R diagnostic criteria for major depression and dysthymia. Criterion-related validity for the Reynolds scales has been supported by significant correlations with depression ratings obtained through structured clinical interviews.[33,34] These correlations were .76 for the RCDS and .83 for the RADS. Correlations of the RCDS with another well-established measure of depression, the Children's Depression Inventory, have been used to support its construct validity. A regression analysis was conducted using the RADS and the BDI as independent variables and the Hamilton Clinical Rating Scale interview scores as the dependent variable. This analysis resulted in a beta of .55 between the RADS and the Hamilton, and a beta of .31 between the BDI and the Hamilton. This indicates more shared variance between the RADS and Hamilton and, therefore, would support the construct validity of the RADS.

The RCDS was normed on a sample of 1620 normal children from the midwestern and western states of the United States.[33] Although the sample was not matched demographically to the census, minorities and divergent socioeconomic groups were relatively well represented. The RADS was normed on a sample of over 8000 adolescents across the country.[34] A three-way analysis of variance of RADS data using grade, sex, and race as independent variables found that RADS scores varied by grade and sex, but not by race. Although not perfect, the normative samples for the RCDS and RADS can be considered quite adequate.

Uses: The RCDS and RADS can be used in clinics, agencies, schools, or hospitals where children or adolescents receive instruction or services. These scales can be used in clinical research exploring treatment efficacy and in investigations aimed at understanding depression and its relationship to other variables, such as stress and eating disorders. The RCDS and RADS appear to be excellent screening instruments for identifying depressed individuals for research or intervention purposes. Although not designed to be diagnostic, the provision of cutoff scores assists in identifying clinically significant levels of depressive symptoms. The RCDS and RADS may also be used to track clinical progress and outcome.

The RCDS and RADS may be administered and scored by nonprofessional staff with minimal training. However, interpretation of RCDS and RADS results should be carried out by those who have adequate knowledge of childhood development, psychopathology, and diagnosis, as well as general psychological testing and interpretation.

8.2.2.3 Symptom Checklist 90 – Revised (SCL-90-R)

Author:	Leonard R. Derogatis
Number of Items:	90
Age Range:	13 through Adult
Time:	15 min
Purpose:	To provide a multidimensional symptom inventory of psychological distress.
Availability:	NCS Assessments
	P.O. Box 1416
	Minneapolis, MN 55440

Description: The SCL-90-R[37] is a 90-item self-report inventory designed to assess psychological symptoms and distress across nine primary dimensions. The items consist of simple statements of symptoms that are rated on a five-point scale (0 to 4), ranging from "not at all" to "extremely." The nine symptom scales of the SCL-90-R are somatization (SOM), obsessive-compulsive (OBS), interpersonal sensitivity (INT), depression (DEP), anxiety (ANX), hostility (HOS), phobic anxiety (PHOB), paranoid ideation (PAR), and psychoticism (PSY). There are also three global indexes derived from the SCL-90-R; the general severity index (GSI), which is a composite score of both number and severity of symptoms; the positive symptom total (PST), which reflects the total number of symptoms; and the positive symptom distress index (PSDI), which is a measure of the intensity of symptoms adjusted for the number of symptoms endorsed.

The SCL-90-R primary scales are scored by summing the ratings for each scale, and then dividing the achieved sums by the number of items answered on that scale. These averaged scale scores are then transformed into T-scores using tables provided in the manual. The manual is extensive and provides a great deal of background and technical information on the SCL-90-R. The SCL-90-R is widely used in both research and clinical settings where assessment of distress and patterns of psychological symptomatology are important.

Psychometrics: Internal consistency and test-retest stability for the SCL-90-R are excellent. Internal consistency reliability was calculated from the responses of 219 symptomatic volunteers using coefficient alpha.[38] For the nine primary scales, reliabilities ranged from a low of .77 for the PSY scale to .90 for the DEP scale. All the internal consistency reliability estimates were .80 or above except for PSY. One week test-retest reliabilities for the primary scales ranged from .78 to .90 for a group of 94 heterogeneous psychiatric outpatients.

Factor analytic studies have confirmed the scale structure of the SCL-90-R. Derogatis and his colleagues[38] also demonstrated convergent validity by showing that the SCL-90-R primary scales correlated most highly with the corresponding scale of the MMPI. Derogatis[37] presents a multitude of studies with the SCL-90-R supporting the convergent validity of the DEP scale in particular, and the ability of this scale to measure change related to psychotherapeutic and psychopharmacologic intervention. Specifically for stress and stress-related medical conditions, the SCL-90-R has proven to be a sensitive instrument. Derogatis, Lobo, Folstein, and Abeloff[39] have shown the SCL-90-R to be capable of differentiating cancer patients in need of psychiatric intervention from those not requiring such intervention. Carrington and colleagues[40] have shown the SCL-90 to be sensitive to positive changes related to meditation and biofeedback interventions. Several other studies have indicated the SCL-90-R to be sensitive to, and useful in, assessing a host of stress related conditions such as tension headache,[41] chronic pain,[42] and sleep disturbance.[43] Also, Kilpatrick, Vernon, and Resick[44] showed systematic alterations in the SCL-90-R profiles of rape victims over a six-month period that clearly differentiated them from non-victims.

The norms for the SCL-90-R are presented in the manual for four large samples, including 974 normal adults, 806 normal adolescents, 1002 heterogeneous psychiatric outpatients, and 310 psychiatric inpatients.[37] The normative sample is further described in the manual with regard to breakdowns in sex, race, marital status, socio-economic status, and religion. Percentages making up each normative cohort are presented for all demographic groups. Means and standard deviations for all scales are also presented for each normative sample. In addition, tables are included for transforming raw scores to T scores for each of the normative samples.

Uses: The SCL-90-R should be considered a good tool for clinical and research applications. Its construction, research base, and normative data make it useful for a broad range of psychiatric and medical populations, as well as with normal populations, when used as a screening instrument or for research purposes.

The SCL-90-R has been used extensively in validating other assessment devices. It can be useful in defining inclusion or exclusion criteria for experimental groups, or to test hypotheses about the relationship of other variables to any of its scale-based constructs.

As a clinical instrument it is ideal for screening purposes, due to its brevity and multidimensional assessment capability. It can be useful in assisting with diagnosis and also, because of its demonstrated sensitivity to change and reactivity to stress, it is a very good instrument for tracking clinical improvement, studying the effects of stress, or monitoring the results of interventions. An additional advantage of the SCL-90-R is that it is one of the few instruments that defines a specific profile for females with anorexia.

8.2.3   Interactional Measures

Interactional theories of stress suggest that stress is best conceptualized in terms of mechanisms or processes within the individual that mediate between environmental events and physical, psychological, and behavioral responses. This view proposes that stress is a result of the interactions among cognitive, perceptual, emotional, and behavioral functions of the individual and the particular configuration or characteristics of the external environment. Such functions are often referred to as coping skills, defense mechanisms, adaptation mechanisms, attributions, belief systems, attitudes, and personality traits. Patterns or habits of interpersonal behavior may also be viewed as interactional processes important to the understanding of stress. How a person perceives and behaves in relation to demands, expectations, conflicts, or need for support from others can be crucial factors, either alone or in conjunction with other stressful events, in the development of stress-related symptoms or illness. Interactional theories, therefore, view measurement only of stressful events, physical symptoms, or emotional responses as inadequate and overly simplistic. Interactive theories of stress have successfully shed light on reactions to general and common environmental stressors,[45] illness,[46] and victimization.[47]

8.2.3.1 Coping Resource Inventory (CRI)

Author:	Allen L. Hammer and M. Susan Marting
Number of Items:	60
Age Range:	14 to Adult
Time:	15 min
Purpose:	To assess personal resources available for coping with stress.
Availability:	Consulting Psychologists Press, Inc. 3803 East Bayshore Road P.O. Box 10096 Palo Alto, CA 94303

Description: The CRI[48] is a 60-item self-report inventory designed to measure coping resources in five domains: Cognitive (COG), Social (SOC), Emotional (EMO), Spiritual/ Philosophical (S/P) and Physical (PHY). These domains are represented by five different corresponding scales, which, when summed, result in a Total Resource Score (TOT).

The coping resources measured by the CRI are differentiated from coping strategies measured by other coping skills assessment inventories. Coping resources are conceptualized as internal characteristics that facilitate coping and become active when a person faces a stressful circumstance. These coping resources allow the individual to deal with stress more adaptively and effectively, experience fewer stress-related symptoms, and recover from stress more quickly.

The COG scale of the CRI measures the degree to which the individual maintains a positive self-concept and optimism about life. The SOC scale reflects the amount of social support the individual has available. EMO relates to the level of acceptance and freedom of expression of emotions. The S/P scale assesses the degree to which personal philosophies, religious, family, and cultural values guide the individual. The PHY scale measures how frequently the respondent engages in health-promoting behavior.

The CRI is scored easily by summing the item ratings (1 to 4) for each scale. The inventories can be hand scored with a template or mailed to the publisher for computer scoring. Raw scores are transformed into T-scores using tables in the manual. Separate tables are provided for males and females. T-scores can be plotted on profile sheets to visually examine the respondent's strengths and weaknesses, as compared to his or her individual responses and to the normative sample. Information regarding interpreting results is also provided in the manual.

Psychometrics: Reliability estimates were derived from a heterogeneous sample of 749 subjects.[48] Median item-scale correlations ranged from .37 for PHY to .46 for COG and EMO. Internal consistency measured by Cronbach's alpha ranged from .72 for PHY to .84 for EMO. The internal consistency reliability for the total resource score was .91. Test-retest reliabilities over a 6-week period ranged from .60 for S/P to .78 for SOC. Overall, the CRI demonstrates adequate but not strong reliability.

Predictive validity for the CRI was demonstrated in a regression analysis in which the CRI added significant incremental variance over that contributed by measures of stressful events in predicting the presence of significant symptoms of stress.[48] In other studies, CRI scores differentiated four clinical groups (physically ill college students, college counseling center clients, adult cardiac and pulmonary patients, and adult stress center clients) from two normal control groups (college resident advisors and high school peer counselors). The CRI does not correlate with the Marlowe-Crown Social Desirability Scale, but has shown significant correlations with related scales of the Myers-Briggs Type Indicator, thus evidencing some concurrent and divergent validity.[48] Normative data for the CRI is based on a heterogeneous sample of 843 individuals.[48] Norms are not corrected for age or education. No attempt was made to provide a census-matched normative sample.

Uses: The CRI is an interesting instrument that is adequate for use in a wide range of practical and research-oriented applications. The CRI is well-suited for research aimed at studying coping resources among various clinical and nonclinical populations, and for research directed toward clarifying relationships between stress-related variables and illness. The CRI can be tentatively used as a tool for targeting treatment interventions or to screen for at-risk individuals. Care should be taken not to place complete confidence in the normative sample and data, due to their size and incompleteness.

8.2.3.2   *Common Belief Inventory for Students (CBIS)*

Authors:	Stephen R. Hooper and C. Clinton Layne
Number of Items:	44
Age Range:	9 to 13
Time:	10 to 15 min
Purpose:	To measure irrational beliefs in children.
Availability:	Stephen R. Hooper, Ph.D.
	Department of Psychology
	Bradley Hospital
	1011 Veterans Memorial Parkway
	East Providence, RI 02915

Description: The CBIS[49] is a 44-item self-report inventory for children, designed to evaluate irrational beliefs based on Albert Ellis' 11 core irrational beliefs. These irrational beliefs are, according to Ellis, held strongly by individuals with various emotional, behavioral, or neurotic difficulties, and are the sources of these individuals' problems. These beliefs are (1) one must be loved by everyone; (2) one must be thoroughly competent; (3) certain people are wicked or evil and warrant punishment; (4) it is horrible and catastrophic when things don't go your way; (5) human happiness is determined by external events and is not under anyone's control; (6) if something is dangerous or fearsome, one should be concerned about it; (7) it is easier to avoid than to face life's difficulties; (8) one should be dependent on others; (9) past history determines one's present behavior; (10) one should become upset about others' problems and disturbances; and (11) there are perfect solutions to human problems, and it is catastrophic if solutions are not found.

Each of these 11 beliefs are represented by four items on the CBIS. Each item is rated by the respondent on a five-point scale (0 to 4) representing the percentage of time the person has held that belief. The ratings for the four items related to each belief can be summed to get a score for that belief. All items can be scored to obtain a total score. The higher the score, the more strongly held the belief and the more irrational the thinking.

Psychometrics: The CBIS demonstrates very good internal consistency.[49] An alpha coefficient of .985 was obtained for the total scale, and split-half reliability was .88.

Test-retest correlations of .84 over a 6-week interval were obtained, indicating very good reliability in terms of stability over time.

Convergent validity has been shown for the CBIS through significant and moderate correlations with a measure of childhood trait anxiety. In two different studies,[49] CBIS scores have been found to change in correspondence to clinical improvements brought about by rational emotive therapy.

The CBIS has been developed from three groups of boys and girls in fourth through seventh grades totaling over 8000.[49] The representativeness of the samples is not described. Means and standard deviations for the total score and 11 beliefs, as well as reliability data, have been presented for a sample of 1226 fourth through seventh graders.

Uses: The CBIS is a promising assessment instrument. It may be useful in researching the relationship of cognition to stress and psychopathology, as well as to adaptation and adjustment to medical illness. The CBIS may also be employed in clinical research related to treatment outcome and therapeutic change. Although no cutoff scores are provided, it can be used as a screening instrument to identify children with emotional problems or at risk for developing them. The generally accepted rule is to use a score one-and-one-half to two standard deviations above the mean as a cutoff. The CBIS can be used clinically to target cognitive intervention and as a measure of treatment efficacy. Until more data are forthcoming regarding the reliability and validity of the 11 irrational belief facets, and also the factor structure of the entire scale, total scores should be utilized for most purposes, with the possible exception of using the CBIS in specifying cognitive interventions. As with many of the instruments reviewed here, the CBIS can be administered and scored by trained technical or paraprofessional staff, but should be interpreted only by an experienced clinician.

References

1. Cox, T., *Stress*, Baltimore, University Park, MD, 1978.
2. Rahe, R.H., Life change measurement as a predictor of illness, *Proceedings of the Royal Society of Medicine*, 61, 1124, 1968.
3. Rahe, R.H. and Lind, E., Psychosocial factors and sudden cardiac death: a pilot study, *Journal of Psychosomatic Research*, 15, 19, 1971.
4. Edwards, M.K., Life Crises and Myocardial Infarction. Unpublished master's thesis, University of Washington, Seattle, 1971.
5. Holmes, T.H. and Rahe, R.H., The social readjustment rating scale. *Journal of Psychosomatic Research*, 11, 213, 1967.
6. Masuda, M. and Holmes, T.H., Life events: perceptions and frequencies, *Psychosomatic Medicine*, 40, 236, 1978.
7. Skinner, H.A. and Lei, H., Differential weights in life change research: useful or irrelevant? *Psychosomatic Medicine*, 42, 367, 1980.
8. Hawkins, N.G., Evidence of psychosocial factors in the development of pulmonary tuberculosis, *American Review of Tubercular and Pulmonary Disease*, 75, 768, 1957.
9. Rahe, R.H., Foistad, R.L., and Beergan, C. A model for life changes and illness research: cross-cultural data from the Norwegian navy. *Archives of General Psychiatry*, 31, 172, 1974.
10. Casey, R.L., Masuda, M., and Holmes, T.H., Quantitative study of recall of life events, *Journal of Psychosomatic Research*, 11, 239, 1967.
11. Rahe, R.H., Recent life change stress and psychological depression, in *Stressful Life Events*, T.W. Miller, ed., International Universities Press Inc., Madison, CT, 1989.
12. Conger, R.D., Burgess, R.L., and Barrett, C., Child abuse related to life change and perception of illness: some preliminary findings, *Family Coordinator*, 28, 73, 1979.

13. Justice, B. and Justice, R., Clinical approaches to family violence. I. Etiology of physical abuse of children and dynamics of coercive treatment, *Family Therapy Collections*, 3, 1, 1982.

14. Schless, A.P., Teichman, A., Mendels, J., and Digiacomo, J.N., The role of stress as a precipitating factor of psychiatric illness, *British Journal of Psychiatry*, 130, 19, 1977.

15. Jacobs, T.J. and Charles, E., Life events and the occurrence of cancer in children, *Psychosomatic Medicine*, 42, 11, 1980.

16. Holmes, T.H. and Masuda, M., Life change and illness susceptibility, *Stressful Life Events and Their Consequences*, B.S. Horenwend and B.P. Dohrenwend, Eds., Rutgers University Press, New Brunswick, NJ, 1974.

17. Stevenson, D.K., Nasbeth, D.C., Masuda, M., and Holmes, T.H., Life change and the postoperative course of duodenal ulcer patients, *Journal of Human Stress*, 5, 19, 1979.

18. Dudley, D.L., Roszell, D.K., Mules, J.E., and Haque, W.H., Heroin vs. alcohol addiction: quantifiable psychological similarities and differences, *Journal of Psychosomatic Research*, 18, 327, 1974.

19. Cohen, S., Tyrell, D.A.J., and Smith, A.P., Psychological stress and susceptibility to the common cold, *New England Journal of Medicine*, 325, 606, 1991.

20. Totman, R., Kiff, J., Reed, S.E., and Craig, J.W., Predicting experimental colds in volunteers from different measures of recent life stress, *Journal of Psychosomatic Research*, 24, 155, 1980.

21. Garrity, T.F., Marks, M.B., and Somes, G.W., The influence of illness severity and time since life change on the size of the life change – health change relationship, *Journal of Psychosomatic Research*, 21, 377, 1977.

22. Meyers, A., The life chart and the obligation of specifying positive data in psychopathological diagnosis, in *Contributions to Medical and Biological Research*, Vol. III, Paul B. Hoeber, New York, 1919.

23. Tennen, H., Affeck, G., and Herzberger, S., Schedule of recent experience, in *Test Criteria*, Vol. I, Keyser, D.J. and Sweetland, R.C., Test Corporation of America, Kansas City, MO, 1983.

24. Coddington, R.D., *Life Event Scale – Children*, Stress Research Company, St. Clairsville, OH, 1981.

25. Coddington, R.D., The significance of life events as etiologic factors in the diseases of children I: a survey of professional workers, *Journal of Psychosomatic Research*, 16, 205, 1972.

26. Coddington, R.D., Measuring the stressfulness of a child's environment, in *Stress in Children*, Humphrey, J.H., ed., AMS Press, New York, 1984.

27. Heisel, J.S., Ream, S., Raitz, R., Rappaport, M., and Coddington, R.D., The significance of life events as contributing factors in the diseases of children III: a study of pediatric patients, *Journal of Pediatrics*, 83, 119, 1973.

28. Cannon, W.B., *The Wisdom of the Body*, Norton, New York, 1932.

29. Selye, H., *The Physiology and Pathology of Exposure to Stress*, Acta, Montreal, 1950.

30. Spielberger, C.D., *Manual for the State-Trait Anxiety Inventory*, Consulting Psychologists Press, Inc., Palo Alto, CA, 1983.

31. Beck, A.T., Ward, C.H., Mendelson, M., Mock, J., and Erbaugh, J., An inventory for measuring depression, *Archives of General Psychiatry*, 4, 561, 1961.

32. Beck, A.T., *Depression: Causes and Treatment*, University of Pennsylvania Press, Philadelphia, 1970.

33. Reynold, W.M., *Reynolds Child Depression Scale (RCDS) Professional Manual*, Psychological Assessment Resources, Inc., 1986.

34. Reynolds, W.M., *Reynolds Adolescent Depression Scale (RADS) Professional Manual*, Psychological Assessment Resources, Inc., 1986.

35. Task Force on DSM-III, *Diagnostic and Statistical Manual of Mental Disorders, Third Edition, Revised*, American Psychiatric Association, 1987.

36. Reynolds, W.M. and Graves, A. Reliability of children's reports of depressive symptomatology. *Journal of Abnormal Child Psychology*, 17, 647, 1989.

37. Derogatis, L.R., *SCL-90-R Administration, Scoring, and Procedures Manual-II*, Clinical Psychometric Research, Towson, MD, 1983.
38. Derogatis, L.R., Rickels, K., and Rock, A., The SCL-90 and the MMPI: a step in the validation of a new self-report scale, *British Journal of Psychiatry*, 128, 280, 1976.
39. Derogatis, L.R., Lobo, A., Folstein, M., and Abeloff, M.D., The SCL-90-R as a psychiatric screening instrument in an oncologic population, *Psychosomatic Medicine*, 46, 53, 1983.
40. Carrington, P., Collings, G.H., Benson, H., Robinson, H., Wood, L.W., Lehrer, P.M., Woolfolk, R.L., and Cole, J., The uses of mediation-relaxation techniques for the management of stress in a working population, *Journal of Occupational Medicine*, 22, 221, 1980.
41. Harper, R.G. and Steger, J.C., Psychological correlates of frontalis EMG and pain in tension headaches, *Headache Journal*, 18, 215, 1978.
42. Pelz, M. and Merskey, H., A description of psychological effects of chronic painful lesions, *Pain*, 14, 293, 1982.
43. Kales, J.D., Kales, A., Soldatos, C.R., Caldwell, A.B., Charney, D.S., and Martin, E., Night terrors: clinical characteristics and personality patterns, *Archives of General Psychiatry*, 37, 1413, 1980.
44. Kilpatrick, D.G., Veronen, L.J., and Resick, P.A., The aftermath of rape: recent empirical findings, *American Journal of Orthopsychiatry*, 49, 658, 1979.
45. Lazarus, R.S. and Folkman, S. *Stress, Appraisal, and Coping*, Springer, New York, 1984.
46. Taylor, S.E., Lichtman, R.R., and Wood, J.V., Attributions, beliefs about control, and adjustment to breast cancer, *Journal of Personality and Social Psychology*, 46, 489, 1984.
47. Taylor, S.E., Wood, J.V., and Lichtman, R.R., It could be worse: selective evaluation as a response to victimization, *Journal of Social Issues*, 39, 19, 1983.
48. Hammer, A.L. and Marting, M.S., *Manual for the Coping Resources Inventory*, Consulting Psychologists Press, Palo Alto, CA, 1988.
49. Hooper, S.R. and Layne, C.C., The Common Belief Inventory for Students: a measure of rationality in children, *Journal of Personality Assessment*, 47, 85, 1983.

Part III

Society and Eating Disorders

9

Family Dynamics

James R. Clopton, Heather L. Haas, and Jan S. Kent

CONTENTS

9.1 Learning Objectives

After completing this chapter you should be able to:

- Identify family characteristics thought to be of clinical significance in contributing to eating disorders;
- Recognize which family variables have been empirically shown to be related to eating disorders, and which variables have been shown to be unrelated;

- Understand the importance of various family characteristics and how they influence the development, maintenance, and treatment of eating disorders;
- Utilize family involvement for the most effective treatment of eating disorders.

9.2   Research Background

The importance of the family's role in eating disorders has been stressed in theoretical and clinical reports for many years. Influential family models were developed by Salvador Minuchin and by Hilde Bruch, clinicians working with young women with anorexia nervosa. Minuchin and his colleagues described five common characteristics found in the families of children with psychosomatic illness (anorexia, diabetes, and asthma): (a) enmeshment, an intense over-involvement among family members that limits the privacy and autonomy of one another; (b) over-protectiveness, a hypersensitivity to distress among family members that leads to excessive nurturing; (c) rigidity, an extreme emphasis on maintaining the status quo, which produces difficulty when changes are needed in the family (e.g., when a child becomes an adolescent); (d) lack of conflict resolution, due either to an avoidance of problems or ineffective ways in dealing with problems; and (e) involvement of a child in the conflicts between parents, with the parents either seeking to have the child take sides, or the avoidance of conflict by focusing on caring for a sick child.[1,2] Working with the entire family to change these five characteristics led to more effective treatment for anorexia nervosa.[3,4]

Bruch's description of the families of young women with anorexia is similar to Minuchin's, especially with respect to the enmeshment that is emphasized in both models.[5,6] In addition to enmeshment, the families of young women with anorexia are described by Bruch as placing inordinate emphasis on appearance, good behavior, and achievement; allowing little expression of feelings, especially negative feelings; and exercising excessive parental control. The family seeks to present itself to others as the picture of normality and happiness when, in reality, much dissatisfaction and disappointment exists. The self-starvation of the young woman makes her special, and allows her to control at least one area of her life, and resist the demands of her parents. From this family description, Bruch concluded that effective treatment should include both individual and family sessions aimed at helping the young woman with anorexia to develop self-confidence and an independent identity.

During the last 20 years, researchers have studied the families of women with eating disorders to determine whether those families do indeed differ in important ways from others. This review of the research literature, which will follow the format of Kog and Vandereycken,[7] will examine three categories of family variables that have been studied extensively: (a) demographic characteristics (social class, birth order, and parental divorce); (b) individual problems in the family (weight and eating problems, mental disorders, physical illness, and sexual abuse and assault); and (c) family relationships (family interaction characteristics as reported by family members or observed by others).

9.2.1   Demographic Characteristics

9.2.1.1   Social Class

Clinical studies have described a higher incidence of anorexia nervosa in upper socio-economic classes.[5,6] One research study found that, compared to patients with other health problems, patients with anorexia nervosa were more likely to come from families with a higher socioeconomic status,[8] and another research study found that patients with bulimia come from families with higher income levels than patients with anorexia.[9] However, several other studies have not made the same correlation.[10–12] For example, one study did not find significant differences in socioeconomic status among young women with bulimia, those with a subclinical-level of symptoms, and those who did not have symptoms of an eating disorder.[13] However, nearly all research participants in that study were from families in the top two levels of Hollingshead's Four-Factor Index of Social Status,[14] and that small range made it difficult to detect group differences in socioeconomic status.

9.2.1.2 *Birth Order*

Clinical reports have hypothesized that young women with eating disorders are likely to be firstborn or lastborn children and are more likely to have sisters than brothers.[5] However, research studies do not support these hypotheses.[15] No significant differences in birth order have been found when women with bulimia have been compared to women who do not have eating disorders,[13,16,17] when women with the restricting type of anorexia have been compared to women with the binge-eating/purging type of anorexia,[18,19] or when normal-weight women with bulimia are compared to women with anorexia.[9] Also no consistent evidence shows that women with eating disorders are more likely to have sisters than brothers.[16] Neither birth order nor the presence of sisters in the family has been found to have any relationship to the success of treatment for anorexia.[20,21]

9.2.1.3 *Incidence of Parental Divorce*

Some evidence in earlier studies suggests that the parents of patients with eating disorders had a lower incidence of divorce than the general population.[22,23] However, a more recent study did not find any differences in parents' marital status when women with bulimia or subclinical bulimia were compared to women who did not exhibit symptoms of eating disorders.[13]

9.2.2 Individual Pathology within the Family

9.2.2.1 *Weight and Eating Problems*

A few studies have examined the possibility of more than one child in a family having an eating disorder. One special way this issue has been studied is by comparing the concordance rates for monozygotic and dizygotic pairs of twins. One study found that the concordance rate for anorexia was much higher for monozygotic twins than for dizygotic twins (68% versus 8%), but the concordance rates for bulimia were similar for monozygotic and dizygotic twins (35% versus 29%).[24] These results suggest that genetic factors play a substantial role in anorexia, but not in bulimia. However, that conclusion has not been confirmed by other studies,[25–27] and as Vandereycken and Van Vreckem have noted,[15] each pairs of twins studied so far has come from the same home. Conclusions about the relative importance of genetic predisposition and family environment in the development of eating disorders must await adoptee studies.

Women with symptoms of bulimia are significantly more likely than asymptomatic women to report problems related to weight and eating among the members of their families.[13] Similarly, the mothers of adolescent girls with a high level of bulimic symptoms are more likely to report that they have symptoms of eating disorders than the mothers of adolescent girls with low levels of symptoms.[28]

9.2.2.2   Mental Disorders

To identify mental disorders in the family members of individuals with eating disorders, researchers have given psychological tests to their parents and have also used more direct methods of identifying mental disorders among family members, such as diagnostic interviews. Psychological test data reveals little evidence of significant psychopathology in the parents of patients with anorexia nervosa.[29,30]

   Much research has been conducted on the incidence of depression and substance abuse in the families of individuals with eating disorders. The first-degree relatives of these patients have been found to have a significantly higher incidence of depression than members of normal or clinical comparison groups.[31–36] A history of substance abuse has often been found in families of individuals with eating disorders.[31,37,38] One study found that women patients with bulimia more often reported both personal and familial substance abuse than women patients with anorexia, obesity, or depression.[39] By contrast, another study found that the first-degree relatives of women with bulimia did not score significantly higher on the Michigan Alcoholism Screening Test than did the first-degree relatives of women without eating disorders.[32] A study that included data from interviews with over 2000 women challenged the notion that there is a strong correlation in families between the occurrence of alcohol dependence and eating disorders.[40] The weak relationship between alcohol dependence and eating disorders occurred mostly when some other mental disorder was also present.

9.2.2.3   Physical Illness

The research evidence concerning the likelihood of physical illness among the families of individuals with eating disorders is inconsistent. A few studies have concluded that a higher rate of physical illness may be found in the families of individuals with bulimia or the binge-eating/purging type of anorexia.[9,41] However, the only study to compare bulimic and symptom-free individuals found no evidence of increased physical illness in the families of the individuals with bulimia.[17]

9.2.2.4   Sexual Abuse and Assault

Research studies have produced contradictory evidence about the relationship between sexual abuse and eating disorders. A recent study compared two large samples of adolescent women, those with a history of sexual abuse, and those who had not been abused. The women who had been abused were more likely to experience several adverse outcomes, including showing symptoms of eating disorders.[42] Living with both biological parents decreased the likelihood of adverse outcomes among abused women, but recent stress in the family increased such a likelihood. Other studies have revealed that sexually abused young women are at a greater risk of developing an eating disorder or other mental disorder.[43,44] Also, women who have been sexually assaulted by family members are more likely to have symptoms of an eating disorder than women who were either sexually assaulted by someone outside the family or were not assaulted at all.[45]

   In contrast to those studies that found a relationship between sexual abuse and eating disorders, some studies have discovered no relationship between childhood sexual abuse and the development of eating disorders later in life.[46,47] One study did not find an overall association between reported sexual abuse and symptoms of bulimia, but among women who reported a history of sexual abuse, binging and vomiting were more frequent for those who had been sexually abused by a family member.[48] Another study conducted at an Austrian university found that although severe physical abuse and an adverse family background increased the likelihood that male students would report symptoms of eating disorders, there was no significant relationship between childhood sexual abuse and symptoms of eating disorders.[49]

Studies conducted in nonclinical settings are especially likely to find no relationship between eating disorders and a history of incest or childhood sexual abuse. However, psychotherapy clients who reported a history of incest were found in one study to be more likely to have attitudes associated with eating disorders.[50] Those attitudes were most likely to be found among the incest survivors exhibiting the poorest social competence and the weakest maternal bonds.

9.2.3   Family Relationships

Numerous controlled studies have been conducted to explore the family relationships of individuals with eating disorders. The focus here will be on the families of individuals with anorexia or bulimia, and the studies for each disorder will be divided into separate sections for internal perceptions (family interaction characteristics as described by a family member, most often the person with the eating disorder) and external observations (family interaction characteristics as described by someone outside the family).

9.2.3.1   *Anorexic Families*

9.2.3.1.1   *Internal Perceptions*

Studies have discovered numerous differences in the perceptions of the families of individuals with anorexia and those of symptom-free individuals. Although the findings are somewhat contradictory, one fairly consistent finding has been the presence of difficulties in the relationships between individuals with anorexia and their mothers, whereas the relationships with their fathers are less likely to be perceived as problematic.[30,51,52] By contrast, one study in which adolescent girls with restricting anorexia and their parents rated their relationships with one another found little evidence of problems in the parent-child relationship but clear evidence of severe marital distress between the parents.[53]

Some research evidence points to the enmeshment and over-protectiveness described by Minuchin as characteristic of families of individuals with anorexia.[51] For example, one study found that the parents of young women with anorexia reported attitudes among family members so undifferentiated as to suggest enmeshment. The parents reported no differences in the attitudes that their respective spouses and their daughters had toward them, and no differences in their own attitudes toward their daughters and spouses.[54] These patterns of nearly identical cross-generational attitudes were not found among the families of symptom-free young women.

9.2.3.1.2   *External Observations*

Researchers who have observed the relationship patterns in the families of individuals with anorexia have reported some common characteristics. The family relationships are enmeshed and overprotective and there appears to be no clear leader within the nuclear family unit.[2,12,55,56] An observational study of relationships in the families of adolescent daughters with the binge-eating/purging type of anorexia and in families whose members did not exhibit any mental disorders found some dramatic differences.[57] Compared to the normal families, the families who had daughters with eating disorders were more likely to be rated as having more conflict (belittling and ignoring) and less mutual support (helping and nurturing). Communications within the families of individuals with eating disorders were also rated as more complex, confusing, and contradictory, especially with respect to the daughters' development of autonomy.

9.2.3.2 Bulimic Families

9.2.3.2.1 Internal Perceptions

Compared to women who do not have eating disorders, women who are in treatment for bulimia have repeatedly been found to report poor family adjustments. Specifically, they have reported more problems with their parents, more conflict, hostility, and over-protectiveness, and less caring, cohesion, and expressiveness.[52,58–66]

Two important cautions need to be made about the perceptions that women with bulimia hold about their families. First, the dramatic differences between the perceptions of women with bulimia and the perceptions of normal women have sometimes tempted researchers to conclude that those differences indicate unique etiological significance for bulimia.[66,67] However, when the perceptions of general psychiatric patients are compared to those of individuals without mental disorders, a similar set of differences has been found, with more conflict and less expressiveness and cohesion.[68] Patients with anxiety disorders and patients with bulimia have described similar levels of dysfunction in their families of origin.[69] In another study, when levels of depressed moods were controlled statistically, there were no differences between the ratings of parents by individuals with eating disorders (bulimia or anorexia) and the ratings by symptom-free individuals.[70] Furthermore, patients in psychiatric treatment tend to report a low level of caring from their parents.[71] So, the family characteristics reported by women with bulimia may help to cause a variety of mental disorders, or they may constitute a common description offered by individuals with various mental disorders.

The second important point to remember about the perceptions bulimic women have about their families is that nearly all of the research studies before 1990 were conducted with women in treatment for bulimia. Even though it is a widespread problem, few women with bulimia seek help.[72–74] The family relationships reported by bulimic women in treatment may differ from those of women who do not seek treatment, especially those whose families are not aware of their bulimia or of its full extent.

Two studies identified college women who were either suffering from bulimia or exhibited subclinical levels of bulimic symptoms, but were not in treatment for their eating problems, and compared them to college women without any symptoms.[13,75] There were few significant differences among those three groups of women. Although women with bulimia reported less expressiveness in their families than symptom-free women, they did not report more family conflict or less parental caring.[13] Those two studies suggested that the family interaction patterns found in previous research may have been a result of studying women in treatment for their bulimia, and that such patterns may not be found among bulimic women not in treatment.

Other studies conducted in nonclinical settings during the past decade have found evidence of increased levels of conflict and turmoil in the families of individuals with bulimia. A recent study identified both bulimic and nonbulimic women in a community sample and found that the bulimic women were significantly more likely to report some type of disruption in their families or social relationships, such as a significant move or change in the structure of the family, during the year before the onset of their eating disorders.[76] Likewise, another study found that female college students who exhibited symptoms of bulimia reported more anger, aggression, and conflict in their families and less commitment, help, and support.[77]

Research on the family relationships of young women with symptoms of bulimia has focused mainly on the perceptions of the young women themselves. A few studies, however, have investigated the relationships between adolescent girls' bulimic symptoms and their parents' attitudes and behavior.[28,78,79] The results of these studies suggest two links between the attitudes and behavior of parents and their daughters' eating disorders. Daughters may model their behavior after parents who are concerned about their own weight and mothers with symptoms of eating disorders. Daughters' symptoms of bulimia may also be brought about or made worse by their parents' criticism of their weight and appearance, as well as their parents' encouragement to diet and exercise more. In comparison to the mothers of low-symptom daughters, one study found that the mothers of high-symptom daughters thought their daughters should lose significantly more weight, and that significant difference remained even after factoring in control statistics accounting for the weight differences in the two groups of daughters.[28] Perhaps the parents of daughters with eating disorders contribute to their daughters' problems by stressing the cultural message that a young woman must be thin to be attractive, and by failing to model healthy eating attitudes and behaviors.

Most of the research on family interaction patterns in eating disorders has involved instructing the participants to describe their current or past family patterns. Additional prospective studies would be helpful. In one such study, interviews with children and their mothers showed that "problem meals" during childhood were associated with symptoms of bulimia during adolescence.[80] Problem meals were characterized as those with a lack of pleasant interaction and with struggles about eating.

9.2.3.2.2 External Observations

In one study, the mothers and fathers of college women who did or did not have bulimia were interviewed about their family relationships, and then judged according to blind ratings of the interviews.[66] Compared to the parents of symptom-free women, the parents of women with bulimia were rated as more demanding and as exhibiting more tension in their relationships with their daughters. The mothers of women with bulimia were rated as being significantly more domineering and controlling, and as holding higher expectations for their daughters than the other mothers. Fathers of women with bulimia were rated as being close to their daughters during childhood, but more distant during adolescence.

9.2.4 Summary of Research Background

The research evidence confirms earlier clinical observations that the families of young women with eating disorders have distinctive characteristics. This evidence supports the clinical observation that enmeshment is often found in the families of individuals with anorexia. The self-reports of both young women and their parents, as well as ratings made by observers, show that conflict and hostility are characteristic of the families of individuals with bulimia. Research evidence also confirms that adolescent girls with symptoms of bulimia often have parents who pressure them to lose weight.

Several important inconsistencies exist in the research literature on the characteristics of families of women with eating disorders (e.g., the possible link between sexual abuse and eating disorders), and certainly no single family pattern is consistent for individuals with anorexia or bulimia. Each family of an individual with an eating disorder has unique characteristics that are important in understanding the disorder and in planning treatment strategies. Table 9.1 summarizes the research evidence on the family characteristics of women with eating disorders.

9.3 Application of Research Question

Two practical issues face the practitioner working with an eating-disordered client: how to assess the family and how to conduct effective family counseling.

TABLE 9.1

Characteristics of the Families of Individuals with Eating Disorders and the Research Evidence[a]

Confirmed Association	No Evidence of Association	Inconclusive Results
Weight and eating problems	Birth order	Social class
Conflict	Having sisters	Parental divorce
Depression		Substance abuse
Enmeshment		Physical illness
Overprotectiveness		Sexual abuse or assault
Lack of mutual support		
Parental criticism of weight and appearance		

[a] The classification of most characteristics in this table was clear-cut. The evidence is inconclusive about the relationship between sexual abuse and eating disorders, but there are several indications that sexual abuse by a family member increases the likelihood of developing symptoms of an eating disorder.[42,45]

9.3.1 Assessment

A number of instruments have been used to assess the family relationships of individuals with symptoms of eating disorders. A few commonly used family measures follow, with information for how to obtain them. The Family Environment Scale consists of 90 true-false items that assess the family's social environment as it is perceived by family members.[84] The Parental Bonding Instrument has 25 items that assess an individual's recollections of his or her parents during the first 16 years of life.[85] The Family Adaptability and Cohesion Evaluation Scale is a self-report measure consisting of 20 items, half measuring adaptability (the extent to which the family's structure can change when faced with new demands) and half measuring cohesion (emotional closeness among family members).[86]

9.3.2 Family Therapy

Before 1970, treatment for eating disorders usually focused exclusively on the individual with the disorder. Since then, family intervention has been used more and more with eating disorders, either as the main focus of treatment or as one aspect of multidimensional treatment.[81] Some family therapists believe that the symptoms of the individual with an eating disorder are responses to family difficulties.[82] However, a clinician may find great value in including family sessions as one component of treatment without necessarily believing that problems in the family have initiated the eating disorder or helped to prolong it. Even if the family of the individual with an eating disorder is not seen in family therapy sessions, it is important that a family systems perspective help guide treatment efforts.[28] Ignoring the influence of the family system is likely to reduce the effectiveness of those efforts, especially if the subject is an adolescent or young adult living with parents.

The value of working with the individual with an eating disorder in the context of family is illustrated by the case study presented later in this chapter. However, including family sessions in the treatment of eating disorders certainly does not ensure successful treatment. A major practical problem is the high drop-out level in family therapy for patients with eating disorders.[83] Furthermore, research in this area has been neglected, so the value of family therapy in the treatment of eating disorders must be evaluated from clinical reports.[3,4,81]

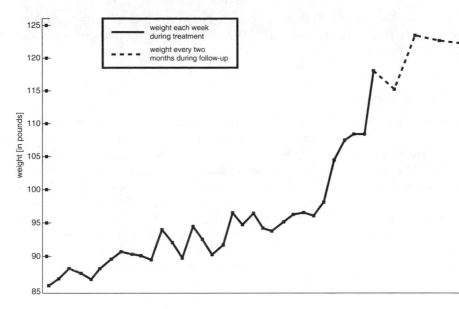

Figure 9.1
Beverly Williams' weight during treatment and follow-up.

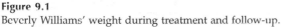

9.4 Case Study

Beverly Williams had the binge-eating/purging type of anorexia nervosa. She was 16 years old, was 5 feet, 6 inches tall, and weighed 85 pounds. Treatment involved individual sessions and sessions with Beverly and other family members. In individual sessions Beverly was encouraged to try different strategies for reducing her self-induced vomiting, consider ways to be less socially isolated at school, and be more direct in communicating her needs to family members.

A key strategy in family sessions was to attempt to increase closeness between Beverly and other family members. A few sessions were spent with Beverly and her three younger sisters attempting, with little success, to identify enjoyable activities they could share. Greater success was achieved in increasing the closeness between Beverly and each of her parents. Mrs. Williams was overweight and found that her difficulties with weight were similar to Beverly's problems. The two of them supported and encouraged each other, and they agreed to shop for clothes together once Beverly had gained enough weight and Mrs. Williams had lost enough weight. The two of them enjoyed working together on weight-related issues; they achieved their goals and made the shopping trip. During a session with Mr. Williams and Beverly, they mentioned a basketball game later that week between the teams of two nearby high schools — the one that Beverly attended and the one that Mr. Williams had attended. Beverly usually went to basketball games alone, but with some encouragement from the therapist, she agreed to go with her father. Attending the basketball game together was an enjoyable experience for both Beverly and her father.

At the start of treatment, Beverly was preoccupied with her weight and fearful of gaining weight. The therapist asked Beverly to put away her scales at home and to stop weighing herself. Instead, the school nurse weighed Beverly and sent the weights to the therapist. Figure 9.1 shows Beverly's weight during treatment and during the following eight months. At the end of treatment, Beverly weighed 118 pounds and no longer had eating binges or episodes of vomiting. During the follow-up period, Beverly reached a stable weight of around 122 pounds and had no symptoms of anorexia or bulimia.

9.4.1 Your Response

Think about the extent to which Beverly and her family exemplify characteristics of adolescents with eating disorders and their families. Were there characteristics of the Williams family that are typical for families in which one member has an eating disorder? Weight and eating problems are often found in the families of individuals with eating disorders, and Mrs. Williams was overweight. However, few of the other characteristics listed in Table 9.1 appear to apply to the Williams family. Beverly's lack of closeness to other family members suggested that she lacked support from family members, but no other evidence demonstrated that mutual support among family members was lacking. Conflict existed in the Williams family over Beverly's binge eating, but little conflict was apparent regarding other issues.

References

1. Minuchin, S., Baker, L., Rosman, B. L., Liebman, R., Milman, L., and Todd, T. C., A conceptual model of psychosomatic illness in children: family organization and family therapy, *Archives of General Psychiatry*, 32, 1031, 1975.
2. Minuchin, S., Rosman, B., and Baker, L., *Psychosomatic Families: Anorexia Nervosa in Context*, Harvard University Press, Cambridge, MA, 1978.
3. Liebman, R., Minuchin, S., and Baker, L., The role of the family in the treatment of anorexia nervosa, *Journal of the American Academy of Child Psychiatry*, 13, 264, 1974.
4. Rosman, B. L., Minuchin, S., and Liebman, R., Family lunch session: an introduction to family therapy in anorexia nervosa, *American Journal of Orthopsychiatry*, 45, 846, 1975.
5. Bruch, H., *Eating Disorders: Obesity, Anorexia Nervosa, and the Person Within*, Basic Books, New York, 1973.
6. Bruch, H., *The Golden Cage: The Enigma of Anorexia Nervosa*, Harvard University Press, Cambridge, MA, 1978.
7. Kog, E. and Vandereycken, W., Family characteristics of anorexia nervosa and bulimia: a review of the research literature, *Clinical Psychology Review*, 5, 159, 1985.
8. Askevold, F., Social class and psychosomatic illness, *Psychotherapy and Psychosomatics*, 38, 256, 1982.
9. Herzog, D., Bulimia: the secretive syndrome, *Psychosomatics*, 23, 481, 1982.
10. Carter, J. A. and Duncan, P. A., Binge-eating and vomiting: a survey of a high school population, *Psychology in the Schools*, 21, 198, 1984.
11. Crowther, J. H., Post, G., and Zaynor, L., The prevalence of bulimia and binge eating in adolescent girls, *International Journal of Eating Disorders*, 4, 29, 1985.
12. Heron, J. M. and Leheup, R., Happy families? *British Journal of Psychiatry*, 145, 136, 1984.
13. Kent, J. S. and Clopton, J. R., Bulimic women's perceptions of their family relationships, *Journal of Clinical Psychology*, 48, 281, 1992.
14. Hollingshead, A. B., *Four-factor Index of Social Status*. Unpublished manuscript, Department of Sociology, Yale University, New Haven, CT, 1975.
15. Vandereycken, W. and Van Vreckem, E. V., Siblings of patients with an eating disorder, *International Journal of Eating Disorders*, 12, 273, 1992.
16. Dolan, B. M., Evans, C., and Lacey, J. H., Family composition and social class in bulimia: a catchment area study of a clinical and a comparison group, *Journal of Nervous and Mental Disease*, 177, 267, 1989.

17. Weiss, S. and Ebert, M., Psychological and behavioral characteristics of normal-weight bulimics and normal-weight controls, *Psychosomatic Medicine*, 45, 293, 1983.

18. Garfinkel, P., Moldofsky, H., and Garner, D., The heterogeneity of anorexia nervosa: bulimia as a distinct subgroup, *Archives of General Psychiatry*, 37, 1036, 1980.

19. Vandereycken, W. and Pierloot, R., The significance of subclassification in anorexia nervosa: a comparative study of clinical features in 141 patients, *Psychological Medicine*, 13, 543, 1983.

20. Casper, R., Personality features of women with good outcome from restricting anorexia nervosa, *Psychosomatic Medicine*, 52, 156, 1990.

21. Hall., A., Slim, E., Hawker, F., and Salmond, C., Anorexia nervosa: long-term outcome in 50 female patients, *British Journal of Psychiatry*, 145, 407, 1984.

22. Halmi, K., Anorexia nervosa: demographic and clinical features in 94 cases, *Psychosomatic Medicine*, 36, 18, 1974.

23. Halmi, K. A., Struss, A., and Goldberg, S. C., An investigation of weights in the parents of anorexia nervosa patients, *Journal of Nervous and Mental Disease*, 166, 358, 1978.

24. Holland, A. J., Sicotte, N., and Treasure, J., Anorexia nervosa: evidence for a genetic basis, *Journal of Psychosomatic Research*, 32, 561, 1988.

25. Fichter, M. M. and Noegel, R., Concordance for bulimia nervosa in twins, *International Journal of Eating Disorders*, 9, 255, 1990.

26. Hsu, L. K. G., Chesler, B. E., and Santhouse, R., Bulimia nervosa in eleven sets of twins: a clinical report, *International Journal of Eating Disorders*, 9, 275, 1990.

27. Waters, B. G. H., Beumont, P. J. V., Touyz, S., and Kennedy, M., Behavioural differences between twin and non-twin sibling pairs discordant for anorexia nervosa, *International Journal of Eating Disorders*, 9, 265, 1990.

28. Pike, K. M. and Rodin, J., Mothers, daughters, and disordered eating, *Journal of Abnormal Psychology*, 100, 198, 1991.

29. Crisp, A. H., Harding, B., and McGuinness, B., Anorexia nervosa. Psychoneurotic characteristics of parents: relationship to prognosis. A quantitative study, *Journal of Psychosomatic Research*, 18, 167, 1974.

30. Garfinkel, P., Garner, D., Rose, J., Darby, P., Brandes, J. S., O'Hanlon, J., and Walsh, N., A comparison of characteristics in the families of patients with anorexia nervosa and normal controls, *Psychological Medicine*, 13, 821, 1983.

31. Bulik, C. M., Drug and alcohol abuse by bulimic women and their families, *American Journal of Psychiatry*, 144, 1604, 1987.

32. Kuntz, B., Groze, V., and Yates, W. R., Bulimia: a systemic family history perspective, *Families in Society*, 73, 604, 1992.

33. Winokur, A., March, V., and Mendels, J., Primary affective disorder in relatives of patients with anorexia nervosa, *American Journal of Psychiatry*, 136, 695, 1980.

34. Gershon, E., Hamovit, J. R., Schreiber, J. L., Dibble, E., Kaye, W., Nurnberger, J., Andersen, A., and Ebert, M., Anorexia nervosa and major affective disorders associated in families: a preliminary report, in *Childhood Psychopathology and Development*, Guze, S., Earls, F., and Barrett, J., Eds., Raven Press, New York, 1983, 279–287.

35. Hudson, J. I., Laffer, P. S., and Pope, H. G., Bulimia related to affective disorder by family history and response to the Dexamethasone Suppression Test, *American Journal of Psychiatry*, 137, 685, 1982.

36. Hudson, J., Pope, H., Jonas, J., and Yurgulun-Todd, D., Family history study of anorexia nervosa and bulimia, *British Journal of Psychiatry*, 142, 428, 1983.

37. Carlat, D. J., Camargo, C. A., Jr., and Herzog, D. B., Eating disorders in males: a report of 135 patients, *American Journal of Psychiatry*, 154, 1127, 1997.

38. Hernandez, J., The concurrence of eating disorders with histories of child abuse among adolescents, *Journal of Child Sexual Abuse*, 4, 73, 1995.

39. Selby, M. J. and Moreno, J. K., Personal and familial substance misuse patterns among eating disordered and depressed subjects, *International Journal of Addictions*, 30, 1169, 1995.

40. Schuckit, M. A., Tipp, J. E., Anthenelli, R. M., Bucholz, K. K., Hesselbrock, V. M., and Nurnberger, J. I., Anorexia nervosa and bulimia nervosa in alcohol-dependent men and women and their relatives, *American Journal of Psychiatry*, 153, 74, 1996.

41. Strober, M., The significance of bulimia in juvenile anorexia nervosa: an exploration of possible etiologic factors, *International Journal of Eating Disorders*, 1, 28, 1981.

42. Chandy, J. M., Blum, R. W., and Resnick, M. D., Female adolescents with a history of sexual abuse: risk, outcome and protective factors, *Journal of Interpersonal Violence*, 11, 503, 1996.

43. Connors, M. E. and Morse, W., Sexual abuse and eating disorders: a review, *International Journal of Eating Disorders*, 13, 1, 1993.

44. Horesh, N., Apter, A., Ishai, J., Danziger, Y., Miculincer, M., Stein, D., and Lepkifker, E., Abnormal psychosocial situations and eating disorders in adolescence, *Journal of the American Academy of Child and Adolescent Psychiatry*, 35, 921, 1996.

45. Baldo, T. D. B., Wallace, S. D., and O'Halloran, M. S., Effects of intrafamilial sexual assault on eating disorders, *Psychological Reports*, 79, 531, 1996.

46. Finn, S. E., Hartmann, M., and Leon, G., Eating disorders and sexual abuse: lack of confirmation for a clinical hypothesis, *International Journal of Eating Disorders*, 5, 1051, 1986.

47. Calam, R. M. and Slade, P. D., Sexual experiences and eating problems in female undergraduates, *International Journal of Eating Disorders*, 8, 391, 1989.

48. Waller, G., Sexual abuse and the severity of bulimic symptoms, *British Journal of Psychiatry*, 161, 90, 1992.

49. Kinzl, J. F., Mangweth, B., Traweger, C. M., and Biebl, W., Eating-disordered behavior in males: the impact of adverse childhood experiences, *International Journal of Eating Disorders*, 22, 131, 1997.

50. Mallinckrodt, B., McCreary, B. A., and Robertson, A. K., Co-occurrence of eating disorders and incest: the role of attachment, family environment, and social competencies, *Journal of Counseling Psychology*, 42, 178, 1995.

51. Owen, S. E. H., The projective identification of the parents of patients suffering from anorexia nervosa, *Australian and New Zealand Journal of Psychiatry*, 7, 285, 1973.

52. Palmer, R. L., Oppenheimer, R., and Marshall, P. D., Eating disordered patients remember their parents: a study using the Parental-Bonding Instrument, *International Journal of Eating Disorders*, 7, 101, 1988.

53. Humphrey, L. L., Relationships within subtypes of anorexic, bulimic, and normal families, *Journal of the American Academy of Child and Adolescent Psychiatry*, 27, 544, 1988.

54. Houben, M., Onderzoek naar enkele relatiekarakteristieken in gezinnen met een anorexia nervosa patient, *Tijdschrift voor Psychiatrie*, 23, 87, 1981.

55. Goldstein, H. J., Family factors associated with schizophrenia and anorexia nervosa, *Journal of Youth and Adolescence*, 10, 385, 1981.

56. Selvini-Palazzoli, M., Boscolo, L., Cecchin, G., and Prata, G., Het gezin van de anorexia-patient en het gezin van de schizfreen: een transactionele studie, *Tijdschrift voor Psychotherapie*, 2, 53, 1976.

57. Humphrey, L. L., Comparison of bulimic-anorexic and nondistressed families using structural analysis of social behavior, *Journal of the American Academy of Child and Adolescent Psychiatry*, 26, 248, 1987.

58. Calam, R., Waller, G., Slade, P. D., and Newton, T., Eating disorders and perceived relationship with parents, *International Journal of Eating Disorders*, 9, 479, 1990.

59. Humphrey, L. L., Family relations in bulimic-anorexic and non-distressed families, *International Journal of Eating Disorders*, 5, 223, 1986.

60. Johnson, C. and Flach, A., Family characteristics of 105 patients with bulimia, *American Journal of Psychiatry*, 142, 1321, 1985.

61. Kog, E., Vertommen, H., and DeGroote, T., Family interaction research in anorexia nervosa: the use and misuse of a self-report questionnaire, *International Journal of Eating Disorders*, 6, 227, 1985.

62. Mitchell, J. E., Hatsukami, D., Eckert, E. D., and Pyle, R. L., Characteristics of 275 patients with bulimia, *American Journal of Psychiatry*, 142, 482, 1985.

63. Norman, D. K. and Herzog, D. B., Bulimia, anorexia nervosa, and anorexia nervosa with bulimia: a comparative analysis of MMPI profiles, *International Journal of Eating Disorders*, 2, 43, 1984.

64. Ordman, A. M. and Kirshenbaum, D. S., Bulimia: assessment of eating, psychological adjustment, and familial characteristics, *International Journal of Eating Disorders*, 5, 865, 1986.

65. Pole, R., Waller, D. A., Stewart, S. M., and Parkin-Fergenbaum, L., Parental caring versus overprotection in bulimia, *International Journal of Eating Disorders*, 7, 601, 1988.

66. Sights, J. R. and Richards, H. C., Parents of bulimic women, *International Journal of Eating Disorders*, 3, 3, 1984.

67. Lacey, J. H., Phil, M., Coker, S., and Birtchnell, S. A., Bulimia: factors associated with its etiology and maintenance, *International Journal of Eating Disorders*, 5, 475, 1986.

68. Moos, R. H. and Moos, B. S., *Family Environmental Scale Manual*, Consulting Psychologists Press, Palo Alto, CA, 1981.

69. Woodside, D. B., Swinson, R. P., Kuch, K., and Heinmaa, M., Family functioning in anxiety and eating disorders — a comparative study, *Comprehensive Psychiatry*, 37, 139, 1996.

70. Wonderlich, S. A. and Swift, W. J., Perceptions of parental relationships in the eating disorders: the relevance of depressed mood, *Journal of Abnormal Psychology*, 99, 353, 1990.

71. Parker, G., *Parental Overprotection: A Risk Factor in Psychosocial Development*, Grune & Stratton, New York, 1983.

72. Fairburn, C. G. and Cooper, P. J., Self-induced vomiting and bulimia nervosa: an undetected problem, *British Medical Journal*, 284, 1153, 1982.

73. Johnson, C. L., Stuckey, M. K., Lewis, C. D., and Schwartz, D., Bulimia: a descriptive survey of 316 cases, *International Journal of Eating Disorders*, 2, 3, 1982.

74. Pyle, R. L., Halvorson, P. A., Neuman, P. A., and Mitchell, J. E., The increasing prevalence of bulimia in freshman college students, *International Journal of Eating Disorders*, 5, 631, 1986.

75. Kent, J. S. and Clopton, J. R., Bulimia: a comparison of psychological adjustment and familial characteristics in a nonclinical sample, *Journal of Clinical Psychology*, 44, 964, 1988.

76. Welch, S. L., Doll, H. A., and Fairburn, C. G., Life events and the onset of bulimia nervosa: a controlled study, *Psychological Medicine*, 27, 515, 1997.

77. Bailey, C. A., Family structure and eating disorders: the Family Environment Scale and bulimic-like symptoms, *Youth and Society*, 23, 251, 1991.

78. Keel, P. K., Heatherton, T. F., Harnden, J. L., and Hornig, C. D., Mothers, fathers, and daughters: dieting and disordered eating, *Eating Disorders*, 5, 216, 1997.

79. Moreno, A. and Thelen, M. H., Parental factors related to bulimia nervosa, *Addictive Behaviors*, 18, 681, 1993.

80. Marchi, M. and Cohen, P., Early childhood eating behaviors and adolescent eating disorders, *Journal of the American Academy of Child and Adolescent Psychiatry*, 29, 112, 1990.

81. Vanderlinden, J. and Vandereycken, W., Guidelines for the family therapeutic approach to eating disorders, *Psychotherapy and Psychosomatics*, 56, 36, 1991.

82. Selvini-Palazzoli, M., *Self-Starvation: From the Individual to Family Therapy in the Treatment of Anorexia Nervosa*, Jason Aronson, New York, 1978.

83. Szmukler, G. I., Eisler, I., Russell, G. F. M., and Dare, C., Anorexia nervosa, parental "expressed emotion" and dropping out of treatment, *British Journal of Psychiatry*, 147, 265, 1985.

84. Moos, R. and Moos, B., *Family Environment Scale Manual (2nd ed.)*, Consulting Psychologists Press, Palo Alto, CA, 1986.

85. Parker, G., Tupling, H., and Brown, L. B., A parental bonding instrument, *British Journal of Medical Psychology*, 52, 1, 1979.

86. Olson, D. H., Portner, J., and Lavee, Y., *FACES-III Manual*, Department of Family Social Sciences, University of Minnesota, St. Paul, 1985.

10

Media Involvement and the Idea of Beauty

Elizabeth Jambor

CONTENTS

10.1 Learning Objectives

After reading this chapter, the reader will be able to:

- Understand the different types of media portraying ideal standards;
- Understand the influence of media on the development of standards of physical appearance, especially for females;
- Understand how the media might negatively impact developing body awareness, especially for females;
- Learn how to counteract the impact of the media on the developing body images of males and females.

10.2 Research Background

10.2.1 Disordered Eating and the Media

The media bombard society with images of the ideal and the idea that good-looking people have better lives and more opportunities. What is an acceptable body image in the media may be unobtainable for many in the general population. Although this may be true for both males and females, the perception that women need to look a certain way (i.e., like Barbie) in order to be accepted in society may lead to inappropriate eating behaviors. This chapter will explore the link between the media and disordered eating behaviors. Included in this discussion will be strategies to help girls and women to filter out the media messages related to acceptable looks so that they might develop better, healthier levels of body image self-acceptance.

Before exploring the impact of the media in developing images of physical acceptance, it is important to distinguish between eating disorders and disordered eating. An eating disorder is defined as compulsive eating behaviors that can be life threatening; examples are anorexia nervosa, bulimia, and compulsive overeating. More common is the occurrence of disordered eating. Disordered eating involves situations wherein an individual develops some ritualistic or structured way of dealing with food or eating and exhibits some unhealthy behaviors related to food and body weight. Although disordered eating may be seen as less severe than eating disorders, it can still lead to complications and consequences for the individual. Disordered eating becomes still more serious when we consider that it can often can go undetected.

Body image and body dissatisfaction play important roles in both eating disorders and disordered eating. These behaviors may stem from a distorted body image, that is, from not seeing the body as it truly appears. This distorted body image may mean that the individual views herself as either larger (fatter) or smaller (thinner) than she is in reality. Where does this body image come from? How does an individual decide what she should look like? The image of an ideal body may come from various sources. However, one common and consistent source is the media.

People are inundated with media images on a daily basis; whether in print, on television, on the ratio, or in some other form. Within these media are messages of what to do, how to be, what products to use, and how to look. Even if the message is not overt, the images within the message suggest what is an acceptable body type. These images produce sociocultural pressures that play an important role in the development of disordered eating and eating disorders.

Historically, culture has dictated the desired female image. At present, the cultural ideal for female body shape in the United States and many other Western cultures is slenderness. The media exploit this image by bombarding consumers with messages that to achieve this ideal body shape is to be in control, happy, attractive, intelligent, wealthy, and successful. To try to conform to this unrealistic idea of thinness, 80% of females are or have been actively dieting.[1]

In the following sections specific forms of media will be discussed with respect to the potential influence they exert on females, in particular, and related research that supports the idea of this influence. This chapter, however, is not meant to be all-inclusive. Its purpose is to provide the reader with a base of information for thoughts on the topic and case studies to which these thoughts can be applied. While going through it, the reader is encouraged to think about and discuss his or her own experiences with media the better to understand its powerful impact on developing images of the ideal self.

10.2.1.1   Print Media

Print media, specifically magazines, feature very few readily available publications that do not picture a slender (or well-muscled), attractive person on the cover. From *Good Housekeeping* and *Redbook,* to *Muscle and Fitness*, from *Shape* to *Details* and *The Rolling Stone*, images of slender people adorn their covers. Even publications that have nothing to do with bodies per se, e.g., *Hot Rod*, display slender women on their covers. Thin is in; thin sells. Because these images are so pervasive within print media, their perception as being the ideal is supported. A 1998 *USA Today* poll suggested that 23% of girls 12 to 17 years old were influenced by magazines in their fashion choices. If these young women are so influenced, do they have the body types to wear that fashion choice, or will they need to attempt some weight-loss tactic to fit in?

Research has supported the idea of visual media influencing the perception of body image.[2] A study conducted by researchers at West Virginia University found that viewing pictures of thin models' ideal body types had a significant impact on females. This was not found to be true for males. Females who looked at pictures of thin models had significantly higher levels of private self-consciousness, body competence, and state anxiety. A related study from Australia found that media and fashion were reported to exert the strongest pressures to be thin on girls ages 14 to 16.[3] These pressures manifested themselves in unhealthy body attitudes and eating behaviors.

Kristen Harrison, a researcher in communications studies, found that magazine reading, especially exposure to thinness-depicting and thinness-promoting media, significantly predicted symptoms of eating disorders in women.[4] Furthermore, women who frequently read fitness magazines for reasons other than an interest in fitness and dieting displayed greater signs of disordered eating than women who rarely read them at all.

10.2.1.2 Television Media

Television enters the homes and minds of millions daily. The images are graphic and surreal at the same time. As with print media, television promotes the idea of what is ideal, and as with print media, larger people typically represent the "before" picture when it comes to pushing weight loss products or medications. Incidences even exist of commercials that support the use of laxatives for weight loss, with a slender woman reporting that taking the product just makes her "feel better."

Even television cartoons are impacted by the ideal body image for females. Examples include Wilma Flintstone, Betty Rubble, Belle of *Beauty and the Beast*, and a host of other cartoon females, as well as voluptuous female superheroes. From a very young age, females are bombarded with images of heroes and heroines that fit a particular body type. Moreover, it is these perfect-looking characters that end up winning the prince or the prize. It is not overtly suggested that these characters' looks allow them to get the best from life. However, in a covert manner, young females are constantly surrounded by images of thin female characters who are portrayed as the ideal.

Research from the University of Southern Florida found that the internalization of social standards of appearance was more powerful than media exposure.[5] However, they added that these social standards are often formulated and supported by media, so for many females it becomes a *Catch-22* situation. What's more, the idea of social standards can be related to body-image disturbance and eating dysfunction. As individuals, and specifically females, are exposed to ideal images from television viewing, disorders can occur. A related study from the University of Michigan demonstrated that being attracted to thin characters in shows like *Ally McBeal* and *Beverly Hills 90210* positively predicted general eating-disorder symptoms — anorexia, bulimia, drive for thinness, perfectionism, and ineffectiveness.[6]

10.2.1.3 Other Media

Many movies and television shows, not to mention books and comic books, feature merchandising tie-ins. Any doubts can be easily dissuaded by a trip to any toy store. Filling the shelves are Disney characters, *Star Wars* action figures, Marvel action figures, and Barbie. Barbie's undersized waist, in conjunction with her oversized breasts, and a plantar flexion stance, do not represent a typical female body size. Naomi Wolf, author of *The Beauty Myth*, stated that a generation ago, the average model weighed 8% less than the average American woman, whereas today, models weigh 23% less.[7] This is a dramatic separation between what the average woman looks like and what the ideal image of a woman looks like. This ideal image is portrayed not only in print and film but also in media-related store merchandise.

10.3 Application of Research Question

Does society have a responsibility to portray body images that are more realistic in the media, and would authentic images have an impact on eating disorders? It is evident from the previous information that the media do exert an impact on the developing ideas and ideals of females. Individuals are inundated with images from print, television, film and other media sources featuring ideal body images and shapes. Information is abundant on the "right look." [Popular culture has set the image for females to achieve.] Unfortunately, the image is more unreal and surreal than achievable.] Not understanding this idea, females endure unhealthy eating and exercise practices to achieve the ideal promoted by the media. In the end, most only achieve a pattern of disordered eating, which may lead potentially to an eating disorder.

What can be done? The possibilities are endless but not easy to achieve. Re-educating the public as to what are appropriate female images would help. Teaching young people that what they see on television or in magazines is not always real, and the achievement of those images is not always healthy, might also have a positive effect. Finding ways to achieve a healthy level of self-esteem that is not dependent on a physical image would go far in helping females to find qualities within themselves that are not related to beauty and body size.

Researchers at the University of Utah supported the idea of using realistic images in portraying attractiveness.[8] These researchers found that exposure to realistic attractiveness is less likely to increase concern about weight, a finding in direct opposition to the attitudes fostered by exposure to unrealistic images. It may thus be asked whether research supports the fact that the drives for thinness and body dissatisfaction are factors in eating disorders. Furthermore, it has been shown that these problems are more common in women than in men. A recent study conducted at Texas Tech University by Jacalyn Robert-McComb, James Clopton, Elizabeth Jambor, and Esther Weekes[9] found that gender, drive for thinness, body dissatisfaction, desired weight and the difference between desired weight and actual weight accounted for 29% of the variance in bulimia, as measured by the BULIT. Furthermore, there was a significant difference between the males and females in the bulimia score, with females scoring significantly higher than males. The important issue to remember is the impact the media have on society. It is powerful and pervasive. What society must remember is that it bears the responsibility to portray images that represent all in a healthy and positive manner.

References

1. Baker-Dennis, A. and Sansone, R. A., Overview of eating disorders, anorexia nervosa, bulimia nervosa, and related disorders, *Laureate*, 2, 57, 1997.
2. Kalodner, C. R., Media influences on male and female non-eating-disordered college students: a significant issue, *Eating Disorders: The Journal of Treatment and Prevention*, 5(1), 47, 1997.

3. Wertheim, E. H., Paxton, S. J., Schutz, H. K., and Muir, S. L., Why do adolescent girls watch their weight? An interview study examining sociocultural pressures to be thin, *Journal of Psychosomatic Research*, 42(4), 345, 1997.
4. Harrison, K., The relationship between media consumption and eating disorders, *Journal of Communication*, 12, 98, 1997.
5. Cusumano, D. L. and Thompson, J. K., Body image and body shape ideals in magazines: exposure, awareness, and internalization, *Sex Roles*, 37(9–10), 701, 1997.
6. Harrison, K., Does interpersonal attraction to thin media personalities promote eating disorders? *Journal of Broadcasting and Electronic Media*, 4, 37, 1997.
7. Wolf, N., *The Beauty Myth*, Vintage Books, Toronto, 1991.
8. Posavac, H. D., Posavac, S. S., and Posavac, E. J., Exposure to media images of female attractiveness and concern with body weight among young women, *Sex Roles*, 38(3–4), 187, 1998.
9. Robert-McComb, J., Clopton, J., Jambor, E., and Weekes, E., Explanatory variance in bulimia. Study conducted at Texas Tech University, Lubbock, 1997.

11

Body Image

Susan Kashubeck-West and Kendra Saunders

CONTENTS

11.1 Learning Objectives

After reading this chapter you should be able to:

- Know how to define body image and its components;
- Understand what factors may affect body image;
- See some consequences of negative body image;
- Recognize differences in body image between men and women;
- Learn strategies for improving body image.

11.2 Research Background

All of us have bodies and all of us have a variety of reactions to our bodies. These reactions comprise what is known as body image. In this chapter, body image is defined as a concept related to physical appearance, specifically, a person's size, shape, and weight. The discussion is organized as follows: (a) the components of body image;

(b) the prevalence of body image disturbance, adjusted for differences in sex, race, and class; (c) the results of research examining factors that are thought to influence body image; and finally (d) ways to improve body image.

11.2.1   Body Image and Its Components

According to Thompson,[1] physical appearance-related body image is generally divided into three components: (1) a perceptual component that relates to how accurately we estimate our body size; (2) a subjective component that involves our feelings, thoughts, and attitudes toward our bodies; and (3) a behavioral component that refers to repetitive checking behavior and the tendency to avoid situations where we might feel uncomfortable about our bodies. Other researchers have defined body image in similar and different manners, and research has seldom focused on the multidimensional nature of body image described above. Rather, in trying to understand the negative body images people often report (called body image disturbance), researchers have tended to focus on body-size distortion and negative attitude toward the body, or body dissatisfaction.

Body-size distortion occurs when a person either over- or underestimates his or her body size. Most of the focus in this field has been on overestimation, and research generally indicates that individuals who have been diagnosed with anorexia nervosa tend to overestimate their body sizes.[2,3] Hilde Bruch, a pioneer in the field of eating disorders, felt that body size distortion is a core feature of anorexia. Interestingly, Slade[4] reported that he and his colleagues believe that individuals with anorexia nervosa have an "uncertain, unstable, and weak body image," so that when asked to estimate body size, they tend to overestimate. Thus, women with anorexia may not really experience body-size distortion. In addition, it appears that individuals with bulimia nervosa and individuals with no eating disorders may also overestimate their body sizes.[5,6] Also, there seems to be little relationship between body-size distortion and reports of body dissatisfaction.[7] These findings have led some individuals to question whether the perceptual component of body image is useful.[8,9] In fact, Smeets and Panhuysen[10] argued that researchers have inappropriate notions about perception, rendering them incapable of explaining disturbances in body-size perception. According to Thompson,[7] research has indicated that numerous methodological factors affect the findings in this area, and those factors need to be investigated before any conclusions can be made. Clearly, more research on body-size distortion is needed.

The second main area of research involves the subjective component of body image disturbance, specifically, the extent of body dissatisfaction. Although this component can be divided into feeling, thinking, and behavioral factors, research has indicated that there is a great deal of overlap among these areas.[11,12] Numerous studies indicate that many women report feeling dissatisfied with various body parts, their whole bodies, and their weight.[13] Indeed, body image disturbance is so pervasive among women that it is normative, rather than unusual, for women to be unhappy with their bodies.[14] However, research indicates that women with eating disorders report much greater levels of body dissatisfaction than women without eating disorders, suggesting that they are exceptionally disparaging of their bodies.[15] In addition, Cash and Deagle's[15] summary of the research literature indicates that women with bulimia nervosa report more body dissatisfaction than women with anorexia nervosa. Thus, women with anorexia (who are underweight) may experience fewer negative feelings about their bodies than women with bulimia, who tend to be of normal weight or overweight.

11.2.2   Prevalence of Body Image Disturbance

It is very common for women to report body image disturbances, especially those relating to body-image dissatisfaction. For example, Cash and Henry[16] reported in a recent national survey that nearly half of American women had negative evaluations of their overall appearance and were preoccupied with their weight. Drewnowski and Yee[17] studied freshman college women and found that 85% of them wanted to lose weight. Alarmingly, body dissatisfaction seems to start very early in life. Collins[18] reported that 42% of a sample of 6- to 7-year-old girls indicated a preference for body figures different from and thinner than theirs. Thompson, Corwin, and Sargent[19] found that 49% of fourth-grade females indicated that an ideal figure would be thinner than their current figure.

Many studies have investigated gender differences in how satisfied people are with their bodies, and the most common finding is that women report greater dissatisfaction than men.[1,20–26] For example, Muth and Cash[24] found that, when compared to men, women had more negative evaluations of their bodies, were more concerned with their appearance, and reported negative feelings about their bodies in more situations. These gender differences also have been noted in young children.[19] However, some studies report that men and women differ as to which parts of their own bodies they regard with dissatisfaction,[27,28] and a few studies have found greater general body image dissatisfaction among men.[29]

To understand these conflicting findings, it is necessary to look at how studies have been carried out. For instance, many studies that investigate gender differences in total-body evaluations find women more dissatisfied than men, while studies that investigate attitudes toward specific body parts find men more dissatisfied with some parts and women more dissatisfied with other parts.[28] More important, however, is whether investigators have taken into account the fact that many men who are dissatisfied with their bodies wish to gain, not lose, weight. As noted by Furnham and Greaves,[21] a discrepancy between how one perceives oneself (actual self) and how one wishes to be (ideal self) seems to be the core of body image dissatisfaction. Studies have shown that many men (often half the sample) feel they should be more muscular and weigh more.[22,23,28,30,31] By contrast, very few women want to gain weight.[32] If studies have not taken into account the direction of men's desired weight change, it is likely that they have a pool of men, half of whom want to gain weight and half of whom want to lose weight. Average these men together, and it will seem as though this pool of men are satisfied with their current weights. Compare these men to a group of women (the vast majority of whom will wish to lose weight) and the women will show greater body dissatisfaction. Interestingly, Kashubeck and Mintz[33] compared men and women who wanted to lose weight, using a body dissatisfaction measure, and found that women still showed greater dissatisfaction with their bodies. Women seem to feel more pressure from society to look a certain way than do men,[34] and so the failure to meet these societal expectations may result in their greater body dissatisfaction.

Regarding racial/ethnic differences in body dissatisfaction, several researchers have postulated that African-American women are less likely to report body dissatisfaction than white women because African American culture places less emphasis on thinness in women.[35] A number of studies have investigated differences between white and black women and found that black women are more satisfied with their bodies,[35–40] despite a higher prevalence of obesity among black women.[36,41] However, other researchers have found comparable levels of body dissatisfaction among black and white women[42–45] and have suggested that stereotypes describing women with eating disorders as white and upper-class may serve to hide eating disorders in women of color.[46] Indeed, Singh[47] found that black women and men did not associate attractiveness with being overweight. Lester and Petrie[48] stated that the available data on culture and eating disorders in African American women suggest that idealization of white cultural values and identity might increase the risk of developing an eating disorder, but that a stronger identification with African American cultural attitudes and beliefs does not seem to offer protection from eating-related problems. Lester and Petrie found that in African American college females, endorsement of specific societal values related to thinness and attractiveness was associated with greater body dissatisfaction.

One confounding factor in the literature examining racial/ethnic differences in body image disturbance is a failure to examine socioeconomic status (SES). Data suggest that class differences exist in body size, preferences for body size, and perceived attractive body size.[49] Failure to examine class in conjunction with race and ethnicity may lead to erroneous conclusions. For example, Caldwell et al.[42] suggested that their failure to find racial differences in body satisfaction among a sample of upper-class white and African American women could have occurred because SES might serve as a more powerful factor than race in understanding body dissatisfaction. Thompson et al.[19] reported that the effect of race was not consistent across SES levels in children's selections of ideal body size. Similarly, Allan, Mayo, and Michel[50] found that black women who were lower in SES held different values concerning actual and attractive body sizes when compared to black women of higher social status and white women of any SES. White and black women of higher social status reported more pressure to be thin and found thinner bodies to be more attractive, whereas black women with lower social status felt less pressure to be thin and selected heavier body sizes as more attractive.

Little work has investigated body image disturbance in women from racial and ethnic groups other than European American and African American. For example, there is little research on Asian American women, who may be at high risk for low self-esteem and poor body image because they experience racism and sexism.[51] Four studies[52-55] report that Asian American women show lower levels of eating disorders when compared to Caucasian women, while two other studies report that Asian American women have higher levels of eating disorders.[56,57] A study done by Mintz and Kashubeck[32] found that gender differences related to body image and disordered-eating variables in Asian American college students were similar to those seen in Caucasian college students. In addition, they found that Caucasian women engaged in more dieting and binging behavior, while Asian American women reported less satisfaction with racially defined body parts (such as eyes and facial features) and lower self-esteem. Both Asian American and Caucasian women were similarly dissatisfied with their abdomens, buttocks, hips, and upper thighs. It appears that there could be race differences in the relationship between body dissatisfaction with lower-torso areas and weight control strategies.[32]

Crago, Shisslak, and Estes[58] and Striegel-Moore and Smolak[59] stated that there are substantial differences among different minority groups in their risks for eating disorders. It is likely that such differences extend to the area of body image as well. Some theorists feel that ethnic cultures may protect against negative body images because their beauty standards do not emphasize thinness.[46,51] By contrast, others argue that "factors associated with racism which may increase vulnerability to EDs (eating disorders) include feeling pressured to look or act 'perfect' in order to be accepted by the dominant culture, and receiving contradictory messages about beauty and weight," as pointed out by Crago, Shisslak and Ests.[58] Acculturation is another factor that needs study. Are individuals who are highly attuned to mainstream culture more at risk for body dissatisfaction than less acculturated individuals, or vice-versa? Much more research is needed in these areas.

Sexual orientation and its relation to body image satisfaction in women has also been investigated. Lesbians are thought to be more likely to reject cultural imperatives regarding female appearance, thus making them less likely to suffer from body dissatisfaction and eating disorders.[60] By contrast, it has been argued that lesbians, like all other women in our culture, are exposed to the same cultural messages regarding thinness and attractiveness, and thus should show the same body dissatisfaction when they fail to meet these societal standards.[61] Heffernan[60] found that lesbians report an endorsement of social norms regarding thinness and attractiveness similar to that of heterosexual women. In addition, Heffernan reported that rates of bulimia nervosa appear similar for heterosexual and lesbian women, although lesbians report higher levels of binge eating. Similar results were reported by Beren, Hayden, Wilfley, and Grilo,[62] who found that lesbians do not differ from heterosexual women in their levels of body satisfaction. The results of these studies suggest that the values of the lesbian community do not protect lesbians from body dissatisfaction, and that lesbians are not immune to the negative effects of failing to meet societal standards for thinness.

11.2.3 Potential Influences on Body Image

11.2.3.1 Demographic Factors

As should already be clear, demographic factors may play a role in the development of body image disturbance. Gender, race, socioeconomic status, and sexual orientation may operate independently and in conjunction with one another to affect body image. Individuals who are different in terms of race, sex, SES, and sexual orientation will likely experience our culture's sociocultural pressures differently, possibly leading to differences in body image disturbance and eating disorders. Research that addresses such demographic factors, and particularly research that examines interactions between gender, race, SES, and sexual orientation, is sorely needed.

11.2.3.2 Developmental Factors

Several developmental factors have been identified as potential contributors to negative body images found among women. Among these factors are puberty, dating, modeling, and teasing/criticism. Smolak, Levine, and Gralen[63] noted that puberty seems to be the time when girls develop weight concerns, body dissatisfaction, dieting habits, and eating disorders. For many adolescent girls, dieting[38] and body dissatisfaction become normative. According to Smolak, Levine and Gralen,[63] two models have been put forward to account for the relationships among puberty, body image disturbance and eating-disordered behavior. The first model suggests that the timing of pubertal maturation is important, in that girls who physically mature early may feel more negative about their bodies and diet more. Supporting this model is a study by Keel, Fulkerson, and Leon,[64] which found that girls who achieved puberty earlier (and were heavier) were more likely to report disordered-eating attitudes and behaviors. Similarly, studies by Attie and Brooks-Gunn[65] and by Killen and colleagues[66,67] indicated that pubertal timing was associated with disordered-eating patterns.

The second model suggests that the impact of several simultaneous events, including puberty, increases the overall stress felt by adolescent girls, resulting in more eating disorder-related distress. Specifically, Levine and Smolak[68] suggested that puberty, with its increase in fat and body size, causes girls to feel their bodies do not meet our culture's ideal of a thin and attractive body. In addition, girls may tie dating success to being thin, and diet to achieve thinner and more attractive figures. If the onset of menstruation and dating occur at the same time (within the same year),

Levine and Smolak argued that girls faced unique stresses with regard to dieting, body image, and eating-disordered attitudes. Smolak et al. investigated this theory and found that simultaneous onset of menstruation and dating was associated with greater body dissatisfaction and stronger eating-disordered attitudes among middle-school girls. In addition, if the onset of menstruation and dating was early, body dissatisfaction and eating-disordered attitudes were even stronger. This finding supports the second model, suggesting a synchrony in the timing of normal developmental events and the onset of eating problems.

Levine, Smolak, Moodey, Shuman, and Hessen[69] continued to evaluate the ability of the second model to explain body dissatisfaction and eating-disordered behavior. Their results suggest that a third factor, intensification of academic demands, is associated with increased risk for disordered eating. They found that if a young woman experienced these three changes (onset of menstruation, dating, and academic pressure) and she placed importance on a thin body, she was at risk for developing eating disturbances. Thus, these studies suggest that biological changes, in concert with social and academic changes, may place young women at risk for the development of a negative body image and eating-disordered behavior.

Paxton,[70] writing about peer influences on body image among adolescent girls, noted that friendship environments constitute a subculture that may place more or less emphasis on thinness and weight-loss behaviors. Friends talk about dieting, losing weight, disdain of fat, and similar topics that indicate the importance of being thin. Levine and colleagues[69,71] found that how strongly friends were perceived to value dieting and how many weight-loss techniques they used were related to an individual's investment in being thin and the number of weight loss strategies used. Thus, peers appear to serve as models for adolescent girls. Family environments may also provide models that emphasize thinness and encourage dieting and body dissatisfaction. For example, Levine and colleagues reported that girls who reported peer and family investment in thinness were at higher risk for body dissatisfaction. Rozin and Fallon[26] reported great similarity in mothers' and daughters' levels of body dissatisfaction and dieting. Rieves and Cash[72] found that college women's reports of maternal body images paralleled their reports of their own body images. If the mothers held negative body images, so did their daughters; positive maternal body images indicated positive body images among their daughters. Thus, peers and family appear to be important influences on body image for adolescent girls.

Similarly, peers and family who tease or criticize young women about their weight may also contribute to the development of negative views of their bodies. Thompson,[7] and Coovert et al.[8] reported that teasing directly influenced body-image disturbance and overall psychological distress in adolescent females. Similarly, Thompson and colleagues[73–75] and Cash and colleagues[72,76] found a history of teasing about appearance during adolescence was strongly related to body dissatisfaction in adults. In a longitudinal study, Thompson, Coovert, Richards, Johnson, and Cattarin[77] found that adolescent girls who were overweight were teased more about their appearance, which in turn was related to the development of both body image disturbances and eating disturbances.

11.2.3.3 Sociocultural Factors

The most common factor thought to influence body image is the sociocultural climate, specifically our society's emphasis on thinness as a necessary component of beauty. Several investigators have demonstrated that this pressure for thinness has intensified over recent years.[78–80] Evidence of the power of sociocultural mores comes from looking at non-Western cultures where thinness is not valued. Nassar[81] reported that in such cultures, eating disorders are much more rare than they are in Western cultures that value thinness. Indeed, for women in Western cultures, being thin represents success, competence, sexual attractiveness, and control.[82]

Women in our society are faced with more pressure than men to be thin and attractive.[83] Rodin, Silberstein, and Striegel-Moore[14] discuss how the female sex-role stereotype has two central features, the pursuit of beauty and preoccupation with beauty. Thus, in order to be a real woman, a woman has to be attractive and focused on her appearance. As noted by Fallon,[84] women in many cultures across time have spent their lives attempting to modify their bodies to fit society's notions of what is attractive and acceptable. Body image has a much greater effect on women's self-concept than it does on men's self-concept, so that happiness and self-esteem are related to how attractive a woman feels.[85]

A variety of sociocultural factors are thought to relate to body image, including the media, gender roles, and pressures from peers, friends, and family. Numerous studies have investigated the relationship between exposure to media (television, magazines, etc.) and body dissatisfaction. Some of these studies have been correlational in nature, establishing that media exposure and body dissatisfaction are related. For example, Tiggeman and Pickering[86] found that the amount of television watched by adolescent women did not relate to body dissatisfaction or drive for thinness. However, the type of program did, so that girls who spent more time watching soap operas and movies and less time watching sports reported greater body dissatisfaction. More time spent watching music videos predicted a greater drive for thinness. Levine et al.[71] reported that reading fashion magazines correlated strongly with a drive for thinness and disordered eating in 10- to 14-year-old girls.

Other studies of the media are experimental in nature (and thus can show cause and effect), and are premised on the idea that exposure to a barrage of thin, idealized women has the effect of promoting standards for thinness that are unattainable for most women, leaving them with greater levels of body dissatisfaction.[87] In an experiment by Hamilton and Waller,[88] eating-disordered women and noneating-disordered women viewed pictures of female bodies in women's fashion magazines. After exposure to the fashion models, the eating-disordered women overestimated their body size to a much greater extent than the noneating-disordered women. Similar findings were reported by Turner, Hamilton, Jacobs, Angood, and Dwyer,[89] who had undergraduate women read fashion magazines or news stories and then rated their body-image satisfaction. Women who read fashion magazines were less satisfied with their bodies, reported more frustration about their weight, were more fearful of getting fat, and were more preoccupied with wanting to be thin than women who read news magazines. Interestingly, men appear susceptible to the negative impacts of models, too. Grogan, Williams, and Conner[90] found that men and women exposed to photos of same-gender models showed a similar decline in body esteem. In a final example of the research on media effects, Heinberg and Thompson[91] found that women who had internalized societal attitudes about the importance of thinness and attractiveness became more angry after exposure to television commercials demonstrating images of thin and attractive women. Women who reported higher levels of body dissatisfaction became even more dissatisfied with their bodies after viewing these commercials. Thus, certain groups of women may be more sensitive to the effects of sociocultural messages about the importance of being thin and attractive. Indeed, Hamilton and Waller[88] suggested that therapists treating women with eating disorders advise their clients to avoid exposure to magazines that portray thin women.

Shaw and Waller[92] explain the connection between media exposure and increased body dissatisfaction with the theory of social comparison. This theory, developed by Festinger[93] states that we evaluate our own attitudes and abilities by comparing them with those of other people. Evidence exists that women compare themselves with women in the media and end up feeling worse about their bodies.[94] This tendency toward social comparison seems to be even stronger in adolescents,[92] adolescence may be a time when body image is more vulnerable to the impact of media images.

Thornton and Maurice[95] wondered if women who had not internalized sociocultural mores about the importance of physical attractiveness (including thinness) would be less likely to evaluate themselves negatively after seeing photos of thin, attractive women. Their results indicated that women who had not internalized the societal emphasis on thinness had higher self-esteem and greater body satisfaction than women who had internalized pressures to be thin. However, there were no differences between the two types of women in how negatively they felt about their bodies after exposure to the photos. In addition, women who strongly believed in the thin ideal were more likely to show evidence of disordered eating.

One explanation for the relationship between media exposure and negative body image could be that women who exhibit eating-disordered behavior and who have internalized the importance of thinness may be more likely to seek out media related to dieting and thinness. Thus, rather than media exposure as the cause of body dissatisfaction, it may be that the desire to be thin and dissatisfaction with body image cause women to expose themselves to media depicting thin ideals. This theory was studied by Harrison and Cantor,[96] who asked college women and men about their media use and disordered-eating symptomatology. Their results did not support the theory that interest in thinness-depicting media would explain the relationship between media exposure and body dissatisfaction. Harrison and Cantor's results were consistent with previous findings which showed that reading fashion magazines was linked to body dissatisfaction and eating-disorder symptomatology in women.

Stice and Shaw[97] explored the relationship between bulimic symptoms and the media's portrayal of the thin ideal. They asked female college students to view neutral pictures, pictures of normal-weight women, or pictures of thin women. After viewing the pictures, participants completed measures of ideal-body stereotype endorsement, body dissatisfaction, negative feelings, and bulimic symptoms. Women who saw the thin models felt more depression, guilt, shame, stress, body dissatisfaction, and less self-confidence than women who saw neutral pictures or pictures of normal-weight women. Body dissatisfaction and internalization of society's thin ideal were found to relate positively to bulimic symptomatology. Stice and Shaw concluded that exposure to the thin ideal leads to negative feelings, which leads in turn to body dissatisfaction, and may trigger bulimic symptoms in certain predisposed women.

A second factor thought to be related to body-image disturbance in women is adherence to society's notions of what women are supposed to be. Women who endorse more feminine traits are thought to be at higher risk for body dissatisfaction, because they will be more concerned with conforming to current images of female beauty, which means being thin and attractive. This reasoning is based on gender schema theory,[98] which posits that masculine males and feminine females are more invested in conforming to cultural standards for physical appearance and thus may be more likely to evaluate themselves in terms of those standards.[99] However, the research in this area has been contradictory. One study[100] found that masculinity, not femininity, was a better predictor of dissatisfaction with body weight in both men and women; however, the results also indicated that femininity was positively associated with concerns about dieting. Kimlicka, Cross, and Tarnai[101] reported that masculine and androgynous women were more satisfied with their bodies than feminine or undifferentiated (no gender type) women. In this study, masculinity, not femininity, was related to positive body images. Jackson et al.[99] found that feminine women rated their physical appearance more negatively than did androgynous women. As in the study by Kimlicka et al.,[101] masculine and androgynous individuals rated their physical appearance more positively than undifferentiated and feminine individuals.

Davis, Dionne, and Lazarus[102] also found that masculinity was positively related to body image in women. Interestingly, this relationship held only for women who had low levels of anxiety-proneness (neuroticism). Thus, levels of masculinity were unrelated to body image for women who reported higher levels of worry, doubt, and self-criticism. It appears that if a woman is a worrier, she will feel anxiety about her weight and shape, and this anxiety will override the positive impact that a higher level of masculinity could impose. It is important to note that the terms masculinity and femininity are not entirely accurate. Rather, masculinity is better defined as instrumentality, or possessing characteristics of being active, intentional, and competitive.[103] Similarly, femininity, as it has been measured, is more accurately characterized as being emotionally expressive, warm, compassionate, nurturant, and helpful.[103] Clearly, men and women can have both instrumental and expressive traits. The research above suggests that having instrumental traits is protective of one's body image, so long as the individual is not highly neurotic.

Martz, Handley, and Eisler[104] suggested that one reason the research literature might be contradictory concerning the relationships between gender-role endorsement and eating disorders is that the measures most commonly used (the Personal Attributes Questionnaire and the Bem Sex Role Inventory) tend to assess desirable aspects of femininity. Martz et al.[104] argue that these positive aspects are not likely to pose significant problems for mental health. Instead, they assert, measuring negative aspects of the feminine gender role would be more helpful. They examined the relations between feminine gender-role stress ("the cognitive tendency among women to appraise specific situations as highly stressful because of commitments, beliefs, and values that are a result of rigid adherence to the traditional feminine gender role"), body image, and eating disorders. They found that feminine gender role stress (FGRS) is higher in women with eating disorders than in women without eating disorders. Martz et al. also reported that women who had high FGRS levels showed cardiovascular stress reactions to having their body fat assessed, unlike women low in FGRS. The authors concluded that stress associated with the more negative aspects of adhering to the feminine gender role may predispose some women to developing problems with body image and disordered eating.

An interesting study by Snyder and Hasbrouck[105] found that neither instrumentality nor expressiveness was related to body image in women. Instead, they found that a strong feminist identity (involving a transcendence of traditional gender roles) was associated with more body-image satisfaction. By contrast, women who expressed traditional gender roles reported more body-image dissatisfaction. The authors stated that rather than a superwoman ideal, wherein a woman expects to meet both feminine and masculine role expectations, feminist identity development may involve moving beyond traditional gender role expectations, thereby reducing women's susceptibility to societal messages emphasizing the importance of thinness and attractiveness. Thus, one way to alleviate body-image disturbance among women might be to encourage the development of a feminist identity.

From the information provided regarding various sociocultural factors related to body dissatisfaction in women, it is clear that sociocultural forces play a large role in determining how women feel about their bodies. Unfortunately, our culture emphasizes a thin ideal that is not attainable for the vast majority of women. Consequently, the majority of women are dissatisfied with their bodies. This dissatisfaction has consequences for some women. One of the most drastic consequences of a negative body image seems to be the development in some women of eating disorders such as anorexia nervosa and bulimia nervosa. Research on body dissatisfaction and eating disorders has established clearly that they are linked,[15,106–108] although not everyone with a negative body image develops an eating disorder.[109]

11.3 Application of Research Question

Our research question is as follows: How can a person's body image be improved? Given all the above research, improving body image in women is an important goal and one that is difficult to achieve. Numerous forces, from the media to family and peer influences to the timing of maturation, are thought to play a role in the development of negative body images in women. However, research does suggest some available strategies aimed at helping someone who has a negative body image.

11.3.1 Treatment

Many authors suggest that using cognitive-behavioral treatment strategies is an effective means of helping reduce body image dissatisfaction. For example, Butters and Cash[110] used cognitive-behavioral therapy that combined education about the prevalence, causes, and consequences of body dissatisfaction, relaxation training, desensitization to reduce anxiety about the body, challenging of automatic negative thoughts about the body, stress inoculation, modification of behavioral avoidance, and relapse prevention. Their findings indicated that individuals receiving this cognitive-behavioral treatment showed significant improvements in body image and overall functioning when compared to a control group that did not receive the treatment. Similar results were reported in a follow-up study by Rosen, Saltzberg, and Srebnik,[111] who also found that education and support alone were not enough to increase satisfaction with body image.

Rosen[112,113] suggested use of a body-image diary to record situations that produce negative thoughts about appearance and to indicate how the thoughts affect mood and behavior. Then each individual could be taught how to replace these negative thoughts with more positive ones, especially if the negative thoughts suggest that she is bad, unlovable, and/or lazy because of her physical appearance. Rosen also suggested including a program of gradual bodily exposure, first in private and then moving slowly to more public situations, such as wearing a swimsuit at a public pool.

Other authors use other theoretical approaches to treat body dissatisfaction. For example, Wooley[114] presents a feminist approach that emphasizes the importance of enabling the individual to choose what kind of body she wants and how she wants to achieve it. Shaw and Waller[92] argue that helping individuals to decrease their social comparison behaviors through individual and/or group therapy is a key to success. Shisslak and Crago[115] suggest a multifaceted approach that includes imagery, drawing or sculpting techniques, mirror work (gradual exposure), positive affirmations, group feedback to correct distorted body images, and moving to music.

Kearney-Cooke and Striegel-Moore[116] believe that helping women to focus on themselves and to develop their own visions of what they value in life will strengthen their intrinsic power, or sense of mastery and potency, in dealing with life. Feeling more intrinsic power will help women develop "a more proactive, life-affirming focus on acceptance of their bodies and a commitment to take care of them." In addition, the authors describe how guided imagery can be an effective strategy in changing clients' body schemas. Finally, Kearney-Cooke and Striegel-Moore suggest that cognitive techniques such as using a positive continuum to evaluate one's body and teaching clients to look for moments in their lives when they feel accepting of their bodies rather than rejecting them is very helpful.

References

1. Thompson, J. K., *Body Image Disturbance: Assessment and Treatment*, Pergamon Press, New York, 1990.
2. Slade, P. D., A review of body-image studies in anorexia nervosa and bulimia nervosa, *Journal of Psychiatric Research*, 19, 255–265, 1985.
3. Slade, P. D. and Russell, G. G. M., Awareness of body dimensions in anorexia nervosa: cross-sectional and longitudinal studies. *Psychological Medicine*, 3, 188–199, 1973.
4. Slade, P. D., What is body image? *Behavior Research, and Therapy*, 32, 497–502, 1994.
5. Pasman, L. and Thompson, J. K., Body image and eating disturbance in obligatory runners, obligatory weightlifters, and sedentary individuals, *International Journal of Eating Disorders*, 7, 759–769, 1988.
6. Thompson, J. K., Berland, N. W., Linton, P. H., and Weinsier, R., Assessment of body distortion via a self-adjusting light beam in seven eating disorder groups, *International Journal of Eating Disorders*, 7, 113–120, 1986.
7. Thompson, J. K., Body image: extent of disturbance, associated features, theoretical models, assessment methodologies, intervention strategies, and a proposal for a new DSM IV diagnostic category – Body Image Disorder, *Progress in Behavior Modification*, vol. 29, Hersen, M., Eisler, R. M., and Miller, P. M., Eds., Sage, New York, 1992, 3–54.
8. Coovert, D. L., Thompson, J. K., and Kinder, B. N., Interrelationships among multiple aspects of body image and eating disturbance, *International Journal of Eating Disorders*, 7, 495–502, 1988.
9. Penner, L. A., Thompson, J. K., and Coovert, D. L., Size estimation among anorexics: much ado about very little? *Journal of Abnormal Psychology*, 100, 90–93, 1991.
10. Smeets, M. A. M. and Panhuysen, G. E. M., What can be learned from body size estimation? It all depends on your theory, *Eating Disorders: The Journal of Treatment and Prevention*, 3, 101–114, 1995.
11. Thompson, J. K., Altabe, M. N., Johnson, S., and Stormer, S., Multiple measures of body image disturbance: are we all measuring the same construct? *International Journal of Eating Disorders*, 16, 311–315, 1994.
12. Williamson, D. A., Barker, S. E., Bertman, L. J., and Gleaves, D. H., Body image, body dysphoria, and dietary restraint: factor structure in nonclinical subjects, *Behavior Research and Therapy*, 33, 85–93, 1995.
13. Whitaker, A., Davies, M., Shaffer, D., Johnson, J., Abrams, S., Walsh, T., and Kalikow, K., The struggle to be thin: a survey of anorexic and bulimic symptoms in a non-referred adolescent population, *Psychological Medicine*, 19, 143–163, 1989.
14. Rodin, J., Silberstein, L. R., and Striegel-Moore, R. H., Women and weight: a normative discontent, in *Nebraska Symposium on Motivation: Psychology and Gender*, Sonderegger, T.B., Ed., University of Nebraska Press, Lincoln, 1985, 267–307.
15. Cash, T. F. and Deagle, E. A., III, The nature and extent of body-image disturbances in anorexia nervosa and bulimia nervosa: a meta-analysis, *International Journal of Eating Disorders*, 22, 107–125, 1997.

16. Cash, T. F. and Henry, P. E., Women's body images: the results of a national survey in the U.S.A, *Sex Roles*, 33, 19–28, 1995.

17. Drewnowski, A. and Yee, D. K., Men and body-image: are males satisfied with their body weight? *Psychosomatic Medicine*, 49, 626–634, 1987.

18. Collins, M. E., Body figure perceptions and preferences among preadolescent children, *International Journal of Eating Disorders*, 10, 199–208, 1991.

19. Thompson, S. H., Corwin, S. J., and Sargent, R. G., Ideal body size beliefs and weight concerns of fourth-grade children, *International Journal of Eating Disorders*, 21, 279–284, 1997.

20. Altabe, M. and Thompson, J. K., Body image changes during early adulthood, *International Journal of Eating Disorders*, 13, 323–328, 1993.

21. Furnham, A. and Greaves, N., Gender and locus of control correlates of body image dissatisfaction, *European Journal of Personality*, 8, 183–200, 1994.

22. McCauley, M. C., Mintz, L. B., and Glenn, A. G., Body image self-esteem and depression: closing the gender gap, *Sex Roles*, 18, 381–391, 1988.

23. Mintz, L. B. and Betz, N. E., Sex differences in the nature, realism, and correlates of body image, *Sex Roles*, 15, 185–195, 1986.

24. Muth, J. L. and Cash, T. F., Body-image attitudes: what difference does gender make? *Journal of Applied Social Psychology*, 27, 1438–1452, 1997.

25. Pliner, P., Chaiken, S., and Flett, G. L., Gender differences in concern with body weight and physical appearance over the life span, *Personality and Social Psychology Bulletin*, 16, 263–273, 1990.

26. Rozin, P. and Fallon, A., Body image, attitudes towards weight, and misperceptions of figure preferences of the opposite sex: a comparison of men and women in two generations. *Journal of Abnormal Psychology*, 97, 342–345, 1988.

27. Gupta, M. A., Schork, N. J., and Dhaliwal, J. S., Stature, drive for thinness and body dissatisfaction: a study of males and females from a non-clinical sample, *Canadian Journal of Psychiatry*, 38, 59–61, 1993.

28. Silberstein, L. R., Striegel-Moore, R. H., Timko, C., and Rodin, J., Behavioral and psychological implications of body dissatisfaction: do men and women differ? *Sex Roles*, 19, 219–232, 1988.

29. Abell, S. C. and Richards, M. H., The relationship between body shape satisfaction and self-esteem: an investigation of gender and class differences, *Journal of Youth and Adolescence*, 25, 691–703, 1996.

30. Cash, T. F. and Brown, T. A., Gender and body images: stereotypes and realities, *Sex Roles*, 21, 361–373, 1989.

31. Jacobi, L. and Cash, T. A., In pursuit of the perfect appearance: discrepancies among self-ideal percepts of multiple physical attributes, *Journal of Applied Social Psychology*, 24, 379–396, 1994.

32. Mintz, L. B. and Kashubeck, S., Body image and disordered eating in Asian and Caucasian college students: An examination of race and gender differences, *Psychology of Women Quarterly*, 23, 781–796.

33. Kashubeck, S. and Mintz, L. B., Gender and body image in people wanting to lose weight, presented at the 105th Annual Convention of the American Psychological Association, Chicago, August, 1998.

34. Rothblum, E. Women and weight: fad and fiction. *Journal of Psychology*, 124, 5–24, 1990.

35. Harris, S. M., Racial differences in predictors of women's body image attitudes, *Women and Health*, 2, 89–104, 1994.

36. Abood, D. A. and Chandler, S. B., Race and the role of weight, weight change, and body dissatisfaction in eating disorders, *American Journal of Health Behavior*, 21, 21–25, 1997.

37. Gray, J. J., Ford, K., and Kelly, L. M., The prevalence of bulimia in a black college population, *International Journal of Eating Disorders*, 6, 733–740, 1987.

38. Rosen, J. C. and Gross, J., Prevalence of weight reducing and weight gaining in adolescent girls and boys, *Health Psychology*, 6, 131–147, 1987.

39. Rucker, C. E. and Cash, T. F., Body images, body-size perceptions, and eating behaviors among African American and White college women, *International Journal of Eating Disorders*, 12, 291–299, 1992.

40. Wilfley, D. E., Schreiber, G. B., Pike, K. M., Striegel-Moore, R. H., Wright, D. J., and Rodin, J., Eating disturbance and body image: a comparison of a community sample of adult black and white women, *International Journal of Eating Disorders*, 20, 377–387, 1996.

41. Kuczmarski, R. J., Flegal, K. M., Campbell, S. M., and Johnson, C. L., Increasing prevalence of overweight among U.S. adults, *Journal of the American Medical Association*, 272, 205–211, 1994.

42. Caldwell, M. B., Brownell, K. D., and Wilfley, D. E., Relationship of weight, body dissatisfaction, and self-esteem in African American and white female dieters, *International Journal of Eating Disorders*, 22, 127–130, 1997.

43. Dolan, B., Lacey, J. H., and Evans, C., Eating behaviour and attitudes to weight and shape in British women from three ethnic groups, *British Journal of Psychiatry*, 157, 523–528, 1990.

44. Pumariega, A. J., Gustavson, C. R., Gustavson, J. C., Motes, P. S. and Ayers, S., Eating attitudes in African-American women: The Essence Eating Disorders Survey, *Eating Disorders: The Journal of Treatment and Prevention*, 2, 5–16, 1994.

45. Rosen, J. C., Silberg, N. T., and Gross, J., Eating Attitudes Test and Eating Disorder Inventory: norms for adolescent girls and boys, *Journal of Consulting and Clinical Psychology*, 56, 305–308, 1988.

46. Root, M. P., Disordered eating in women of color, *Sex Roles*, 22, 525–536, 1990.

47. Singh, D., Body fat distribution and perception of desirable female body shape by young black men and women, *International Journal of Eating Disorders*, 16, 289–294, 1994.

48. Lester, R. and Petrie, T. A., Physical, psychological, and societal correlates of bulimic symptomatology among African American college women, *Journal of Counseling Psychology*, 45, 315–321, 1998.

49. Sobal, J. and Stunkard, A. J., Socioeconomic status and obesity: a review of the literature, *Psychological Bulletin*, 105, 260–275, 1989.

50. Allan, J. D., Mayo, K., and Michel, Y., Body size values of white and black women, *Research in Nursing and Health*, 16, 323–333, 1993.

51. Hall, C. C. I., Asian eyes: body image and eating disorders of Asian and Asian American women, *Eating Disorders: The Journal of Treatment and Prevention*, 3, 8–19, 1995.

52. Akan, G. E. and Grilo, C. M., Sociocultural influences on eating attitudes and behaviors, body image, and psychological functioning: a comparison of African-American, Asian American and Caucasian college women, *International Journal of Eating Disorders*, 18, 181–187, 1995.

53. Johnson, C. Lewis, C., Love, S. Lewis, L. and Stuckey, M., Incidence and correlates of bulimic behavior in a female high school population, *International Journal of Youth and Adolescence*, 13, 15 –26, 1984.

54. Lucero, K., Hicks, R. A., Bramlette, J., Brassington, G. S., and Welter, M. G., Frequency of eating problems among Asian and Caucasian college women, *Psychological Reports*, 71, 255–258, 1992.

55. Nevo, S., Bulimic symptoms: prevalence and ethnic differences among college women. *International Journal of Eating Disorders*, 4, 151–168, 1985.

56. Gross, J. and Rosen, J., Bulimia in adolescents: prevalence and psychosocial correlates, *International Journal of Eating Disorders*, 7, 55–61, 1988.

57. Story, M., French, S. A., Resnick, M. D., and Blum, R. W., Ethnic/racial and socio-economic differences in dieting behaviors and body image perceptions in adolescents, *International Journal of Eating Disorders*, 18, 173–179, 1995.

58. Crago, M., Shisslak, C. M., and Estes, L. S., Eating disturbances among American minority groups: a review, *International Journal of Eating Disorders*, 19, 239–248, 1996.

59. Striegel-Moore, R. and Smolak, L., The role of race in the development of eating disorders, in *The Developmental Psychopathology of Eating Disorders: Implications for Research, Prevention, and Treatment*, Smolak, L., Levine, M. P., Striegel-Moore, R., Eds., Lawrence Erlbaum Associates, Mahwah, NJ, 259–284, 1996.

60. Heffernan, K., Eating disorders and weight concern among lesbians, *International Journal of Eating Disorders*, 19, 127–138, 1996.

61. Dworkin, S. H., Not in man's image: lesbians and the cultural oppression of body image, *Women and Therapy*, 8, 27–39, 1989.

62. Beren, S. E., Hayden, H. A., Wilfley, D. E., and Grilo, C. M., The influence of sexual orientation on body dissatisfaction in adult men and women, *International Journal of Eating Disorders*, 20, 135–141, 1996.

63. Smolak, L., Levine, M. P., and Gralen, S., The impact of puberty and dating on eating problems among middle school girls, *Journal of Youth and Adolescence*, 22, 355–368, 1993.

64. Keel, P. K., Fulkerson, J. A., and Leon, G. R., Disordered eating precursors in pre- and early adolescent girls and boys, *Journal of Youth and Adolescence*, 26, 203–216, 1997.

65. Attie, I. and Brooks-Gunn, J., Development of eating problems in adolescent girls: a longitudinal study, *Developmental Psychology*, 25, 70–79, 1989.

66. Killen, J. D., Hayward, C., Litt, I., Hammer, L. D., Wilson, D. M., Miner, B., Taylor, C. B., Varady, A., and Shisslak, C., Is puberty a risk factor for eating disorders? *American Journal of Diseases of Children*, 146, 323–325, 1992.

67. Killen, J. D., Hayward, C., Wilson, D. M., Taylor, C. B., Hammer, L. D., Litt, I., Simmonds, B., and Haydel, F., Factors associated with eating disorder symptoms in a community sample of 6th and 7th grade girls, *International Journal of Eating Disorders*, 15, 357–367, 1994.

68. Levine, M. P. and Smolak, L., Toward a developmental psychopathology of eating disorders, in *The Etiology of Bulimia: The Individual and Familial Contexts*, Crowther, J. Hobfoll, S. Stephens, M., and Tennenbaum, D., Eds., Hemisphere Publishers, Washington, D.C., 1992, 59–80.

69. Levine, M. P., Smolak, L., Moodey, A. F., Shuman, M. D., and Hessen, L. D. Normative developmental challenges and dieting and eating disturbances in middle school girls, *International Journal of Eating Disorders*, 15, 11–20, 1994b.

70. Paxton, S. J., Prevention implications of peer influences on body image dissatisfaction and disturbed eating in adolescent girls, *Eating Disorders: The Journal of Treatment and Prevention*, 4, 334–337, 1996.

71. Levine, M. P., Smolak, L., and Hayden, H., The relation of sociocultural factors to eating attitudes and behavior among middle school girls, *Journal of Early Adolescence*, 14, 471–490, 1994a.

72. Rieves, L. and Cash, T. F., Social developmental factors and women's body-image attitudes, *Journal of Social Behavior and Personality*, 11, 63–78, 1996.

73. Thompson, J. K., Body shape preferences: effects of instructional protocol and level of eating disturbance, *International Journal of Eating Disorders*, 10, 193–198, 1991.

74. Thompson, J. K., Fabian, L. J., Moulton, D. O., Dunn, M. F., and Altabe, M. N., Development and validation of the physical appearance related testing scale, *Journal of Personality Assessment*, 56, 513–521, 1991.

75. Thompson, J. K. and Psaltis, K., Multiple aspects and correlations of body figure ratings: a replication and extension of Fallon and Rozine (1985), *International Journal of Eating Disorders*, 7, 813–818, 1988.

76. Cash, T. F., Developmental teasing about physical appearance: retrospective descriptions and relationships with body image, *Social Behavior and Personality*, 23, 123–130, 1995.

77. Thompson, J. K., Coovert, M. D., Richards, K. J., Johnson, S., and Cattarin, J., Development of body image, eating disturbance, and general psychological functioning in female adolescents: covariance structure modeling and longitudinal investigations, *International Journal of Eating Disorders*, 18, 221–236, 1995.

78. Garner, D. M., Garfinkel, P. E., Schwartz, D., and Thompson, M., Cultural expectations of thinness in women, *Psychological Reports*, 47, 483–491, 1980.

79. Silverstein, B., Peterson, B., and Perdue, L., Some correlates of the thin standard of bodily attractiveness for women, *International Journal of Eating Disorders*, 5, 895–905, 1986.

80. Wiseman, M. A., Gray, J. J., Mosimann, J. E., and Ahrens, A. H., Cultural expectations of thinness in women: an update, *International Journal of Eating Disorders*, 11, 85–89, 1992.

81. Nassar, M., Culture and weight consciousness, *Journal of Psychosomatic Research*, 32, 573–577, 1988.

82. Wilfley, D. E. and Rodin, J., Cultural influences on eating disorders, in *Eating Disorders and Obesity: A Comprehensive Handbook*, Brownell, K. D. and Fairburn, C. G., Eds., Guilford Press, New York, 78–82, 1995.

83. Fallon, A. E., Body image and the regulation of weight, in *Psychological Perspectives on Women's Health*, Adesso, V. J., Reddy, D. M., and Fleming, R., Eds., Taylor and Francis, Washington, D.C., 1994, 127–180.

84. Fallon, A. E., Culture in the mirror: sociocultural determinants of body image, in *Body Images: Development, Deviance and Change*, Cash, T. and Pruzinsky, T., Eds., Guilford Press, New York, 1990, 80–109.

85. Wadden, T. A., Brown, G., Foster, G. D., and Linowitz, J. R., Salience of weight-related worries in adolescent males and females, *International Journal of Eating Disorders*, 10, 407–414, 1991.

86. Tiggeman, M. and Pickering, A. S., Role of television in adolescent women's body dissatisfaction and drive for thinness, *International Journal of Eating Disorders*, 20, 199–203, 1996.

87. Nemeroff, C. J., Stein, R. I., Diehl, N. S., and Smilack, K. M., From the Cleavers to the Clintons: role, choices and body orientation as reflected in magazine article content, *International Journal of Eating Disorders*, 16, 167–176, 1994.

88. Hamilton, K. and Waller, G., Media influences on body size estimation in anorexia and bulimia: an experimental study, *British Journal of Psychiatry*, 162, 837–840, 1993.

89. Turner, S. L., Hamilton, H., Jacobs, M., Angood, L. M., and Dwyer, D. H., The influence of fashion magazines on the body image satisfaction of college women: an exploratory analysis, *Adolescence*, 32, 603–614, 1997.

90. Grogan, S., Williams, Z., and Conner, M., The effects of viewing same-gender photographic models on body-esteem, *Psychology of Women Quarterly*, 20, 569–575, 1996.

91. Heinberg, L. J. and Thompson, J. K., Body image and televised images of thinness and attractiveness: a controlled laboratory investigation, *Journal of Social and Clinical Psychology*, 14, 325–338, 1995.

92. Shaw, J. and Waller, C., The media's impact on body image: implications for prevention and treatment, *Eating Disorders: The Journal of Treatment and Prevention*, 3, 8–19, 1995.

93. Festinger, L., A theory of social comparison processes, *Human Relations*, 7, 117–140.

94. Richins, M. L., Social comparison and the idealized images of advertising, *Journal of Consumer Research*, 18, 71–83, 1991.

95. Thornton, B. and Maurice, J., Physique contrast effect: adverse impact of idealized body images for women, *Sex Roles*, 37, 433–439, 1997.

96. Harrison, K. and Cantor, J., The relationship between media consumption and eating disorders, *Journal of Communication*, 47, 40–67, 1997.

97. Stice, E. and Shaw, H. E., Adverse effects of the media-portrayed thin ideal on women and linkages to bulimic symptomatology, *Journal of Social and Clinical Psychology*, 13, 288–308, 1994.

98. Bem, S. L., Gender schema theory: a cognitive account of sex typing, *Psychological Review*, 88, 354–364, 1981.

99. Jackson, L. A., Sullivan, L. A., and Rostker, R., Gender, gender role, and body image, *Sex Roles*, 19, 429–443, 1988.

100. Hawkins, R. C., Turell, S., and Jackson, L. J., Desirable and undesirable masculine and feminine traits in relation to students' dieting tendencies and body image dissatisfaction, *Sex Roles*, 9, 705–718, 1983.

101. Kimlicka, T., Cross, H., and Tarnai, J. A., A comparison of androgynous, feminine, masculine, and undifferentiated women on self-esteem, body satisfaction, and sexual satisfaction, *Psychology of Women Quarterly*, 7, 291–294, 1983.

102. Davis, C., Dionne, M., and Lazarus, L., Gender-role orientation and body image in women and men: the moderating influence of neuroticism, *Sex Roles*, 34, 493–505, 1996.

103. Spence, J. T. and Helmreich, R. L., *Personal Attributes Questionnaire (PAQ) and Extended Personal Attributes Questionnaire (EPAQ)*. Unpublished manuscript, 1996.

104. Martz, D. M., Handley, K. B., and Eisler, R. M., The relationship between feminine gender role stress, body image, and eating disorders, *Psychology of Women Quarterly*, 19, 493–508, 1995.

105. Snyder, R. and Hasbrouck, L., Feminist identity, gender traits, and symptoms of disturbed eating among college women, *Psychology of Women Quarterly*, 20, 593–598, 1996.

106. Nelson, C. L. and Gidycz, C. A., A comparison of body image perception in bulimics, restrainers, and normal women: an extension of previous findings, *Addictive Behaviors*, 18, 503–509, 1993.

107. Williamson, D. A., Cubic, B. A., and Gleaves, D. H., Equivalence of body image disturbance in anorexia and bulimia nervosa, *Journal of Abnormal Psychology*, 102, 177–180, 1993.

108. Veron-Guidry, S., Williamson, D. A., and Netemeyer, R. G., Structural modeling analysis of body dysphoria and eating disorder symptoms in preadolescent girls, *Eating Disorders: The Journal of Treatment and Prevention*, 5, 15–27, 1997.

109. Santonastaso, P., Favaro, A., Ferrara, S., Sala, A., and Zanetti, T., Prevalence of body image disturbance in a female adolescent sample: a longitudinal study, *Eating Disorders: The Journal of Treatment and Prevention*, 3, 342–350, 1995.

110. Butters, J. W. and Cash, T. F., Cognitive-behavioral treatment of women's body-image dissatisfaction, *Journal of Consulting and Clinical Psychology*, 55, 889–897, 1987.

111. Rosen, J. C., Saltzberg, E., and Srebnik, D., Cognitive behavior therapy for negative body image, *Behavior Therapy*, 20, 393–404, 1989.

112. Rosen, J. C., Assessment and treatment of body image disturbance, in *Eating Disorders and Obesity: A Comprehensive Handbook*, Brownell, K. D. and Fairburn, C. G., Eds., Guilford Press, New York, 1995, 369–373.

113. Rosen, J. C., Cognitive-behavioral body image therapy, in *Handbook of Treatment for Eating Disorders*, 2nd ed., Garner, D.M. and Garfinkel, P.E., Eds., Guilford Press, New York, 1997, 188–201.

114. Wooley, S. C., Feminist influences on the treatment of eating disorders, in *Eating Disorders and Obesity*, Brownell, K. D. and Fairburn, C. G., Eds., Guilford Press, New York, 1995, 294–297.

115. Shisslak, C. M. and Crago, M., Toward a new model for the prevention of eating disorders, in *Feminist Perspectives on Eating Disorders*, Fallon, P., Katzman, M. A., and Wooley, S. C., Eds., Guilford Press, New York, 1994, 419–437.

116. Kearney-Cooke, A. and Striegel-Moore, R., The etiology and treatment of body image disturbance, in *Handbook of Treatment for Eating Disorders*, 2nd ed., Garner, D. M. and Garfinkel, P. E., Eds., Guilford Press, New York, 1997, 295–306.

12

Eating Disorders and Sexuality

Jan S. Richter

CONTENTS

12.1 Learning Objectives

Upon completion of this chapter you should be able to:

- Understand the risk factors contributing to an eating disorder;
- Describe sexuality's biological, social, and experiential correlation to fatness;
- Analyze the dynamics that characterize the anorexic's psychosexual development;
- Articulate the socialization of the female anorexic's as it relates to gender roles and gender identity;
- Examine the sexist ideals of body size with relation to eating disorders;
- Differentiate bulimia nervosa's biological, experiential and social correlation to fatness from that of anorexia nervosa;
- Compare and contrast the sexual behavior and attitudes of the bulimic to those of the anorexic;
- Explain sexual orientation and its relationship to males with eating disorders.

12.2 Research Background

Two of life's most basic instincts are sex and eating. The two are commonly linked through literary allusion, sexual slang and innuendo, and jaunty humor.[1] Communal gatherings such as marriages, anniversaries and births link celebratory eating with occasions that exude subtle undertones of sexual intimacies. Sexual humor associated with eating saturates our social dialogue. Ravenous appetites after lustful bouts of lovemaking or a sexually sparked courtship ignited over succulent food, wine, and candlelight are the hallmarks of cliché. This characterization is accentuated by the kitchens in our homes. Although the kitchen symbolizes platonic, affectionate nurturance, it offers what is most needed by our families: bodily sustenance. The presence of an eating disorder suggests the inability of the one who suffers to attain gratification through love and to convert that love into life-enhancing sexuality.[2]

In North American culture, there is an uneasiness with the body in its natural state. Western cultures have a long history of regarding the human body as licentious.[3] This prevailing attitude influences the ways in which evolving adolescents regard their bodies, a concern that extends to the parts that are sexual. Contemporary psychoanalysts believe sexuality has a role in the most serious distortions of body image, such as those seen in anorexia nervosa and bulimia nervosa.[4] However, current research supports the fact that sexuality alone is not always the single substantive issue for many anorexics and bulimics. More central to eating disorders is sexuality's biological, social, and experiential correlation to fatness.[2]

Theoretically, the biological emergence of adolescent sexuality cannot be divorced from pubertal development and the development of body fat. The linkage is significant.[5] The onset of the menstrual cycle is critically connected to the fat threshold necessary for menstruation to occur. Furthermore, the development of secondary sex characteristics is dependent upon the development of a certain percentage of body fat. Hence, the emerging sexuality of the adolescent female is critically linked physiologically to fat. Because, today's adolescents develop physically earlier than any preceding generation of women, and do so in a society that does not protect them, eating disorders are unnatural consequences of this radical development. In some cases, eating disorders are attempts by adolescents to regress to a pre-adolescent state in which sexuality and sexual feelings are effectively banished.[6] Thereby, they render themselves biologically asexual, while simultaneously creating a façade of protection against society's psychological molestation of their bodies.

The young adolescent female in Western culture finds no relief from the unrelenting self-scrutiny on which the media and their markets thrive. Contemporary culture exacerbates normal adolescent self-consciousness and encourages precocious sexuality.[7] Socially, our culture places a heavy emphasis on physical attraction, particularly during adolescence and young adulthood. To be sexually appealing, women may enlarge their breast size, subject themselves to severe diet restrictions, suction fat from their buttocks and thighs, wear constricting and uncomfortable shoes and clothes, and alter their hair colors. Most fear of fat is centered not on health but on physical appearance.[8] The answer to the prevailing adolescent angst of, "Who am I? What do I want to be?" centers on the body.[5]

The body has become an obsession, and our contemporary culture is especially preoccupied with a passion to be thin that has been subconsciously internalized.[5] This rage to be thin is a recent phenomenon, emerging in Western culture in only the last 60 years. For over six centuries before that, the maternal woman's soft body was idealized, and the fatness of her supple body considered fashionable and sexually erotic.[9]

This current widespread adolescent preoccupation with curbing body shape and appetite is socially connected to a world that worships a new definition of physical perfection.[10] Ideal body shape and size are culturally relative concepts, and the cultural norm in the United States for both men and women is becoming slimmer and slimmer. Television portrays our deities as slim, sexy, perfectly muscled actors, models, and athletes. Female centerfolds are taller today than in any past decade, but instead of depicting normal weight gain appropriate to height, the models have drastically and abnormally reduced their weight in relation to their height.[11] The objectification of women in our society has never been as pervasive as it is at present.

An adolescent may subconsciously feel that by accepting the curves of her body she accepts the objectification of the true self[5], and thereby accepts the traditional gender role expected of her. Becoming asexual through excessive thinness can be a means of retreat from a hypersexual environment.[12] It is not unusual for adolescents to experience fear and feelings of powerlessness as their bodies and roles change. Refusing to eat can be viewed as rebellion against models of femininity, female subservience, and gender ineffectiveness. Acquiring an asexual body is a means of retreating from the powerful sources of sexuality.[13] For some females, manipulation of their own bodies may be the only area over which they feel control and strength.

For adolescents, sexuality can appear dangerous and wicked on the one hand, and desirable and beautiful on the other. The conflict thus generated can result in sexuality becoming disembodied from the person.[12] Compounding this adolescent paradox is today's beleaguered parents. Parents expect their children to be autonomous, competent, and sophisticated by the time they reach adolescence.[14] This expectance of pseudo-sophistication has caused extreme stress among young people trying to adjust emotionally to their developing bodies and new social roles in a hypersexual culture in which most parental figures, are physically and emotionally inaccessible to their adolescent children. And, the bodies of adolescent daughters have borne the brunt.

Ultimately, the general relaxation of sexual mores that occurred during the 1960s has had a more powerful influence on females. Studies of sexual behaviors in the past three decades indicate that female adolescents are becoming more sexually active at an earlier age with their sexual experiences now differing little from those of their male counterparts.[5] Furthermore, the current cultural climate points in the direction of sexual permissiveness. The eroticization of our homes by television, sexualized pre-adolescent fashion models, and pornography has not been healthy. In some cases, vulnerable adolescents have developed a symptom — eating disorders — that represents a radical avoidance and withdrawal from the implications of sexuality.[2] Adolescents are trying to find order in a sexual environment in which traditional middle-class sexual self-regulation has unraveled.[15] Eating disorders may represent the need to control this state of sexual chaos. The ones who suffer regress to a pre-pubertal state in which sexual feelings and experiences are effectively banished, thereby allowing the victims to feel a sense of control and a means to power over their sexual-social environment while negating the cultural ideals of femaleness.

Contemporary psychoanalysts are cognizant of the association between experiential sexuality and eating disorders for adolescents. However, rather than seeing sexuality at the core of the problem, most psychoanalysts see unwanted or negative sexual experience as the trigger that sparks a crisis in adolescent self confidence, which tends to precipitate restrictive dieting.[16] Early sexual and physical abuse may trigger feelings of being unclean or unworthy when the innate sexual drive intensifies at puberty. Abused individuals often feel empty and demoralized, with a full response to sexuality engendering even greater feelings of self-fragmentation. Patients with eating disorders tend to have concerns, questions, and problems about hurtful past sexual experiences, as well as ideas about sex that lead them to hide their suffering from others. They tend to restrict their normal sexual interests and pleasures as much as they restrict adequate and normal eating. By inhibiting their sexual responses, individuals with eating disorders feel in greater control over themselves and their partners. This control may be especially important if they feel a lack of competence in other areas of their lives. In some cases, consensual first intercourse is viewed as disgusting or painful. This view can exacerbate an already vulnerable self-concept. To a vulnerable adolescent in some instances first intercourse can be as drastic an experience as sexual assault or sexual abuse. Perceived or real, experiences of sexual violation and body vulnerability are experientially connected and implicated in anorexia nervosa and bulimia nervosa and represent the victim's method of ridding the body of every emerging sign of femaleness.[15]

Correspondingly, clinical experience suggests an unusually high rate of sexual abuse among adolescents with eating disorders. Theoretically, sexuality and its link to experiential encounters cannot be ignored. More often than not, clinicians who work with eating disorders often find clients with histories of incest or sexual abuse. These adolescents have been raised to be fearful of sex and to view the body as dirty or sinful.[16] Sexual dysfunction and inhibitions are very common occurrences among those with eating disorders.

As we enter the millennium, living in a female body is more complicated than it was 100 years ago. Diet and exercise programs designed for women, body sculpturing, liposuction, and breast augmentation, indicate that the female has internalized the contemporary absolute of a perfect body. On one hand, society tells females that their gender role is not a barrier to achievement, yet females of this generation have learned very early that their power is linked to what they look like and how sexy they are. This generation of females spends exorbitant amounts of time denying hunger and working on their bodies. They walk the precipice between normal and pathological; they live in a culture of unrelenting objectification. As a community, we have not yet seen the crest of this millennial phenomenon.[20]

12.3   Application of Research Question

Why are women with eating disorders so victimized by the cultural ideal of beauty, power, and sex as glamorized by societal expectations? What type of backgrounds do they come from; how do they feel about their sexual instincts, and what do their striking thinness and sexual behaviors signify? Are males also victims of unrealistic demands made by society for a sexy body and the power the attainment of this ideal has to offer?

12.3.1   Anorexia Nervosa and Sexuality

Anorexics frequently come from religious backgrounds characterized by strict puritanical attitudes toward female sexuality. Anorexics see their sexual instincts as unacceptable. They feel dirtiness inculcated by messages about menstrual staining and sanitation through deodorization. They feel a need to be punished for any acknowledgment of sexual drive. They must control sexuality to the greatest degree possible, for fear they will be rejected for being sexually interested or punished for becoming sexually out of control.[2]

Among adolescents concerned with the transition to adulthood, these intense concerns with appetite control and their bodies work in tandem. With increasing anxiety over sexuality and the implications of changing gender roles, sex is the second important arena of social change (the first being the shift away from the maternal body ideal) that may contribute to the rising number of anorexics. There are in fact, some justifiable social reasons why contemporary young women fear adult womanhood. The anorexic generations, particularly those born after 1960, have been subject to a set of insecurities that make heterosexuality an anxious rather than pleasant prospect.[5] From childhood on, family insecurity reflected in the frequency of divorce and changing sex and gender roles has become a fact of life for this group. These youngsters have grown up with men and women on different sides of the bargaining table. They have heard angry voices, and they have seen relationships torn asunder and families renegotiated. Although no positive correlation between divorced families and anorexia nervosa is evident, family disruption is a part of the world-view of the anorexic generation. Its members understand implicitly that not all heterosexual relationships have happy endings.[17]

Therefore, anorexics articulate their socialization as females in terms of confusion about gender roles and female identity. Many report having grown up with secret fantasies about being male, which began at puberty.[9] This fantasy is not analogous with conflicts related to sexual identity, biological genitalia assignment, or with issues related to sexual orientation. This fantasy more correctly illustrates the anorexic's identification with an ideal, asexual intellectuality related to traditional and non-traditional roles that are socially and culturally assigned to males and females.[18]

Accordingly, anorexia is a desire to escape womanhood and to achieve a certain type of masculine ideal. Anorexics will attempt to disengage themselves from their own bodily feelings of femaleness to bond with their father's expectations of them, thereby provoking the emotional disconnections they have from their mothers. Theirs is an ideal of intellectual and spiritual puberty, rather than physical puberty, as the central theme within the dynamics of their families.[18]

This quandary mirrors the real-world situation in which the female role is changing, and therefore, sexist ideals of body size are imposed even more insistently in order for the anorexic to attain a sense of control. The making of the thinness ideal reflects a conspiratorial effort to keep women in their places, and the anorexic female colludes and joins in the conspiracy by internalizing the misogynistic hatred of female fatness exhibited by women's round breasts, hips, and curves. The current epidemic of eating disorders is a reflection of the ambiguity of female sexual roles and sexual identity in a century rife with ambiguity.[17] Ironically, as women's gender relationships with males change, more and more cases of anorexia nervosa are diagnosed.

It is interesting that anorexic females tend to be popular with males. They long for male power and intellectualization, yet through their eating disorder, they dangerously epitomize the ideal cultural definition of femaleness, which is thin, pampered, weak, and eager to please. These young women report that up until hospitalization, they are often complimented by males on their appearance. Anorexia nervosa is a metaphor. It is a young woman's statement that she will become what she believes the culture asks of its women. She will be thin and non-threatening. Anorexia signifies she is so delicate she needs a male to shelter and protect her from a world she cannot control. Anorexics, with their bodies, tell society they will take up only a small amount of space; they won't intimidate or threaten anyone. Who is afraid of a 70-pound adult or, to be more exact, an adult-child? [15]

Therefore, the cultural ideal of female thinness to which anorexics aspire may be related to aspirations for equal power with men.[8] Conflicts between new cultural ideals and traditional identification with eating disorders in women reinforce the dilemma of the anorexics who have difficulty reconciling their own intellectual aspirations with their femaleness. Their solution to the dilemma is to diminish the female characterization of the body, which can be interpreted on one level as a means to control their conflict and on another as an their internalization of cultural misogyny.[13]

In friendlier terms, eating is an expression of the libido or sexual drive, and generally, anorexics are not sexually active adolescents.[3] Psychoanalysts consider the contemporary anorexic unprepared to cope with the psychological and social consequences of adulthood, as well as adult sexuality. Anorexics make their bodies serve as substitutes for the lives they cannot control. By refusing food, anorexics slow the process of sexual maturation by stopping menses and maintaining childlike bodies.[4]

Since, adult sexuality frightens anorexic females, starving is a way to stay small, asexual, and dependent, and, so they can avoid psychological maturity, which requires independent judgments.[10,18] Anorexic females restrict their sexual interests and pleasures as much as they restrict adequate and normal eating.[2] Anorexia is their triumph over impulses and passions.

12.3.2   Bulimia Nervosa and Sexuality

While anorexia often begins in junior high, bulimia tends to develop in later adolescence. It is called the "girls' disease" because so many young women develop it in sororities and dorms. While anorexic females are perfectionistic and controlled, bulimic young women are impulsive, and they experience themselves as chronically out of control. They are more vulnerable to alcoholism than their anorexic peers. Unlike anorexics, bulimics come in all shapes and sizes. Bulimic young women are like their anorexic sisters in that they are oversocialized to the feminine role. They are ultimate people pleasers; most are attractive and have good social skills. Often they are the cheerleaders, homecoming queens, the straight-A students and prides of their families. Bulimic women have lost their true selves. In their eagerness to please, they have developed an addiction that destroys their central core. They have lost their souls in their attempts to have perfect bodies. They have a long road to recovery.[19]

Bulimics tend to have difficulty with impulse control, which is exhibited through compulsory alcohol or drug abuse and indiscriminate sexual behavior. The family histories of bulimics are replete with open conflict and turmoil. The bulimics' relationships with others tend to be intensely dependent and emotionally stormy. The disorder rarely emerges at puberty, and usually surfaces in late high school or early college years. Whereas anorexics tend to be phobic about sexuality and avoid sexual encounters, bulimics tend to be sexually active and engage in heterosexual relationships.[9] Bulimics tend to have more partners and sexual involvements and tend to be more sexually active than individuals who do not have eating disorders. Some bulimics use sex to find comfort and connection with an available partner. Their behavior may appear overtly sexual, but it masks a childlike plea for nuturance.[15]

Sexuality is a means to draw close to a mother substitute. A bulimic looks for a compatible and complementary partner; gender is irrelevant. By doing so, she is attempting to feel whole and alive. Sex, like binging, is an attempt to fill a void. It alleviates anxiety and brings physical closeness through a union of bodies. Such fusion can blur the boundaries between bulimics and their sexual partners. Many bulimics have multiple sex partners, but they do not enjoy sexual relationships. Their ardent search for partners develops the fragmentation of their inner selves by providing them with a soothing and caring presence. What appears as a ploy for sexual fulfillment is not sexual at all. It is an attempt to feel alive while anchored to another person.[15]

Like the anorexic, the bulimic is typically an achiever in school and work, and appears to be an independent and competent individual. However, underneath this façade, bulimics are profoundly troubled by feelings of neediness, dependency, and low self-esteem. There is a split in identity, which leaves little room for expressions of dependency or rebellion, due to the unavailability of parental figures in their lives. This lack leads to the development of a pseudo-maturity characterized by a façade of perfection. Only in the privacy of the kitchen or bathroom can this façade be dropped and the dependency and rebellion can be expressed through gorging and purging.[15] This false-self type represents an extremely common pattern in bulimics and is interchangeable with a host of self-destructive symptoms including alcoholism, self-mutilation, and sexual indiscretions.[20]

In contrast to anorexics, bulimics maintain a strong conscious identification with the traditional female sex role. They are often in non-traditional adolescent roles, acting as the adult figure in their households. Most bulimics have a history of early sexual involvement and are oriented to pleasing males. Many times, they have very ambivalent relationships with their fathers.[15] Typically fathers of bulimics are extraordinarily critical and overtly absent both physically and emotionally. Bulimics see their fathers as both mysterious and fascinating, while simultaneously remaining enormously sensitive to male criticism and rejection. This makes relationships with all males turbulent and volatile.[17] Bulimics tend to distance themselves from their mothers, who are usually physically present in their lives, and choose to admire and idealize their fathers. Their attitudes toward their male role models are initially connected with their ideas about size. They associate thinness with gaining masculine power via the male, and they associate fatness with social, economic, and political weakness. Therefore, bulimics are caught between trying to integrate ambition and the need to be powerful with the traditional female role based on placating, compliance, and unassertiveness in the face of the powerful male. To bulimics, thinness is the ideal that brings these two social dichotomies together. Thinness shows that they are powerful, competent, and in control, but at the same time tiny, small, nurturing, and pleasing to men. They conclude that if their males are pleased, they will gain the power they desire.[13]

12.3.3 Males, Eating Disorders, and Sexuality

Male anorexics and bulimics do exist, and clinically they closely resemble female patients, with the exception of amennorrhea.[15] Male patients manifest uncharacteristic sex role behavior. Many males feel stigmatized as having a female disorder, and the result is a sense of shame, thereby making males reluctant to seek help.[12] Males with eating disorders, who have been studied, tend to have explicit conflicts with their sexual identities. Sexual identity is the process of discovery, defining who we are as sexual beings and involves issues related to gender identity, male and female gender roles, and sexual orientation, as opposed to conflicts in social gender roles experienced by females. Some males with eating disorders manifest conflicts about achievement and autonomy, have feelings of external determination, and display low self-esteem, all of which are more central to the issues of eating disorders than sexual identity.

Many males with eating disorders have explicit homosexual conflicts, and documentation exists showing a higher prevalence of male anorexics and bulimics in the male homosexual population than are found among heterosexual males.[6] Nevertheless, as males, both homosexuals and heterosexuals become more preoccupied with appearance, and as they internalize messages of validation through sexual objectification, they very well may experience an increase in eating disorders. Projections indicate, however, that a growing incidence of eating disorders among males appears unlikely.[15]

References

1. Benjamin, J., *The Bonds of Love*, Pantheon, New York, 1988.
2. Zerbe, K. J., *The Body Betrayed: A Deeper Understanding of Women, Eating Disorders, and Treatment*, Gurzee Publishers, Carlsbad, CA, 1993.
3. Schwartz, H., *Never Satisfied: A Cultural History of Diets, Fantasies, and Fats*, Free Press, New York, 1986.
4. Fisher, S., *Body Consciousness*, Prentice-Hall, Englewood Cliffs, NJ, 1973.
5. Pipher, M., *Hunger Pains: The Modern Woman's Tragic Quest for Thinness*, Ballantine Books, New York, 1995.
6. Rost, W., Newhaus, M., and Florin, I., Bulimia nervosa sex roles, sex role behavior, and sex role related levels of control in bulimanexic women, *Journal of Psychosomatic Research*, 26, 403–408, 1982.
7. Bruch, H., Anorexia nervosa: therapy and theory, *American Journal of Psychiatry*, 139, 1531–1538, 1982.
8. Rosenweig, M. and Spruill, J. J., Twenty years after Twiggy, *International Journal of Eating Disorders*, 6, 59–66, 1987.
9. Brumberg, J. J., *Fasting Girls: The History of Anorexia Nervosa*, Harvard University Press, Cambridge, MA, 1988.
10. Brumberg, J. J., *The Body Project: An Intimate History of American Girls*, Harvard University Press, Cambridge, MA, 1997.
11. Casky, N., Interpreting anorexia nervosa, in *The Female Body in Western Culture*, Sulieman, S., ed., Harvard University Press, Cambridge, MA, 1986.
12. Orbach, S., *Hunger Strike: Anorexia Nervosa as a Metaphor for Our Time*, W. W. Norton, New York, 1986.
13. Orbach, S., *Fat Is a Feminist Issue: The Anti-Diet Guide to Permanent Weight Loss*, Paddington Press, New York, 1978.
14. Elkind, D., *Ties that Stress: The New Family Imbalance*, Harvard University Press, Cambridge, MA, 1994.
15. Gordon, R. A., *Anorexia and Bulimia: Anatomy of a Social Epidemic*, Blackwell Publishers, Malden, MA, 1991.
16. Jacobson, A. and Herald, C., The relevance of childhood sexual abuse to adult psychiatry in patient care, *Hospital and Community Psychiatry*, 41, 154–158, 1990.
17. Kommarovsky, L., *Women in College*, Basic Books, New York, 1985.
18. Crisp, A. H., *Anorexia Nervosa: Let Me Be*, Academic Press, London, 1980.
19. Herzog, D., Bulimia: the secretive syndrome, *Psychosomatics*, 23, 481–487, 1982.
20. Whitaker, L. C. and Davis, W. N., *The Bulimic College Student: Evaluation, Research, and Prevention*, Hayworth Press, New York, 1989.

Part IV

Primary Prevention of
Eating Disorders in Children

13

Factors Associated with Eating Disorders in Children

John Rohwer and Marilyn S. Massey-Stokes

CONTENTS

13.1 Learning Objectives

After completing this chapter you should be able to:

- Recognize eating disorders as a significant problem in recent years among children and youth, especially girls and young women;
- Comprehend the complex relationship between the onset of eating disorders and the transition from childhood to adolescence;
- Identify the risks that lead to increased vulnerability to eating disorders.

0-8493-2027-5/01/$0.00+$.50
© 2001 by CRC Press, Inc.

13.2 Research Background

13.2.1 Dieting: An Unhealthy Behavior for Many Girls and Some Boys

Far too many of America's children, particularly girls, are growing up afraid to eat, afraid to gain weight, and afraid to mature normally. These concerns are linked to the sociocultural forces that strongly equate female desirability with appearance, and desired appearance as a thin, pre-pubescent body. The media, family, peers, and other significant adults (e.g. coaches, teachers, counselors) all contribute messages to support these concepts.

Given this cultural ideal, it is not surprising that as girls enter puberty and begin to gain weight, they do not have, nor are they encouraged to have, realistic expectations of normal physical changes. Therefore, they do not accept natural genetic diversity in weight and shape. Given the adolescent's heightened need for peer inclusion (and interest in desirability), it is logical that girls become anxious and dissatisfied with their naturally developing curves and roundness.

An increasing number of adolescent females tend to perceive themselves as too fat and as needing to diet to lose weight. Such body dissatisfaction is extending to every-younger age groups and is now occurring in significant numbers even among girls in the third to fifth grades.[1,2] Weight concerns, dieting for weight loss, and binge eating increase with age, as girls move through elementary and middle school and into high school.[3,4] As many as 70% of normal-weight adolescent girls feel fat and engage in unhealthy eating practices to lose weight.[5,6] Alarmingly, up to 35% of children as young as third-graders now feel they should go on diets.[2] Dissatisfaction with their bodies may also be increasing in boys.[7] Yet, boys' teasing and other negative remarks about weight and shape directed at girls play an important role in girls' body-image attitudes.[8] Sadly, as this powerful sociocultural concept clashes with human biology, casual and aggressive measures of weight control (through restricted eating, etc.) have become the norm among adolescent girls and young women.

Various unhealthy and counterproductive effects of calorie restriction for weight loss are well documented. Dieting is associated with other chronic disturbances in eating, such as obsession with food, anxiety about eating, interference with natural hunger regulation, binge-eating, hoarding, hiding and avoiding food, and malnourishment, along with more acute effects such as irritability, social withdrawal, inability to concentrate, and fatigue. Of primary concern are the effects of inadequate nutrition in growing children and an increasing rate of unnatural, reactive weight gain and obesity.[9,10]

The glorification of thinness and fear of fat that leads to dieting is a primary risk factor for eating disorders, which represent the third most common chronic illness among American adolescent females.[11] A review of the research literature indicates that although full-blown eating disorders occur in about 3% of adult women, the prevalence of partial eating disorders is at least twice as high.[12] These serious illnesses are of grave concern.

However, most agree that the eating-disorder risk factors themselves (such as low self-esteem, the desire for perfection, and parental attitudes toward weight) provide the greatest threat to public health and the social fabric. Several theorists have addressed the ways in which chronic weight and shape concerns (i.e., the dieting mentality) contribute to self-objectification, to unhealthy competition among women, and to consumption of physical and psychological energy that could be allocated to more life-enhancing personal, social, and political concerns.[13,14] Although the majority of children and youth will not develop diagnosable eating disorders, it is clear that excessive anxiety about appearance, self-consciousness, obsessive inner dialogues about weight and shape, and the consequences of restricted eating interfere significantly with the developmental needs and resiliency of adolescents.[14,15]

13.2.2   Development of Eating Disorders

Eating disorders most commonly begin sometime during adolescence. Anorexia nervosa does occur in prepubertal children[16] but it increases dramatically after puberty, with the majority of cases beginning before age 25.[17,18] Bulimia nervosa is virtually unheard of prior to adolescence[16] and the vast majority of women clinically diagnosed with bulimia nervosa display symptoms before age 25.[18] Problematic eating at young ages is probably due to the onset of factors associated with eating disorders, such as weight and shape consciousness, body dissatisfaction, and the belief in the worth of dieting. Often these concerns are related to normative events of early adolescence, such as going through puberty, beginning to date, and making the transition to middle school or junior high. Furthermore, females, who are at greater risk for eating disorders, appear to be affected more negatively by these normative changes.[3]

13.2.3   Transition: Growth and Developmental Changes

Several critical developmental challenges occur during adolescence, including dealing with the physical and psychological effects of puberty, moving toward increasing independence, developing peer relationships, internalizing achievement values, and achieving an integrated sense of self.[19,20] Furthermore, the transition from childhood to adolescence involves reorganization in personality and in cognitive and relationship structures, as well as changes in social roles and cultural expectations. Subsequently, the transition leads to new dynamics among behaviors, beliefs, concepts, and attitudes. This change period suggests that eating behaviors only become problematic when a reorganization occurs that ties eating to attractiveness, success, control, and self-worth.[21]

   Adolescence is broken down into three stages: early, middle, and late adolescence. The timing of these stages differs between genders, with girls typically entering adolescence earlier than boys. For girls, early adolescence usually encompasses the ages 11 through 13 (middle school/junior high).[20] Typically, adolescence is a more difficult transition for girls than for boys. As an example, girls experience greater drops in self-esteem, particularly in body esteem. Moreover, early adolescence involves special risk periods for the development of eating disorders.[17,22,23] This is evidenced by the increase in associated eating problems, such as body dissatisfaction and dieting.[3,24,25] Even in elementary school, girls exhibit some of the behaviors, attitudes, and beliefs that may lead them to emerge from the early adolescence transition with eating problems. What follows offers a brief overview of some of the developmental issues that need to be considered in the prevention of eating disorders among early adolescents.

   Puberty, the onset of the physical capacity to reproduce, is a long process that includes numerous physical and emotional changes. It usually takes 4 to 5 years for boys and 3 to 4 years for girls to complete puberty. Changes that accompany puberty can occur as early as age 7 and as late as age 18. However, nearly 50% of all boys and girls reach puberty before age 13.[26] The physical changes that occur throughout puberty include development of secondary sex characteristics. For girls, these changes involve gains in height and weight, widening of hips, breast enlargement, growth of pubic and underarm hair, and menarche. Many young females are startled and unbalanced by these physical changes, particularly the ones that cause their bodies to become naturally heavier and differently shaped (i.e., rounder and more curvaceous, as opposed to thin and boyish). Early maturers may be at greater risk for unhealthy dieting behaviors because they generally are heavier than their peers,[19] possess poorer self-concepts, and experience more emotional distress.[20] It is very important that parents, teachers, coaches, and other significant adults clearly explain the process of puberty, so that girls and boys understand that weight gain is necessary and to be expected. In addition, children need to understand that each individual is different and may begin puberty earlier or later. They need to understand that this is normal and they are not freaks if they develop more quickly or more slowly than most (or all) of their same-age peers. Adults need to take the time to discuss pubertal changes with girls and boys and allow them to express their feelings and concerns about the physical and emotional turmoil they are experiencing. If a girl or boy indicates that she or he is developing an unhealthy body image that could lead to harmful dieting behaviors, then appropriate preventative action can be taken. A later chapter entitled "The Role of Parents, School Personnel, and the Community in the Primary Prevention of Eating Disorders among Children" offers tips for the prevention of eating disorders in children. (See Table 13.1 for growth and developmental characteristics and related needs of children ages 5–14.)

Moving toward autonomy is an essential developmental need that begins in early adolescence. Research shows that during this period, the time spent with parents decreases,[20] and children tend to disengage emotionally from the family as they pursue outside relationships.[19] This is a particularly troublesome transition for girls whose families are enmeshed or overprotective, and in which separation and independence are discouraged.

Peer relationships become increasingly important during this period of development, and conformity to peer expectations is a strong motivator for behavior.[20] Peers send powerful messages regarding weight and body shape, often through teasing and ostracizing. Another salient aspect of these relationships is the onset of dating. Early dating, along with menarche and entering middle school all appear to make early adolescent girls more vulnerable to eating problems.[20]

Early adolescence marks a major transition from elementary to middle school (or junior high); therefore, many girls put a great deal of pressure on themselves to excel, which can feed into perfectionistic tendencies and create a vicious cycle of achievement-perfectionistic strivings. These tendencies often transfer to the area of physical appearance and body image and can lead to eating disturbances.

Then, too, early adolescence is a crucial period for achieving an integrated sense of self, which includes development of self-esteem, self-efficacy, and self-control,[20] as well as coping skills. Problems can arise when a young adolescent girl sees herself as a body rather than **a** total person with unique and diverse attributes.

13.3 Application of Research Question

What factors may make individuals vulnerable to eating disorders? Through education and shared knowledge, can society prevent children's natural weight and body image concerns from progressing clinically diagnosed eating disorders?

TABLE 13.1

Growth and Developmental Characteristics and Needs of Children Ages 5–13

Years of Age	Growth and Developmental Characteristics	Needs
5–7	Growth is relatively slow Large muscles are better developed than small ones Hungry at brief intervals; may overeat and gain inappropriate weight if physical activity is inadequate Susceptibility to respiratory infections and childhood diseases Tires easily When starting school, tendency is to engage in regressive behavior (e.g., thumbsucking, toilet lapses). Eager to learn, energetic, restless Attention span short, but increasing; learns best through experiential activities Thrives on encouragement Strongly identifies with parents and teachers	A great deal of sleep and rest Regular large-muscle physical activity Balanced nutrition Some responsibilities without pressure to adhere to rigid standards Freedom to perform various tasks Help making adjustments to new situations Positive peer relationships to provide sense of belonging Encouragement, praise, warmth, and patience from caring adults Build self-confidence and feel sense of accomplishment
8–10	Growth is slow and steady Small muscles are developing Poor posture may develop Some girls may begin menstruation at age 9 or 10 Boys begin puberty cycle around 10–13 years Sensitive to criticism and teasing Strong peer relationships; best friends highly valued	Friends and group membership Opportunity to develop skills without undue pressure Praise, encouragement, and warmth from caring adults Patient guidance from caring adults 10–12 hours of sleep and rest Physical activity involving the whole body Balanced nutrition
11–13	Rapid and often uneven growth Development of secondary sex characteristics Wide range of individual differences and maturity levels, with girls maturing faster than boys Groups or gangs important Developing an interest in sex Competitive in nature Shows restraint in expressing feelings (e.g., does not openly show love to parents) Emotional instability; mood swings Self-conscious Socially insecure Very peer conscious	To understand normal developmental changes of puberty To experience success To develop a positive self-image Warm affection and approval from caring adults Increased opportunities for independence A sense of belonging and positive relations with peers Values development 9–11 hours of sleep and rest Participation in individual and team sports/activities Balanced diet and enough calories to support physical activity To express difficult emotions (e.g., anger, fear, frustration, etc.) To identify with a significant adult (parent, teacher, coach, older friend)

13.3.1 Risk Factors

Risk factors can be defined as circumstances or predispositions that result in increased levels of vulnerability to harmful health behaviors. For eating disorders, the risk factors are intricate and varied. While anorexia and bulimia have been considered purely biological or psychological, they are now viewed as more complex, resulting from the interaction of biological, psychological, and social factors. In fact, it appears that risk factors leading to the onset of eating disorders cross social, environmental, biological, and cultural lines. A number of empirical studies have attempted to isolate various risk factors associated with eating disorders. These risk factors can be categorized as follows: (a) demographics (age, gender, socio-economic status, ethnic backgrounds, particularly outside of Anglo ethnic groups, and family factors, such as parental attitudes toward weight); (b) biological factors (gender, age at onset of menarche, body type); (c) psychological and behavioral factors (low self-esteem, low self-efficacy, distorted body image, restrained eating or dieting, binge-purging behaviors, and the desire for perfection); and (d) social and cultural factors (attitudes and practices of the peer group that promote harmful norms, influence of mass media, teasing, and perception of society's glamorization of thinness).

13.3.1.1 Demographic Characteristics

13.3.1.1.1 Age, Gender, and Socio-Economic Status

Eating disorders in youth occur predominantly among females between the ages of 12 and 20 from middle- or upper-class social backgrounds.[27,28] An inverse relationship between weight and social background demonstrates that a higher social background is associated with lower desired and current body weights for 18-year-old women. This relationship leads to higher levels of dieting, binge eating, and exercise for weight control.[29]

Eating disorders are more common in females than in males. Several possibilities have been proposed to explain this phenomenon. The most plausible argument centers on the fact that females and males receive different messages about appropriate attitudes, characteristics, and behaviors.[30] For example, females are more likely to be judged for their attractiveness in the dating culture, and they are supposed to eat less than their male counterparts, especially on a first date.[30,31] Research also has found that body dissatisfaction and restrictive eating practices are much more common among females than among males.[30,31]

13.3.1.1.2 Ethnic Background

Changes are beginning to occur in the ethnic distributions of eating disorders. They now appear in the black youth population, whereas eating disorders among this ethnic group were almost unheard of before the 1980s.[27,32,33] Several studies have shown that white high-school girls still exhibit greater body dissatisfaction and diet more than females in non-white groups.[1,34,35] Differing gender roles may offer one possible explanation for this. Black children apparently are not as gender-stereotyped in their beliefs as white children[36] and black girls are more satisfied with their weights than their white counterparts.[37-39] By the same token, black children have been found to be less likely than white children to fear becoming fat.[39]

Research also found that black girls experience less social pressure to conform to the thin ideal than do their white counterparts.[39-41] For example, black schoolchildren are reportedly less likely to feel that they look fat to others. One study found that black adolescent girls were more likely to report that their friends and families viewed them as thin, even though the two groups did not differ on a measure of current body size.[42] While black girls make it clear that physical appearance is important in black culture, they are not obsessed with thinness. Rather, the emphasis is on developing pride in one's body regardless of its physical appearance. Black girls are encouraged to emphasize their assets through grooming and clothing selections. This cultural norm may serve as a protective barrier to eating-disordered behaviors.[43]

13.3.1.1.3 Family Characteristics

Eating disorders seem to be unrelated to religious affiliation, family size, proportion of females to males in the family, birth order, or family dissolution due to separation, divorce, or death.[27] This can be attributed to the tremendous variability in cases of eating disorders, to the inherent limitations of verbal reports gathered after the onset of a serious illness, and to the paucity of studies that compare the families of patients with eating disorders to the families of patients with no disorders or with equally serious psychiatric problems. However, based on case histories of eating disorders and on investigations of success-oriented families, it is reasonable to hypothesize that the family is the principal communicator of cultural values.

Maternal attitudes about weight seem influential; mothers' perceived investments in slenderness are predictors of dieting in middle-school-aged girls.[8] Parents who dieted were significantly more likely to propose weight-loss methods to their children than were non-dieting parents.[44] Several carefully designed studies[45] have revealed very few differences between the parents of young women with eating disorders and the parents of normal young women, when matched only for age and social background.

13.3.1.1.4 Biological Characteristics

Female Gender: Females are genetically programmed to have proportionately higher body fat composition than males, a sex difference that holds throughout all races and cultures. The gender differences in fatness increase across the life span. In attempts to understand eating disorders, it is crucial to examine biological and genetic factors. Recent research in genetic epidemiology has suggested some degree of family risk for eating disorders. High childhood body mass is one often-cited etiological precursor of eating problems.[46]

Body Type and Shape: A number of studies have reported that females of a particular body type seem most vulnerable, namely that women with higher weights and levels of body fat than their peers exhibit more body dissatisfaction, dieting, and eating-disorder symptoms.[47,48]

Body shape and weight, including obesity, are typically considered to have significant genetic components.[49,50] That may be evidenced under varying environmental circumstances. Although genetics may contribute to a tendency to gain weight easily, an individual's weight does not simply reflect this genetic predisposition.[50] Childhood body mass index is only moderately predictive of adult body mass index.[51]

Onset of Menarche: Early menarche, which involves having to contend with a different, fuller-looking body, has been cited as a risk factor in some reports,[31,48] although other researchers suggest that the timing of menarche does not seem to be a predictor.[3,47,52,53]

The work of Gralen et al.[3] suggests that risk factors may be different for different developmental levels. For example, Gralen et al.[3] and Levine et al.[8] found that menarche and dating were significant predictors of dieting and eating problems in sixth and eighth graders. By the ninth grade, however, these predictors were beginning to be displaced by more abstract concepts such as body image, body ideal, and current shape. Stress of adolescent transitions, including menarche, may have other implications as well. Gralen et al.[3] also found that when menarche coincided with a sense of increased academic pressure and worry over school performance, eating disorders increased significantly.

Genetic Trait: In addition to the genetic predisposition to a specific body weight, a predisposition to an eating disorder may be genetically transmitted. Research on this issue is in the early stages but initial findings suggest familial clustering of eating disorders. Studies have documented a significantly higher incidence of anorexia and bulimia among the first-degree female relatives of anorexic patients than in the immediate families of control subjects.[53,54]

13.3.2.1 Psychological and Behavioral Factors

13.3.2.1.1 Self-Esteem and Self-Concept

Similar psychological and behavioral factors can be contributing elements to and the consequences of eating disorders. Psychological and behavioral factors that increase vulnerability include personality predispositions such as perfectionism and low self-esteem.[55] While these factors may contribute, the process becomes a vicious cycle, as dieting causes stress[56] and may place females at risk for depression and, at the same time, decreases self-esteem.[57] Also, the typical ineffectiveness of diets as a means of weight control[58,59] can lead to frustration, feelings of failure, and lowered self-esteem.[31] Fisher et el al.[35] found an association between disordered-eating attitudes and lower self-esteem and higher anxiety among high school students. Girls' strong investments in social relationships may also render them vulnerable as they move into middle school, where such relationships change dramatically.[55,60] For example, girls are relatively silenced (in terms of assertively expressing opinions, desires, etc.) in middle school and may find attractiveness to be one of the few available pathways to success.[55]

Differences in self-concept are already evident in children. For instance, when asked to describe themselves, girls as young as seven refer more to the views of other people in their self-depictions than do boys.[61] It seems that self-concept is an interpersonal construct for girls more than for boys. In addition, although the role of body image in children's self-concepts has not been studied extensively, body build is correlated with self-esteem for girls, but not boys, in the fourth, fifth, and sixth grades.[62,63] Furthermore, even among these young girls, weight was critical in the relationship between body image and self-concept. The thinner the girl, the more likely she was to report feeling attractive, popular, and academically successful. In addition, studies have found that even as children, females are more dissatisfied with their bodies than are males. Although non-obese girls have more positive attitudes toward their bodies than obese girls, they still express more concerns about their appearance than both non-obese and obese boys. Indeed, Tobin-Richards, Boxer, and Petersen[64] found that perceived weight and body satisfaction were negatively correlated with weight for girls. By contrast, boys valued being of normal weight and expressed equal dissatisfaction with being underweight or overweight.

13.3.2.1.2 Perfectionism

Perfectionism has long been linked to adult eating problems.[9] Indeed, the original image of the anorexic was that of the "best little girl in the world."[32] Steiner-Adair[65] studied adolescent girls' images of the ideal woman and their own goals for themselves, and then looked at the relationship between these views with performance on the Eating Attitudes Test (EAT), a widely used measure of disordered eating.[27] Interestingly, all girls had a similar picture of the ideal "superwoman" (career, family, beauty); but those girls who saw the superwoman as consistent with their own goals had elevated eating pathology scores. Noneating-disordered girls had more modest goals. A girl's ability to put distance between the societal ideal and her own expectations for herself pointed toward decreased evidence of eating disturbance. Thus, perfectionism may be linked to eating problems through the superwoman ideal.[64,65]

Brown and Gilligan[56] documented the existence of perfectionism among some elementary school girls. These girls demonstrated their desire to always be pretty, always be nice, and always be good in school. Such unrealistic goals may set the stage for a loss of self-esteem as it becomes clear that they are falling short of the ideal. These goals also may be driven by a need for social approval, which has been associated with eating problems in adults. This pattern may be especially insidious for minority girls who adopt white middle-class ideals, when their race or ethnicity guarantees that they will never find full acceptance, even if they do become thin, earn good grades, and so forth.[55,66]

13.3.2.1.3 Dieting Behaviors

The risks of dieting, then, are not solely attributable to real weight problems. Body image and eating concerns begin in girls between the ages of 9 and 11, but appear to increase dramatically during the transition to junior high school.[21] Many grade school and high school girls diet to lose weight even if they are normal or underweight.

Research has established that repeated dieting, especially with weight fluctuations, is a risk factor for eating disorders. Early onset of dieting is also associated with an increased risk.[67] Children and adolescents who diet tend to be heavier than nondieters, but they usually are not obese or even overweight by medical standards.[21,68] It is possible that the risk is due to dieting itself, which can lead to a metabolic slowing that requires more extreme methods to lose weight and maintain weight loss.[69] As the body struggles to escape starvation, binge eating may develop.[14] Given this possible path toward the development of eating problems, it is worrisome that up to 40% of elementary school girls report trying to lose weight.[1,21]

Many middle-school girls live in a culture of dieting in which their mothers and friends diet and worry about weight. These girls also read the teen magazines that send the broader culture's slenderness messages. Such girls tend to have higher Eating Attributes Test scores, diet more frequently, and express greater body dissatisfaction.[68] They may also develop a thinness scheme emphasizing the importance of thinness to attractiveness, the importance of attractiveness to social and career success, the dangers of fat, methods of becoming thin, and the importance of attractiveness to self-esteem. This thinness scheme may lead to selective processing of information that supports these girls' assessments of thinness and its importance.[52]

Gralen et al.[3] found that dieting and disordered eating varied across age levels. Younger girls (sixth and eighth graders) were influenced more heavily by the concrete events of menarche and dating. For many developing girls, dieting seems to be part of an adjustment to the fat increase associated with menarche[70] and the attractiveness demands associated with dating. By the ninth grade, events such as dating and menarche (including the timing of menarche) no longer predict dieting or eating problems. This strongly suggests that even though an adjustment is made at the time of menarche and dating, few long-term effects will remain.[71] Nevertheless, the dieting cycle persists.

Research suggests that young children know that it is undesirable to be fat.[72] Not all elementary school children believe that thinness is important to attractiveness,[21] but girls who equate the two may be especially susceptible to the peer and media pressure that is part of the early-adolescent world, and that may serve as the impetus for the development of problematic eating.

TABLE 13.2

Risk Factors Associated with Eating Disorders in Children

Demographics	Age and gender
	Socioeconomic status
	Ethnic background
	Family factors
Biological Factors	Female gender
	Onset of menarche
	Body type
Psychological and	Low self-esteem and low self-efficacy
Behavioral Factors	Distorted body image
	Drive for thinness
	Restrained eating or dieting
	Binge-purging behaviors
	Desire for perfection
Sociocultural Factors	Attitudes and practices in peer group that promote harmful behavior
	Teasing
	Influence of mass media
	Perception of society's glamorization of thinness

13.3.3.1   *Social and Cultural Factors*

13.3.3.1.1   *Gender Message Differences*

Little girls learn from their families that they should be pretty and serve as aesthetic adornments in their environments.[73] Young girls learn that attractiveness is intricately interwoven with pleasing and serving others and, in turn, will secure the love of others. Beyond the family environment, schools also promote their strong societal message. For example, more teachers provide positive feedback to boys specifically regarding their intellectual performance, whereas girls are more often praised for characteristics that are intellectually irrelevant, such as neatness and appearance.[74]

During early adolescence, girls particularly value opportunities to seek advice and support from friends about personal issues, such as attractiveness and self-control. It appears that adolescent girls talk to one another about body shape, eating, and weight loss, all of which may contribute to unhealthy attitudes and behaviors. One peer trait that may contribute to the development of body dissatisfaction and promotion of the slender ideal is teasing about weight.[69] When students tease each other about being overweight, they are reflecting beliefs and attitudes they have learned from parents, educators, counselors, and the media.

13.3.3.1.2   *Media Messages*

Mass media regularly promote the ideal body, especially the ideal female body. Television teaches girls a singular feminine ideal of thinness, beauty, and youth, set against a world in which men are more competent and more diverse in appearance.[75,76] Television programs seldom include children or adults who are large or overweight. Some of the few adult television stars who are overweight have experienced scathing media critiques of their weight, and others have undergone highly publicized weight-loss campaigns, only to regain the weight. What do these kinds of painful experiences exemplify for children, especially those who are larger than average?

13.3.4   Summary

Risk factors leading to eating disorders appear to cross social, environmental, biological, and cultural lines, and they are extremely intricate, varied, and complex. Table 13.2

summarizes the risk factors discussed in this chapter; however, the identification of risk factors in eating disorders does not necessarily provide a clear sense of what particular strategies are needed to reduce the risks. The determination of those factors that can be most effectively targeted for prevention offers a key challenge that still needs to be answered.

References

1. Gustafson-Larson, A.M., and Terry, R.D., Weight-related behaviors and concerns of fourth-grade children, in *The Developmental Psychopathology of Eating Disorders: Implications for Research, Prevention and Treatment*, Smolak, L. Levine, M.P., and Striegel-Moore, R., Eds., Lawrence Erlbaum Associates, Mahwah, NJ, 1996, 207.
2. Pierce, J. and Wardle, J., Cause-and-effect beliefs and self-esteem of overweight children, *Journal of Child Psychology and Psychiatry Allied Disciplines*, 38, 645, 1997.
3. Gralen, S.J., Levine, M.P., Smolak, L., and Murnen, S.K., Dieting and disordered eating during early and middle adolescence: do the influences remain the same? *International Journal of Eating Disorders*, 9(5), 501, 1990.
4. Thelen, M.H., Powell, A.L., Lawrence, C., and Kuhnert, M.E., Eating and body image concerns among children, *Journal of Clinical Child Psychology*, 21(1), 41, 1992.
5. Ferron, C., Body image in adolescence in cross-cultural research, *Adolescence*, 32, 735, 1997.
6. Rierdan, J. and Koff, E., Weight, weight-related aspects of body image, and depression in early adolescent girls, *Adolescence*, 32, 615, 1997.
7. Grange, D., Tibbs, J., and Slibowitz, J., Eating attitudes, body shape, and self-disclosure in a community sample of adolescent girls and boys, *Eating Disorders*, 3(3), 253, 1995.
8. Levine, M.P., Smolak, L., Mordey, A.F., Shuman, M.D., and Hessen, L.D., Normative developmental challenges and dieting and eating disturbances in middle school girls, *International Journal of Eating Disorders*, 15(1), 11, 1994.
9. Garner, D. and Wooley, S., Confronting the failure of behavioral and dietary treatment for obesity, *Clinical Psychological Review*, 11, 729, 1991.
10. Story, M. and Neumark-Sztainer, D., School-based nutrition education programs and services for adolescents, *Adolescent Medicine: State of the Art Reviews*, 7(2), 287, 1996.
11. Fisher, M., Golden, N.H., and Katzman, D.K., Eating disorders in adolescents: a background paper, *Journal of Adolescent Health*, 16(6), 420, 1995.
12. Shisslak, C., Crago, M., and Estes, L., The spectrum of eating disturbances, *International Journal of Eating Disorders*, 11(3), 209, 1995.
13. Roden, J., Silberstein, L.R., and Striegel-Moore, R.H., Women and weight: a normative discontent, in *Psychology and Gender*, Sandergger, T.B., Ed., Nebraska Symposium on Motivation, Lincoln, University of Nebraska Press, 1985, 267.
14. Steiner-Adair, C., The politics of prevention, in *Feminist Perspectives on Eating Disorders*, Fallon, P., Katzman, M., and Wooley, S., Eds., Guilford Press, New York, 1993.
15. Cash, R.F., The psychology of physical appearance: aesthetics, attributes, and images, in *Body Images: Development, Deviance, and Changes*, Cash, T.F. and Pruzinsky, T., Eds., Guilford Press, New York, 1990, 51.
16. Gislason, I.L., Eating disorders in childhood, in *The Eating Disorders: Medical and Psychological Basis of Diagnosis and Treatment*, Blinder, B., Chitin, B., and Goldstein, C.R., Eds., PMA, New York, 1988, 285.
17. Halmi, K., Casper, R., Eckert, E., Goldberg, S., and Davis, J., Unique factors associated with age of onset of anorexia nervosa, *Psychiatry Research*, 1, 209, 1979.
18. Woodside, D.B. and Garfinkel, P., Age of onset in eating disorders. *International Journal of Eating Disorders*, 12, 31, 1992.
19. Attie, I. and Brooks-Gunn, J., The development of eating regulation across the life span, in *Developmental Psychopathology*, Dante, C. and Cohen, D. J., Eds., John Wiley & Sons, New York, 1995, chap. 10.

20. Shisslak, C. M., Crago, M., Estes, L. S., and Gray, N., Content and method of develop-
    mentally appropriate prevention programs, in *The Developmental Psychopathology of Eating
    Disorders: Implications for Research, Prevention, and Treatment*, Smolak, L., Levine, M. P.,
    and Striegel-Moore, R., Eds., Lawrence Erlbaum Associates, Mahwah, NJ, 1996, chap. 14.
21. Smolak, L., and Levine, M.P., Toward an empirical basis for primary prevention of eating
    problems with elementary school children, *Eating Disorders*, 2(4), 283, 1994.
22. Abramowitz, R., Petersen, A., and Schulenberg, J., Changes in self-image during early
    adolescence, in *Patterns of Adolescent Self-Image*, Offer, D., Ostrov, E., and Howard, K.,
    Eds., Jossey-Bass, San Francisco, 1984, 19.
23. Wooley, S. and Wooley, O.W., Intensive outpatient and residential treatment for bulimia,
    in *Handbook of Psychotherapy for Anorexia Nervosa and Bulimia*, Garner, D. and Garfinkel, P.,
    Eds., Guilford Press, New York, 1985, 392.
24. Koff, E. and Rierdan, J., Perceptions of weight and attitudes toward eating in early
    adolescent girls, *Journal of Adolescent Health Care*, 11, 203, 1991.
25. Richards, M.H., Casper, R.C., and Larson, R., Weight and eating concerns among pre-
    and young adolescent boys and girls, *Journal of Adolescent Health Care*, 11, 203, 1990.
26. Miller, D.F., Telljohann, S.K., and Symons, C.W., *Health Education in the Elementary and
    Middle-Level School*, 2nd Ed., McGraw-Hill, Boston, 1996.
27. Garfinkel, P.E. and Garner, D.M., *Anorexia Nervosa: A Multidimensional Perspective*, Brunner/
    Mazel, New York, 1982.
28. Maloney, M.J. and Klykylo, W.M., An overview of anorexia nervosa, bulimia, and obesity
    in children and adolescents, *Journal of the American Academy of Child Psychology*, 22, 99, 1982.
29. Drewnoski, A., Kurth, C., and Krahn, D., Body weight and dieting in adolescence: impact
    of socioeconomic status, *International Journal of Eating Disorders*, 16, 639, 1994.
30. Worell, J. and Todd, J., Development of the gendered self, in *The Developmental Psychopa-
    thology of Eating Disorders: Implications for Research, Prevention, and Treatment*, Smolak, L.,
    Levine, M.P., and Striegel-Moore, R.H., Eds., Lawrence Erlbaum Associates, Mahwah, NJ,
    1996, 135.
31. Striegel-Moore, R., Silberstein, L.R., and Rodin, J., Toward an understanding of risk
    factors for bulimia, *American Psychologist*, 41, 246, 1986.
32. Levenkron, S., *Treating and Overcoming Anorexia Nervosa*, Scribner, New York, 1982.
33. Silber, T.J., Anorexia nervosa in blacks and Hispanics, *International Journal of Eating
    Disorders*, 5, 121, 1986.
34. Abrams, K.K., Allen, L., and Gray, J.J., Disordered eating attitudes and behaviors,
    psychological adjustment, and ethnic identity: a comparison of black and white college
    students, *International Journal of Eating Disorders*, 14, 49, 1993.
35. Fisher, M., Pastore, D., Schneider, M., Pegler, C., and Napolitano, B., Eating attitudes in
    urban and suburban adolescents, *International Journal of Eating Disorders*, 16, 67, 1994.
36. Rand, C. and Kuldan, J., The epidemiology of obesity and self-defined weight problems
    in the general population: gender, race, age, and social class, *International Journal of Eating
    Disorders*, 9, 329, 1990.
37. Bardwell, J.R., Cochran, S.W., and Walker, S., Relationship of parental education, race, and
    gender to sex role stereotyping in five-year-old kindergartners, *Sex Roles*, 15, 275, 1986.
38. Chandler, S.B., Akord, D.A., Lee, D.T., Cleveland, M.Z., and Daly, J.A., Pathogenic eating
    attitudes and behaviors and body dissatisfaction differences among black and white
    college students, *Eating Disorders*, 2, 319, 1994.
39. Harris, S.M., Family, self, and sociocultural contributions to body-image attitudes of
    African-American women, *Psychology of Women Quarterly*, 19, 129, 1995.
40. Powell, A.D. and Kahn, A.S., Racial differences in women's desires to be thin, *Interna-
    tional Journal of Eating Disorders*, 17, 191, 1995.
41. Children, A.C., Brewerton, T.D., Hodges, E.L., and Jarrell, M.P., The kids' eating disorders
    survey (KEDS): a study of middle school students, *Journal of the American Academy of
    Child and Adolescent Psychiatry*, 32, 843, 1993.
42. Streigel-Moore, R.H., Schreiber, G.B., Pike, K.M., Wilfley, D.E., Schreiber, G., and Rodin, J.,
    Drive for thinness in black and white preadolescent girls, *International Journal of Eating
    Disorders*, 18, 59, 1995.

43. Kemper, K.A., Sargent, R.G., Drane, J.W., Valois, R.F., and Hussey, J.W., Black and white females' perceptions of ideal body size and social norms, *Obesity Research*, 2, 117, 1994.

44. Streigel-Moore, R. and Smolak, L., The role of race in the development of eating disorders, in *The Developmental Psychopathology of Eating Disorders: Implications for Research, Prevention and Treatment*, Smolak, L., Levine, M.P., and Striegel-Moore, R., Eds., Lawrence Erlbaum Associates, Mahwah, NJ, 1996, 259.

45. Striegel-Moore, R.H. and Kearney-Cooke, A., Exploring determinants and consequences of parents' attitudes about their children's physical appearances, *International Journal of Eating Disorders*, 15, 337, 1994.

46. Garfinkel, P., Garner, D., Rose, J., Darby, P., Brandes, J.S., O'Hanlon, J., and Walsh, N., A comparison of characteristics in the families of patients with anorexia nervosa and normal controls, *Psychological Medicine*, 17, 821, 1983.

47. Zerbe, K., *The Body Betrayed*, American Psychiatric Press, Washington, D.C., 1993.

48. Attie, I. and Brooks-Gunn, J., Development of eating problems in adolescent girls: a longitudinal study, *Developmental Psychology*. 25, 70, 1989.

49. Killen, J., Hayward, C., Wilson, D., Tyalor, C., Hammer, L., Litt, S., Simmonds, B., and Haydal, F., Factors associated with eating disorder symptoms in a community sample of 6th and 7th grade girls, *International Journal of Eating Disorders*, 15, 357, 1994.

50. Brownell, K. and Rodin, J., The dieting maelstrom: is it possible and advisable to lose weight? *American Psychologist*, 49, 781, 1994.

51. Meyer, J. and Stunkard, A., Genetics and human obesity, in *Obesity: Theory and Therapy*, Stunkard, A. and Wadden, T., Eds., Raven, New York, 1993, 137.

52. Guo, S., Roche, A., Chumlee, W., Gardner, J., and Siervogel, R., The predictive value of childhood body mass index values for overweight at age 35 years, *American Journal of Clinical Nutrition*, 59, 810, 1994.

53. Smolak, L. and Levine, M.P., Adolescent transitions and the development of eating problems, in *The Developmental Psychopathology of Eating Disorders*, Smolak, L., Levine, M. P., and Striegel-Moore, R., Eds., Lawrence Erlbaum Associates, Mahwah, NJ, 1996, 207.

54. Gershon, E.S., Schreiber, J.L., Hamouit, J.R., Dibble, E.D., Kaye, W., Nurnbroger, J.I., Andersen, A.E., and Ebert, M., Clinical findings in patients with anorexia nervosa and affective illness in their relatives, *American Journal of Psychiatry*, 141, 1419, 1984.

55. Strober, M. and Humphrey, L.L., Familial contributions to the etiology and course of anorexia nervosa and bulimia, *Journal of Consulting and Clinical Psychology*, 55, 654, 1987.

56. Brown, C. and Gilligan, C., *Meeting at the Crossroad*, Harvard University Press, Cambridge, MA, 1992.

57. Rosen, J., Tacy, B., and Howell, D., Life stress, psychological symptoms, and weight reducing behavior in adolescent girls: a prospective analysis, *International Journal of Eating Disorders*, 9, 17, 1990.

58. McCarthy, M., The thin ideal, depression, and eating disorders in women, *Behavioral Research and Therapy*, 28, 205, 1990.

59. Bennett, W. and Gurin, J., *The Dieter's Dilemma*, Basic Books, New York, 1982.

60. Polivy, J. and Herman, P., *Breaking the Diet Habit*, Basic Books, New York, 1983.

61. Eccles, J. and Midgley, C., Changes in academic motivation and self-perception during early adolescence, in *From Childhood to Adolescence: A Transitional Period?* Montemayor, R., Adams, G., and Gullota T., Eds., Sayer, Newbury Park, CA, 1990, 134.

62. McGuire, W.J. and McGuire, C.V., Significant others in self-space: sex differences and developmental trends in the social self, in *Social Psychological Perspectives on the Self*, Suls, J., Ed., Lawrence Erlbaum Associates, Hillsdale, NJ, 1982, 71.

63. Guyot, G.W., Fairchild, L., and Hill, M., Physical fitness, sport participation, body build, and self-concept of elementary school children, *International Journal of Sports Psychology*, 12, 105, 1981.

64. Tobin-Richards, M., Boyer, A., and Petersen, A., The psychological significance of pubertal change: sex differences in perceptions of self during early adolescence, in *Girls of Puberty: Biological and Psychosocial Perspectives*, Brooks-Gunn, J. and Petersen, A., Eds., Plenum, New York, 1983, 127.

65. Steiner-Adair, C., The body politic: normal female adolescent development and the development of eating disorders, *Journal of the American Academy of Psychoanalysis*, 14, 95, 1986.

66. Levine, M.P. and Smolak, L., Toward a model of the developmental psychopathology of eating disorders: the example of early adolescence, in *The Etiology of Bulimic Nervosa: The Individual and Familial Context*, Crowther, J., Tenninbaum, D., Hobfoll, S., and Stephens, M., Eds., Hemisphere, Washington, D.C., 1992, 59.

67. Thompson, B., *A Hunger So Wide and So Deep*, University of Minnesota Press, Minneapolis, 1994.

68. Tobin, D., Johnson, C., Steinberg, S., Stacts, M., and Dennis, A., Multi-factorial assessment of bulimia nervosa, *Journal of Abnormal Psychology*, 100, 14, 1991.

69. Emmons, L., Predisposing factors differentiating adolescent dieters and nondieters, *Journal of the American Dietetic Association*, 94, 725, 1994.

70. Levine, M.P., Smolak, L., and Hayden, H., The relation of sociocultural factors to eating attitudes and behaviors among middle school girls, *Journal of Early Adolescence*, 14, 471, 1994.

71. Brooks-Gunn, J. and Warren, M., Effects of delayed menarche in different contexts: dance and nondance students, *Journal of Youth and Adolescence*, 14, 285, 1985.

72. Simmons, R. and Blyth, D., *Moving in Adolescence: The Impact of Pubertal Change and School Context*, Aldine, Hawthorne, NJ, 1987.

73. Yuker, H. and Allison, D., Obesity: sociocultural perspectives, in *Understanding Eating Disorders*, Alexander, L. and Lunsden, D.B., Eds., Taylor and Francis, Washington, D.C., 1994, 243.

74. Barnett, R.C. and Baruch, G.K., *The Competent Woman: Perspectives on Development*, Irvington, New York, 1980.

75. Dweck, C.S., Davidson, W., Nelson, S., and Enna, B., Sex differences in learned helplessness: II. The contingencies of evaluative feedback in the classroom; and III. An experimental analysis, *Developmental Psychology*, 14, 268, 1978.

76. Schwartz, L.A. and Markham, W.T., Sex stereotyping in children's toy advertisements. *Sex Roles*, 12, 157, 1985.

14

Educational Programs Aimed at Primary Prevention

John Rohwer

CONTENTS

14.1 Learning Objectives

After completing this chapter you should be able to:

- Identify the various dimensions of prevention and determine when they are most appropriately applied in program development;
- Recognize how the comprehensive prevention model can be incorporated into an eating disorder prevention program;

- Understand the various components for each of the health behavior change theories and how they might be applied to an eating disorder prevention program.

14.2 Research Background

In contrast to the vast numbers of published reports regarding the prevalence and treatment of eating disorders, very little research has been conducted regarding their prevention. However, a number of authors have proposed greater emphasis on prevention, suggesting the most appropriate prevention levels, the target populations, the theoretical framework, and the program content.

14.2.1   Levels of Prevention

Prevention is multifaceted and broad in focus. Its overall goal is to foster a climate in which a systematic attempt is made to change the circumstances that promote, sustain or intensify problems. Primary intervention occurs when a teacher, parent, or counselor first begins to notice signs of an eating disorder. Prevention, therefore, means creating optimum conditions and developing skills to promote the well-being of the young person. Three levels of prevention have been classified: primary, secondary and tertiary (see Table 14.1).

Primary prevention aims at reducing the incidence of a disorder. Its objective is to help individuals avoid problems before signs or symptoms occur. This implies eliminating or reducing the sociocultural factors (such as the stigma attached to being overweight or misconceptions about weight reduction) that increase the risk of eating disorders and involves changing the behaviors that influence body image, self-esteem, eating habits, coping skills, etc. Therefore, one of the reasons for designing elementary-school primary prevention programs is the relatively low prevalence of serious eating problems in that environment, and hence the opportunity to prevent their onset, or at the very least decrease their rate and severity.

Secondary prevention focuses on reducing the duration of a disorder through early diagnosis and effective treatment. The objective is to facilitate identification and correction of a disorder in its early stages when it is less likely to be a lifestyle and associated with other significant problems, such as depression. Secondary prevention involves knowing the (a) warning signs, (b) effective ways to reach out to people in distress, and (c) sources of treatment.

Tertiary prevention directs efforts at the stage when a disorder has become established or an unwanted behavior has become fixed. These prevention efforts are directed at reducing the consequences in case a disorder or negative behavior cannot be completely controlled. The appropriate levels of prevention with regard to eating disorders are diagrammed in Table 14.1.

14.2.2   Primary Prevention

Most of the professional literature on eating disorders recommends primary prevention.[1,2] Shisslak et al.[3] have indicated that neglect of primary prevention may result in

TABLE 14.1

Three Levels of Prevention

Levels	Distinctions	Examples
Primary prevention attempts to forestall the onset of unwanted behavior.	Precedes the earliest signs of a disease and involves efforts directed at a time before the disease or unwanted behavior occurs.	Educational programs designed to encourage students to understand the determinants of body size and weight; develop healthy, balanced eating and activity patterns; and develop social and cultural resiliency skills.
Secondary prevention attempts to reduce the extent of the unwanted behavior.	Identifies diseases at their earliest stages and when the unwanted behavior manifests itself or is believed to be a threat.	The early identification via the DSM-IV diagnostic criteria; accurate referral; emphasis on social alternatives.
Tertiary prevention attempts to prevent relapse following recovery in a treatment program.	Maintains appropriate treatment through its full course to complete rehabilitation. Efforts are directed at reducing the consequences of the disease or behavior.	Full-scale treatment of severe eating disorders, including psychotherapy; hospitalization; re-education on body image; dieting and exercise.

an even greater increase in eating disorders among young people. These same experts have indicated that elementary, middle school and junior-high students are the most appropriate target populations for both primary and secondary prevention efforts. School is by far the most recommended site for these efforts because schools have large captive audiences. In addition, the school is also a place for early identification of eating disorders and a place where referrals to health professionals should be made.

While the necessity of developing some type of primary prevention program for eating disorders has received attention for some time, some researchers have questioned whether a primary prevention program for eating disorders is possible. Vandereycken and Meermann,[4] for example, contend that not enough is known about the etiology of these disorders to develop primary prevention programs and that it would be difficult, if not impossible, to modify sociocultural influences, such as the emphasis on thinness in women. However, Katz,[5] Yager[6] and Neumark-Sztainer[1] consider sociocultural factors to be the most appropriate targets for primary prevention efforts. They believe that enough is known to develop prevention programs and begin research on approaches such as social influence.

Smead[7] has also outlined some of the problems to be faced when designing a primary prevention program for eating disorders, e.g. the influence of the media, fashion, dietetic, and physical fitness industries. These industries have proven to be powerful antagonists. Because the media teach women what the ideal female body should be and how to attain the ideal by diet, exercise, cosmetics, and clothing, these billion-dollar industries are only concerned about marketing products.[8] Therefore, efforts at primary prevention, which may threaten vested economic interests and the established customs and mores of society, are often not encouraged or supported, monetarily or otherwise.

While evidence of dieting, body dissatisfaction, and fear of fat is present among elementary school children (ages 6 to 11), data suggest that these attitudes and behaviors are not as interconnected or ingrained as they are in adolescents.[2] If indeed, these attitudes and behaviors are not yet fully developed in elementary school children, then early intervention may prevent the onset of eating disorders. The focus in such intervention might, for example, place an emphasis on developing a positive body image, as well as identifying the dangers of caloric-restrictive dieting.

A third problem faced by those attempting to develop a primary prevention program for eating disorders is the concern that programs to increase public awareness through education may actually encourage eating disorders.[9,10] If, for example, a teacher were to show a video on eating disorders to a fifth grade class, this might likely lead one or more students to experiment with dieting. Some people compare this to ineffective drug-prevention programs that suggest behavior change is possible through videos demonstrating the use and administration of drugs, or the use of law enforcement officers to show students how to recognize different drugs. This same argument suggests that eating disorders cannot be prevented and that children and youth are not capable of responding appropriately to such information.[7] The question then becomes whether society protects children and youth more by withholding information about eating disorders than by disseminating it through prevention education programs. However, rather than directing curious young minds toward eating disorders, effective prevention efforts place the emphasis on ways to develop a positive body image; that is, an acceptance of heredity and the bodily changes being experienced.

Perhaps the most widely developed and researched prevention programs in the mental health field are those aimed at reducing substance abuse among grade-school and high-school students. These programs have received mixed reviews and have been subjected to some of the same criticisms that have been directed toward the prevention of eating disorders.

Some reviewers of substance-abuse-prevention programs in the schools have concluded that these programs have effected only minor changes in behavior.[11,12] Hochheimer[13] emphasizes that many prevention programs have not delivered their messages effectively and should utilize more interpersonal-persuasion techniques. Other reviewers have emphasized the importance of peer-group leaders in bringing about positive behavioral changes through these programs.[14,15] Recommendations have included the use of trained teachers employing a variety of strategies, including cognitive and behavioral techniques, as well as interventions at the family and community levels.[16] Perhaps because of these recommendations, a number of recent studies of substance-abuse prevention programs have yielded more positive results.

Because substance-abuse prevention programs in the schools are aimed at adolescents, the age group most likely to develop eating disorders, some methods suggested by reviewers of these programs might work in developing prevention programs for eating disorders, for example, (a) the use of peer-group leaders in discussion groups (especially those who have recovered from eating disorders); (b) the use of various persuasion techniques to deliver the messages of these programs more effectively; and (c) the use of interventions at the family and community levels to help generalize and maintain the effects of these programs.

Finally, not all aspects of eating disorders are amenable to change within the context of a school-based prevention program. While personality disorder and family dysfunction probably contribute to the development of at least some cases, these factors are not likely to be affected by educational interventions. Similarly, classroom lessons are not likely to alter existing behavior.[1,17] Therefore, some children will need to be referred to health professionals for diagnosis and/or treatment when warranted.

Primary prevention programs for eating disorders must be comprehensive and involve many systems, educational, medical, business, etc. Prevention efforts must focus on programs and strategies that deal with risks and environmental conditions. They should be collaborative efforts involving multiple strategies to reduce specific risk factors contributing to the incidence of eating disorders among children and youth and encourage them to develop the personal and social skills employed by many of the effective drug education prevention programs.

TABLE 14.2

Models for Primary Prevention

Models	Distinctions	Examples
Information	Knowledge will change attitudes. Knowing the harmful consequences will cause a less positive attitude toward a behavior. Didactic instruction common.	Knowledge that bad breath, yellow teeth, and smelly hair caused by smoking will be prevented. Short-term or current problems such as making friends.
Affective	Improving personal growth results in desired behavior. Attitudes determine behavior.	Focuses on clarifying values, exploring feelings and enhancing self-esteem. Presents idea that poor self-esteem or body image increases the risk for eating disorders.
Social Influence	Resisting social environmental influences that promote unhealthy behaviors. Teaching personal and social skills.	Resisting peer pressure to diet prevents or delays the onset of an eating disorder. Use of peer-group leaders, rejection of society's standard of beauty, and use of various persuasion techniques.
Comprehensive	Incorporating key components from each of the other three models.	Use of sound research base for factual information. Skills for countering environmental influences; e.g., decision-making and communication. Developing healthy weight regulation practices.

14.2.3 Some Models for Primary Prevention in the Schools

A number of different theoretical models aimed at primary prevention of eating disorders have been proposed. Levine, Smolak, and Striegel-Moore[18] state that existing substance-abuse models for primary prevention could be modified to fit the prevention of eating disorders. Hansen[19] reviewed the substance-abuse prevention research literature and identified four basic prevention models: the information model, the affective education model, the social influence resistance model, and the comprehensive prevention approaches (see Table 14.2). Of these, the comprehensive prevention model was deemed to be generally the most effective.

14.2.3.1 Information Model

The information model is based on the theory that an increase in knowledge will change an individual's attitudes. The assumption is that more knowledge about the harmful consequences of chemical use or smoking will prompt a less positive attitude toward that behavior and that a negative attitude will lessen chances of its occurring. Research evidence suggests that, for at least the short term, this process works with children, though with decreasing frequency as their ages increase.

Much drug education, including tobacco education, has been based on the information model, which assumes that people are rational and do not want to suffer harm, and if they are told about the dangers of a behavior, they will avoid it. This approach works to a limited degree with adults, but much less so with children and adolescents. Young people have a normal sense of invulnerability; they think death and disease happen only to old people. Presenting the health hazards of smoking has little personal relevance to most youth. Furthermore, young people may even be enticed by danger. Being told that something is dangerous may be appealing. They know other kids who smoke, and their friends or acquaintances have not had smoking-related illnesses. They do not expect to smoke permanently, at least not long enough to contract any smoking-related diseases.

Instead, experience has taught us that adolescents are much more motivated by the immediate, short-term consequences of smoking. These consequences include limited endurance in sports, bad breath, yellow teeth, smelly hair, and the perception that people like them do not smoke. In the long run, these issues may seem trivial, but they are very influential with teens. The flip side is that many teen girls smoke because they believe it will help them control their weight. This perception, which is a false one, has been nurtured by tobacco ads (e.g., Virginia Slims) and popular lore. In any event, tobacco prevention programs targeting adolescents must prominently feature these negative short-term effects of smoking.

The information model of drug education is generally presented by a teacher in an instructional setting. A lecture format, usually with audiovisual aids, commonly serves as the information model. Occasionally an outside expert, such as a police officer or health-care professional, may be invited into the classroom as a presenter. The information shared generally covers both the short-term and long-term physiological effects of chemical use, with frequent emphasis on the detrimental consequences. The information model is most appropriately designated as "teaching the facts."

In addition, given the nature of adolescent concern with short-term or current problems like making friends, the didactic information model of drug education which emphasizes long-term consequences, such as cirrhosis of the liver or lung cancer, may tend to fall on uninterested ears. However, information that addresses short-term tobacco-related issues such as polluted breath and stained teeth, the possibility of damaging a parent's car while alcohol impaired, or the risk of losing a driver's license, etc., can have more impact.

In summary, "teaching the facts" or the information model alone, while having the potential to be helpful, has not proven to be an efficient means of reducing adolescent chemical use. Researchers conclude from empirical data on this model that adolescents may know about the harmful consequences of chemical use, and display negative attitudes toward the behavior, but still choose to take the risks.

14.2.3.2 Affective Education Model

The affective education model is based upon the theory that improving an individual's personal growth will mean he or she is less likely to use or abuse chemicals. A major assumption is that the problem of chemical use lies within the child, that is, using drugs is compensation for a lack of self-esteem or a lack of adequate tools for making rational decisions. Research is not conclusive in demonstrating the relationship between self-esteem and drug use. Proponents of affective education, a model of the 1970s, believed that young people's attitudes toward alcohol, tobacco, and other drugs (ATOD) determined whether they would use them. Practitioners and researchers suggested that young people's values were not thoroughly grounded, and they were unable to express their feelings adequately. Research showed that people who used drugs often had difficulty identifying and expressing feelings and exhibited poorly developed senses of values and life goals. Affective education efforts focused on clarifying values, exploring feelings, and enhancing self-esteem. Through educational strategies and techniques, students received opportunities to clarify their values about ATOD. Teachers served as catalysts to help students determine their values, but the teachers remained value free. Proponents believed that students who had high self-esteem chose abstinence, so improving a student's self-esteem resulted in reduced ATOD use.

Opponents of this model believed that teachers needed to instill society's values rather than allowing students to develop their own. They said that society valued total abstinence, and students were too young to know right from wrong.

So the battle erupted over who should teach values. Some parents wanted values taught only in the home and religious institutions, not in the schools. Other parents wanted school personnel involved in teaching values, because most parents communicated inadequately with their children.

Research indicated that some affective education efforts were successful in changing values, but evidence did not link changes in values with changes in behavior. Thus, affective education efforts alone were not effective in preventing ATOD use.

14.2.3.3 Social Influence Resistance Model

Social influence resistance approaches are designed to prepare children and youth to resist the various socio-environmental influences that promote unhealthy behaviors. Research in the field of substance use prevention suggests that interventions that enhance skills to resist social and environmental influences that promote tobacco use may prevent or delay the onset of cigarette smoking.[19] Methods for teaching social influence resistance skills are derived from McGuire's[20] Social Inoculation Theory, which has been used in smoking and alcohol prevention, to expose young people to arguments in favor of alcohol or tobacco use that they are likely to encounter in the future. By familiarizing students with the arguments before they hear them in life situations, they are better able to resist. The term *inoculation* derives from the concept of inoculating individuals with germs (social pressures to use tobacco) in order to facilitate development of antibodies (skills for resisting pressures to adopt unhealthy behaviors).[21] The primary objectives are to acquaint students with the powerful social influences that may trigger smoking (e.g. advertising, peer pressure) and to provide them with coping skills and the strong sense of self-efficacy that will enable them to resist such influences. Social influence resistance is recognized as the single most effective component in the substance-abuse prevention research literature.

Neumark-Sztainer[1] recommends the use of social influence mechanisms when discussing unrealistic and unhealthy attitudes about body weight. In her opinion, it is necessary to reduce the value associated with a thin body shape and to increase the value of a healthy diet and physical activity for young people. Emphasis should be placed on helping youth to perceive the negative consequences of excessive dieting and other disordered-eating behaviors. Children need to know that rejection of society's standard for beauty will not produce important negative effects.

Shisslak et al.[8] recommend including other techniques used in substance abuse programs, such as the use of peer-group leaders in discussion groups, the use of various persuasion techniques to deliver the messages more effectively, and the use of interventions at the family and community, levels to help generalize and maintain the effects of these programs. In addition, behaviors of all those involved in the school, community and home must be motivated to become more health enhancing. All must understand and master the number of coping skills available and use them to resist the various social influences promoting dieting and overconcern with weight and shape. Although dieting appears to be pandemic in our culture, it may be possible to teach adolescents to develop healthful eating and exercise patterns.

14.2.3.4 Comprehensive Intervention Model

The comprehensive intervention framework has shown the most promise in the area of drug prevention efforts. As this approach incorporates key elements from each of the other programs. These programs typically use a combination of information and skill-building strategies that include developing problem-solving and decision-making skills, developing cognitive skills for resisting interpersonal and media-based messages, and increasing self-awareness and self-esteem. Because many of the current eating-disorder prevention programs are following the lead from substance-abuse research efforts, further discussion will center on the psychosocial approaches to explaining health-related behaviors as they pertain to the prevention of eating-disorder symptoms.

14.2.4   Other Change Models

A number of health-behavior change models have been developed and evaluated for both community and school health programs. Several have helped to prevent such problems as pregnancy, STD/HIV infection, substance abuse, violence, sexual abuse, suicide, and eating disorders. The following section contains a brief summary of the three most commonly used model, with special attention to the social cognitive model.

14.2.4.1   *Health Belief Model*

The health belief model (HBM) proposes that actions are based on beliefs and that individuals choose behaviors on the basis of their (a) readiness to minimize health risks; (b) environmental influences; and (c) behaviors and skills designed to facilitate the change. Readiness is based on perceived susceptibility (it can happen to me), perceived severity (it has potentially serious consequences), and the desire to change (this behavior's benefits outweigh its costs). The health belief model has broad implications for teachers, counselors, coaches, and parents, because the model provides the opportunity to influence the behaviors and perceptions of young people. In essence, this model postulates that underlying human needs, attitudes, and cognitive processes must be identified and understood before a successful preventive intervention program can be designed.

14.2.4.2   *Precede Model*

This model suggests that there are three major determinants of health behavior: predisposing, enabling, and reinforcing factors. Predisposing factors are the ones a person brings to the situation, such as life experiences, knowledge, cultural and ethnic inheritance, and current beliefs and values. Some of them come from accurate and reliable sources and tend to have a positive impact. Others, however, are picked up through advertisements, articles or popular magazines, as well as conversations with well-meaning relatives and friends. Those beliefs, many of which may have no scientific basis, often become intertwined with more reliable health tenets and values. Enabling factors (such as skills and resources necessary to espouse a healthy behavior) can make health decisions more convenient or more difficult. Educational strategies could be designed, for example, to help children recognize the social pressures to diet, and/or teach them assertiveness skills to cope and resist those pressures. Reinforcing factors relate to the presence or absence of support, encouragement, or discouragement offered by friends and relatives in any situation. These three factors, work together in a cyclical manner to influence behaviors. As a person interacts with others and the environment, the feedback thus received affects the decisions made relative to his or her health status.

14.2.4.3   *Social Cognitive Theory*

Social cognitive theory (SCT) is particularly suitable for programs aimed at preventing excessive weight-loss behaviors. This theory stresses the importance of addressing socio-environmental, personal, and behavioral influences. It states that it is not only events but also the perceptions of events that influence behavior and recognizes the strong influences of positive and negative consequences arising from both the social and the physical environment. However, it places more emphasis on internal factors such as knowledge, attitudes, skills, and values as behavioral determinants.

Behavioral change in this paradigm can be achieved directly by reinforcement of particular behaviors, indirectly through social modeling or observing someone else being reinforced for the behavior, and through self-reward. According to this theory, lifestyle changes will occur if the individual believes: (a) his or her current behaviors pose a threat to a personally valued outcome, for example, health or appearance; (b) the specific behavior change will be likely to reduce these threats; and (c) the person is competent to perform the desired behavior.

14.3 Application of Research Question

14.3.1 Program Content

Specific topics suggested for primary prevention of eating disorders include (a) information about normal physiological, social, and psychological changes during puberty, the increased deposition of fat tissue, and the diversity among individuals; (b) information about nutrition, meal skipping and other eating habits, and the connection between food and emotions; (c) information about physical activity, its importance and appropriate levels; (d) information about weight control, including an understanding of the physiological and psychological effects of food restriction and chronic dieting, discouragement of drastic weight-loss techniques, an understanding of the facts and myths of dietary fads, realistic and safe methods of weight control, and realistic goals for weight change and maintenance; (e) information about body image, including discussions of the role of the media in suggesting slimness as the answer to social concerns and of student images of the ideal body, and an offer of help in determining one's appropriate body weight; (f) information about women-related issues, including the role of women in society, media portrayal of women, and the balance between femininity and competence/autonomy; (g) information related to self-esteem and personal identity; (h) activities focused on skills for coping with stress and with social pressures (i.e., being assertive); and (i) information on anorexia and bulimia nervosa in a manner that discourages their glamorization.

14.3.2 Prevention Strategies

Specific strategies to help prevent the development of eating disorders or risk factors in children have been suggested by various investigators.[2,3,22,23] Suggested strategies for children (see Table 14.3) include teaching them (a) acceptance of a wide range of body shapes; (b) interests and skills that lead to success and fulfillment that are not based on appearance; (c) healthy eating and exercise habits, emphasizing the negative effects of dieting; (d) ways to resist teasing about weight and pressure to diet; and (e) an acceptance of weight gain as a normal, necessary part of development.

14.3.3 Learning Strategies

For the most effective learning to take place, program implementers should seek student-centered strategies that provide for group involvement, and use more than

TABLE 14.3

Recommendations for Child Prevention Programs

The prevalence of body dissatisfaction and dieting among elementary school children are causes for concern in their own rights and as possible precursors to disordered eating. Even without dieting, it is likely that the basis of some adolescent and adult eating disorders is established in childhood. Add to this the consistent failure of middle and high school prevention programs, and one finds compelling arguments for introducing eating disorder prevention in elementary schools. These programs should have several goals, many of which are similar to those found in adolescent prevention programs.

- Acceptance of diverse body shapes. This requires discussion of the causes of body size and shape and of prejudice against heavy people. It should also include, especially among older elementary school age children, information concerning pubertal changes.
- Understanding that body shape is not infinitely mutable.
- Understanding proper nutrition, including the importance of dietary fat and minimum caloric intake.
- Discussion of the negative effects of dieting, as well as the lack of long-term positive effects.
- Consideration of the positive effects of moderate exercise and the negative effects of excessive or compensatory exercise.
- Development of strategies to resist teasing, pressure to diet, propaganda about the importance of slenderness, etc.

Source: From Smolak, L. and Levine, M.P. Toward an Empirical Basis for Primary Prevention of Eating Problems with Elementary School Children, *Journal of Eating Disorders and Prevention,* Winter, 2(4), 301, 1994.

one strategy or activity for each major concept to address the full variety of student abilities and aptitudes. The objective should be to select those strategies that are most appropriate and effective with the target audience, based on student learning styles.

Learning strategies include the following, which have been incorporated into many of the current eating disorder prevention curricula: (a) conflict resolution skill training, which can help ease the tensions children experience during the transition to adolescence; (b) peer group involvement, especially the use of older peer facilitators who can correct unrealistic attitudes and misperceptions regarding weight and appearance;[24] (c) group exercises utilizing role-playing techniques to learn to cope with teasing;[25] (d) assertiveness training, which can teach coping skills, as well as how to deal with increased peer pressures to diet; and (e) problem-solving and time-management skills, which can help children and youth to set realistic goals balancing achievement and relaxation.

The goal, therefore, of prevention intervention should be to help each child or youth develop a strong, positive sense of self-worth, self-respect, and integrity regarding body image. The strategies should be used to assist youngsters in recognizing the importance of eating for health and satisfaction of hunger, not to manipulate weight. Children should learn that choices can be made about which, when, and how food will be eaten, and about a sedentary versus active lifestyle. Children should also learn how healthy bodies progress through puberty. They should learn critical thinking skills, how to resist messages contradicting realistic body diversity, and how to select positive role models.

14.3.4   School-Based Primary Prevention Programs

Although many recommendations have been made with regard to the implementation of school-based programs, and although various eating-disorder programs have been integrated into school curricula, published results and evaluations of their effects have been scant. In general, however, suitable programs should include teaching some or all of the following: (a) signs, symptoms, and health consequences of eating disorders; (b) treatment options; (c) risk factors (sociocultural emphasis on thinness in women, low self-esteem, family problems, and dieting); (d) healthy versus unhealthy weight regulation; and (e) enhancement of life skills (i.e. problem-solving, decision-making, communication, and assertiveness training).

14.3.4.1 Early Prevention Programs

Killen et al.[26] published one of the first long-term controlled studies in which they evaluated the effectiveness of a prevention curriculum designed to modify the eating attitudes and unhealthful weight regulation practices of adolescent girls. Their 18-lesson prevention intervention was delivered via slide show presentations that illustrated the stories of seven girls who demonstrated healthy and unhealthy approaches to weight regulation. Lessons were developed around the assumptions that (a) weight gain is a normal and necessary part of pubertal growth in females; (b) excessive caloric restriction is not an effective long-term weight-control strategy; (c) caloric restriction may actually foster weight fluctuations; (d) adolescents can learn to counteract the cultural pressures promoting dieting and a thin body ideal; and (e) adolescents can be trained to adopt more healthful nutrition practices and physical activity regimens. The impact of the intervention demonstrated an increase in knowledge. Among high-risk students, there was a small effect on body mass index. The authors concluded that it may be more cost effective to target prevention interventions toward high-risk students.

14.3.4.2 Weigh-to-Eat

Neumark-Sztainer[1] recently developed and conducted a program aimed at the prevention of eating disturbances based on psychosocial theory with a strong behavioral approach. The educational program entitled, *The Weigh to Eat*, includes ten sessions addressing topics such as knowledge of nutrition, weight loss and eating disorders, attitudes toward weight-loss methods, and issues of body image and self-esteem. The results indicate a moderate effect with regard to the prevention of unhealthy dieting and binging behaviors.

14.3.4.3 Eating Smart

Smolak[27] developed a ten-lesson primary prevention school-based curriculum for fourth- and fifth-graders entitled *Eating Smart, Eating for Me*. The lessons, aimed at reducing the influence of risk factors and introducing the impact of protective factors, addressed the following concepts: (a) healthy eating without counting calories or fat; (b) exercising for fun, fitness, and friendship; (c) reduction of ignorance and prejudice toward body fat and fat people; (d) greater acceptance of natural diversity in weight and shape; (e) development of a positive body image; (f) the dangers of calorie-restricted dieting; and (g) a critical evaluation of media messages pertaining to body image and nutrition. The program was relatively successful at imparting knowledge. The children learned that (a) there should be no forbidden foods; (b) puberty and genetics significantly contribute to body fat; and (c) dieting to reduce weight has more negative than positive effects. Negative attitudes about fat people appeared to decrease as a result of curriculum participation. The results of the program suggested that contextual differences, perhaps related to school environment, might influence the likelihood of dieting among elementary school children, as they do with young adolescents.

14.3.4.4 Teaching Kids to Eat and Love Their Bodies Too!

In 1997, Kater developed a school-based curriculum program aimed at developing healthy body images and preventing disordered eating for fourth- and sixth-graders

entitled, *Teaching Kids to Eat and Love Their Bodies Too!* The curriculum contains ten separate lessons with specified goals and objectives, rationale, and elaboration on background concepts. Four of the ten lessons emphasize the biology of what cannot be
controlled regarding body size, shape, and hunger. Four additional lessons emphasize factors influencing weight and body image that offer choices: eating well to satisfy hunger, energy and nutritional needs, limiting sedentary activities, embracing a
balanced sense of identity (versus placing undue focus on any single aspect, such as
appearance), and choosing realistic role models. Two lessons are sociocultural in
nature. Preliminary results of this pilot study indicate that the curriculum produces
an increase in knowledge, positive attitudes, and healthful intentions, relative to
(a) body image, (b) influences controlling body size and shape, (c) the hazards of
weight-loss dieting, and (d) unrealistic media images.*

14.4 Summary

Program evaluation research and the prevalence of dieting and body dissatisfaction
in young children emphasize the need for new prevention programs. For this reason,
preventionists propose that focusing programs on elementary school children rather
than on adolescents may be more effective. Elementary school prevention programs
may be able to prevent the impacts of messages that support the thinness schema,
while encouraging realistic expectations of the normal physical changes of maturation. Finally, school prevention programs can teach children about the normality of
body fat and the futility and danger of dieting to achieve below-normal weight.

References

1. Neumark-Sztainer, D., School-based programs for preventing eating disturbances,
   Journal of School Health, 66, 64–71, 1996.
2. Smolak, L. and Levine, M.P., Toward an empirical basis for primary prevention of eating
   problems with elementary school children, *Eating Disorders*, 2, 293–307, 1994.
3. Shisslak, C.M., Crago, M., and Neal, M.E., Prevention of eating disorders among
   adolescents, *American Journal of Health Promotion*, 5, 100–106, 1990.
4. Vandereyaken, W. and Meermann, R., Anorexia nervosa: is prevention possible?
   International Journal of Psychiatry and Medicine, 14, 191–205, 1984.
5. Katz, J.L., Some reflections on the nature of the eating disorders: on the need for humility,
   International Journal of Eating Disorders, 4, 617–626, 1985.
6. Yager, J., Afterward, in *Psychiatry Update: Annual Review*, R. Hales and A. Frances, Eds.,
   American Psychiatric Association, Washington, D.C., 4, 1985, 516–521.
7. Smead, V.S., Considerations prior to establishing preventive interventions for eating
   disorders, *Ontario Psychologist*, 17, 12–17, 1985.
8. Shisslak C.M., Crago, M., Estes, L.S., and Gray, N., Content and method of developmen-
   tally appropriate prevention programs, in *The Developmental Psychopathology of Eating
   Disorders: Implications for Research, Prevention and Treatment*, L. Smolak, M.P. Levine, and
   R. Striegal-Moore, Eds., Mahwah, NJ, Lawrence Erlbaum Associates, 1996, 341–363.

* For grades 4–6. Available from K. Kater, Franklin Center, Suite 109, 2397 Seventh Avenue East, North
St. Paul, MN 55109.

9. Garner, D.M., Iatrogenesis in anorexia nervosa and bulimia nervosa, *International Journal of Eating Disorders*, 4, 701–726, 1985.

10. Chiodo, J. and Latimer, P.R., Vomiting as a learned weight-control technique in bulimia, *Journal of Behavior Therapy and Experimental Psychiatry*, 14, 131–135, 1983.

11. Nathan P.E., Failures in prevention, *American Psychologist*, 38, 459–467, 1983.

12. Schaps, E., Bartolo, R., Moskowitz, J., Palley, C.S., and Churgin, S., A review of 127 drug abuse prevention program evaluations, *Journal of Drug Issues*, 11, 17–43, 1981.

13. Hochheimer, J.L., Reducing alcohol abuse: a critical review of educational strategies, in *Alcohol: A Public Policy*, M.H. Moore and D.R. Gerstein, Eds., National Academy Press, Washington, D.C., 1982, 186–235.

14. Botvin, C. J., Baker, E., Renick, N.L. Filazzola, A.D., and Botvin, E.M., A cognitive-behavioral approach to substance abuse prevention, *Addictive Behaviors*, 9, 137–147, 1984.

15. Luepker, R.V., Johnson, C.A., Murray, D.M., and Pechauk, T.F., Prevention of cigarette smoking: three-year follow-up of an educational program for youth, *Journal of Behavioral Medicine*, 6, 53–62, 1983.

16. Saylor, K.E., Coates, J.J., Killen, J., Slinkard, L.A., Nutrition education research: feast or famine? *Promoting Adolescent Health: A Dialogue in Research and Practice*, T.G. Coates Ed., Academic Press, Orlando, FL, 1982, 355–380.

17. Swisher, J., Early adolescent belief systems and substance abuse, in *Early Adolescence: Perspectives on Research, Policy and Intervention*, R.M. Lerner, Ed., Lawrence Erlbaum Associates, Mahwah, NJ, 1993, 369–382.

18. Smolak, L., Levine, M.P., and Striegel-Moore, R., *The Developmental Psychopathology of Eating Disorders: Implications for Research Prevention and Treatment*, Lawrence Erlbaum Associates, Mahwah, NJ, 1996.

19. Hansen, W.B., School-based substance abuse prevention: a review of the state of the art in curriculum, 1980-1990, *Health and Education Research*, 7, 403–430, 1992.

20. McGuire, W., Inducing resistance to persuasion, in *Advances in Experimental Psychology*, L. Berkowitz Ed., Academic Press, New York, 1964, 191–229.

21. McAlister, A.L., Perry, C., and Maccoby, N., Adolescent smoking, onset and prevention, *Pediatrics*, 63, 15–28, 1979.

22. Levine, M.P. and Hill, L., *A 5-Day Lesson Plan for Eating Disorders: Grades 7–12*, NEDCO, Tulsa, OK, 1991.

23. Striegel-Moore, R.H., Prevention of bulimia nervosa: questions and challenges, in *The Developmental Psychopathology of Eating Disorders: Implications for Research, Prevention, and Treatment*, L.S. Smolak, M.P. Levine, and R. Striegel-Moore Eds., Lawrence Erlbaum Associates, Mahwah, NJ, 1996, chap. 14.

24. Shisslak, C.M. and Crago, M., Toward a new model for the prevention of eating disorders, in *Feminist Perspectives on Eating Disorders*, P. Fallon, M.A. Katzman, and S.C. Wooley Eds., Guilford Press, New York, 1994, 419–437.

25. Cattarin, J.A. and Thompson, J.K., A three-year longitudinal study of body image, eating disturbance, and general psychological functioning in adolescent females, *Eating Disorders: Journal of Treatment and Prevention*, 2, 114–125, 1994.

26. Killen, J.D., Taylor, C.B., Taylor, C.B., Hammer, L.D., Litt, I., Wilson, D.M., Rich, T., Hayward, C., Simmonds, B., Kramer, H., and Verady, A., An attempt to modify unhealthful eating attitudes and weight regulation practices of young adolescent girls, *International Journal of Eating Disorders*, 13, 369–384, 1993.

27. Smolak, L., Levine, M.P., and Shermer, F., Lessons from lessons: an evaluation of an elementary school prevention program, *The Prevention of Eating Disorders*, Van Noordenboss, G. and Vandereycken, W., Eds., Athlone, London, 1998.

28. Kater, K., Teaching kids to eat, and love their bodies too! North St. Paul, MN, 1997.

15

The Role of Parents, School Personnel, and the Community in the Primary Prevention of Eating Disorders in Children

Marilyn Massey-Stokes

CONTENTS

15.1 Learning Objectives

After completing this chapter, the reader will be able to:

- Explain the concept of primary prevention;
- Discuss the roles of parents in the primary prevention of eating disorders in children;
- Discuss the roles of school personnel in the primary prevention of eating disorders in children;

0-8493-2027-5/01/$0.00+$.50
© 2001 by CRC Press, Inc.

- Explain the role of the community in the primary prevention of eating disorders in children;

- Discuss the significance of stress management in the prevention of eating disorders in children;

- Develop a personal action plan to help prevent childhood eating disorders.

15.2 Research Background

15.2.1 Primary Prevention

In recent years, much discussion has revolved around the concept of primary prevention along with the numerous definitions, models, and theories explaining its meaning and how it relates to the promotion of individuals' health and well-being. Fundamentally, primary prevention involves more than reducing or eliminating factors that contribute to a particular condition. It also includes developing personal attributes and creating environmental conditions that promote health and wellness.[1] According to Pransky,[1] research demonstrates that a wide array of social-behavioral problems, including alcohol and drug abuse, child abuse and neglect, eating disorders, and teen suicide, stem from general contributing causes. He explains, "We can do more than just respond to these symptoms. We can ensure that common factors that contribute to the creation of each of these problems are reduced or eliminated and that a set of healthy conditions is built that will serve to prevent them all." For example, Pransky's conceptual framework* for the prevention of eating disorders depicts contributing factors (risk factors) as cultural influences, socio-environmental stressors, organic factors, lack of opportunity, and family dysfunction. Protective factors within the individual, family, school, peers, and community that promote resilience and offset these risk factors include healthy self-perceptions, social skills, awareness, and social support. This process is summarized in Table 15.1.

All of these elements interact synergistically, a fact that often overwhelms people when it comes to learning how to take the first step in prevention. Similarly, Bloom[2] constructed a prevention framework illustrating that relevant prevention strategies need to be considered in terms of increasing strengths (protective factors) and decreasing limitations (risk factors). Bloom's model depicts interaction among these key actions: *increasing* individual strengths, social supports, and physical environmental resources, and *decreasing* individual limitations, social stressors, and physical environmental pressures.[2]

Although numerous health education and prevention programs for children and adolescents focus on risk behaviors, a more positive pathway to prevent young people from adopting unhealthy attitudes and behaviors is through helping them to acquire protective assets. Extensive research conducted by the Search Institute** reveals 40 developmental assets that constitute the building blocks young people need to make wise decisions, choose positive paths, and grow into healthy, competent, and caring adults.[3] These are classified in eight primary categories: support, empowerment, boundaries and expectations, constructive use of time, commitment to learning, positive values, social competencies, and positive identity. The categories

---

* Available from NEHRI Publications, Cabot, VT.
** 700 South Third Street, Minneapolis, MN 55415.

TABLE 15.1

The Conceptual Framework of Eating Disorders

Factors Contributing to Eating Disorders

Cultural Influences

Cultural demands for/image of thinness
Appear predominantly in women (10:1 ratio)
Most appear in adolescence, a time of developmental pressures, identity and boundary searching
in world that gives mixed messages about future productive roles, particularly for female
adolescents

Social Stresses

Appear during transition and separation periods, like entering high school or college
External avoidance behaviors
Weight gains shown during stress, particularly life-stress situations
Poor diet increases stress on the body

Organic Factors

Difficulty recognizing hunger/disturbance in hunger awareness
Constitutional impulsivity/self-regulation difficulties
Perfectionistic, overly compliant and overconscientious personality
May be constitutionally heavy but tries to fight it with constant dieting
Binging-purging or excessive dieting produces imbalance (blood-sugar roller coaster)
Serotonin deficiencies related to depression

Lack of Opportunity

Perception of lack of opportunity to make major life decisions
Feelings of helplessness related to being overachiever

Family Dysfunction

Difficulties in maternal bonding (hostile-dependent mother-child relationship)
Forced feeding based on other than biological needs, often present in infancy
Obesity related to disturbances in family relationships
Overrestrictiveness (especially around food); parent makes most decisions
"Best little girl in the world" syndrome
Poor boundary definitions
Characteristics of enmeshment, overprotectiveness, conflict avoidance, and rigidity

Factors Building Resistance to Eating Disorders

Healthy Self-perceptions

Capability and success (related to sense of failure; not in step with others)
Self-worth (related to low self esteem and belief that worth depends on weight)
Control over life (related to lack of control in life)
Self-image (related to distorted perception of self and negative self-statements)

Social Skills

Getting in touch with feelings
Impulse control
Self-motivation
Self-evaluation
Alternative ways of achieving relief and comfort (instead of gaining it through substitute of binging
and vomiting)

TABLE 15.1 (*continued*)

The Conceptual Framework of Eating Disorders

Awareness

Knowledge that there's no need to live up to others' expectations
Effects of lack of food and binging
Vomiting cycle's effect on body

Support

Eating disorder support group

Source: From Pransky, J., *Prevention: The Critical Need*, Burrell Foundation, Springfield, MO, 1991, p. 24. With permission.

are further divided into two major dimensions: (1) *external assets* — the positive developmental environments and experiences that surround and protect children and youth, and (2) *internal assets* — the skills and values necessary for strong character development (see Table 15.2.) The more of both types of assets children and adolescents acquire, the more likely they are to thrive and reach their fullest potential.[3]

Everyone can play a proactive role in the asset-building process. Parents, school personnel, child care providers, and community members can all work together to assure that young children have opportunities to learn life skills and acquire the competencies, relationships, and values they need for healthy development.

15.2.2 Dieting and Weight Concerns in Children

It has been widely reported that adolescent females (and males) have concerns about body weight and shape and engage in dieting behaviors. What is less clear is the extent to which preadolescents possess similar weight concerns and use dieting to control body weight. Studies have shown that girls as young as 9 years old use dieting and exercise to lose weight, even those who do not consider themselves to be overweight.[3-7] Collins[8] reported that body-figure perceptions and expectations pertaining to thinness among females may begin as early as 6 to 7 years of age. In addition, Thelen, Lawrence, and Powell[7] noted that beginning at the age of 6, children exhibit a developmental progression of internalizing cultural ideals regarding physical attractiveness. Childress, Brewerton, Hodges, and Jarrell[9] used the Kids' Eating Disorders Survey with 3175 students (1610 females and 1565 males) in grades 5 to 8. Their findings revealed that more than 40% of the students reported "feeling fat" and/or the desire to lose weight. Another study that examined body image in preadolescent and adolescent females showed that both groups wanted to look thinner than they actually were.[10] Although preadolescent girls are concerned about their body images, they have not developed such critical levels of body dissatisfaction as their adolescent peers.[10] Therefore, many experts recommend implementing primary prevention at the elementary school level.[11-17]

Furthermore, because research points to the early years — birth to age 5 — as an extremely crucial developmental period, it is essential to begin prevention efforts in early childhood. Although some studies have targeted body image, body dissatisfaction, and eating attitudes and behaviors of elementary school children, research involving children at the preschool and kindergarten levels is scarce. Nevertheless, the strategies and tips presented in this chapter can be modified to address the needs of children at various stages of development, including the early childhood years.

TABLE 15.2

Forty Developmental Assets of Healthy Communities

40 Developmental Assets

Search Institute has identified the following building blocks of healthy development that help young people grow up healthy, caring, and responsible.

	CATEGORY	ASSET NAME AND DEFINITION
External Assets	Support	1. **Family support** — Family life provides high levels of love and support. 2. **Positive family communication** — Young person and her or his parent(s) communicate positively, and young person is willing to seek advice and counsel from parent(s). 3. **Other adult relationships** — Young person receives support from three or more nonparent adults. 4. **Caring neighborhood** — Young person experiences caring neighbors. 5. **Caring school climate** — School provides a caring, encouraging environment. 6. **Parent involvement in schooling** — Parent(s) are actively involved in helping young person succeed in school.
	Empowerment	7. **Community values youth** — Young person perceives that adults in the community value youth. 8. **Youth as resources** — Young people are given useful roles in the community. 9. **Service to others** — Young person serves in the community one hour or more per week. 10. **Safety** — Young person feels safe at home, at school, and in the neighborhood.
	Boundaries & Expectations	11. **Family boundaries** — Family has clear rules and consequences and monitors the young person's whereabouts. 12. **School boundaries** — School provides clear rules and consequences. 13. **Neighborhood boundaries** — Neighbors take responsibility for monitoring young people's behavior. 14. **Adult role models** — Parent(s) and other adults model positive, responsible behavior. 15. **Positive peer influence** — Young person's best friends model responsible behavior. 16. **High expectations** — Both parent(s) and teachers encourage the young person to do well.
	Constructive Use of Time	17. **Creative activities** — Young person spends three or more hours per week in lessons or practice in music, theater, or other arts. 18. **Youth programs** — Young person spends three or more hours per week in sports, clubs, or organizations at school and/or in the community. 19. **Religious community** — Young person spends one or more hours per week in activities in a religious institution. 20. **Time at home** — Young person is out with friends "with nothing special to do" two or fewer nights per week.
Internal Assets	Commitment to Learning	21. **Achievement motivation** — Young person is motivated to do well in school. 22. **School engagement** — Young person is actively engaged in learning. 23. **Homework** — Young person reports doing at least one hour of homework every school day. 24. **Bonding to school** — Young person cares about her or his school. 25. **Reading for pleasure** — Young person reads for pleasure three or more hours per week.
	Positive Values	26. **Caring** — Young person places high value on helping other people. 27. **Equality and social justice** — Young person places high value on promoting equality and reducing hunger and poverty. 28. **Integrity** — Young person acts on convictions and stands up for her or his beliefs. 29. **Honesty** — Young person "tells the truth even when it is not easy." 30. **Responsibility** — Young person accepts and takes personal responsibility. 31. **Restraint** — Young person believes it is important not to be sexually active or to use alcohol or other drugs.
	Social Competencies	32. **Planning and decision making** — Young person knows how to plan ahead and make choices. 33. **Interpersonal competence** — Young person has empathy, sensitivity, and friendship skills. 34. **Cultural competence** — Young person has knowledge of and comfort with people of different cultural/racial/ethnic backgrounds. 35. **Resistance skills** — Young person can resist negative peer pressure and dangerous situations. 36. **Peaceful conflict resolution** — Young person seeks to resolve conflict nonviolently.
	Positive Identity	37. **Personal power** — Young person feels he or she has control over "things that happen to me." 38. **Self-esteem** — Young person reports having a high self-esteem. 39. **Sense of purpose** — Young person reports that "my life has a purpose." 40. **Positive view of personal future** — Young person is optimistic about her or his personal future.

Source: From Search Institute, *Healthy Communities: Healthy Youth Tool Kit*, 1998. With permission.

15.2.3   Sexual Abuse and Eating Disturbances

Although results on the relationship between abuse and eating disturbances have been equivocal,[18,19] research indicates that a disproportionate number of women who seek treatment for eating disorders have personal history of abuse or sexual assault.[18–20] Therefore, it is imperative that primary prevention of problematic eating should coexist with prevention programs that target prevention of sexual, emotional, and physical abuse. These programs need to begin in early childhood (e.g., lessons concerning body boundaries and "good touch" vs. "bad touch"), and should be implemented regularly throughout the school years. In addition, community programs need to be available for adults who are struggling with these problems and issues related to abuse. Health care providers, hospital emergency personnel, police officers, and those who work with battered women and children should serve as sentinels looking for signs of problematic eating in children and women who live with domestic violence. Finally, an organized referral system should be in place, so that these women and children can receive the help they need.

15.2.4   The Role of Stress Management in the Prevention of Eating Disorders in Children

A growing concern exists concerning the impact of stress on the lives of children. Numerous life events can produce varying degrees of childhood stress, including domestic violence; death of a family member, friend, or pet; marital conflict, marital separation, and divorce; remarriage of a parent; birth of a brother or sister; loss of a job by a parent; and illness of a child or other family member. Other stressors include a dysfunctional family life, school pressures, exposure to violence, exposure to a pervasive drug culture, and poverty and crowded housing.[21] Children need to learn personal and social skills to help them successfully meet life's demands and challenges. Stress management and coping skills are fundamental personal and social skills that children need to learn at a young age. Without these life skills, children are, in effect, going on a survival trip without a backpack. Maladaptive coping mechanisms adversely influence all dimensions of health and wellness and greatly diminish overall quality of life. For example, lack of stress management skills can upset children's mental and emotional well-being, harm their interpersonal relationships, and negatively impact their performance in school and various activities. In addition, eating disturbances in children have been associated with a lack of coping skills. In their examination of the development of restrictive eating throughout the life span, Attie and Brooks-Gunn[22] cite research studies that link several stress-related factors to childhood eating disorders, for example, low self-esteem manifested in interpersonal problems, perfectionistic behavior, depression, family stress, and major life events. Other authors have identified similar findings.[11,23,24]

Stress management and relaxation techniques are valuable tools to help prevent eating disturbances. Benson's[25] seminal work regarding the relaxation response undergirds the significant impact that relaxation techniques can have on health and well-being. These techniques include deep breathing, meditation, repetitive prayer, progressive muscle relaxation, and imagery. Comprehensive stress management includes relaxation techniques, plus an arsenal of other powerful strategies, including effective communication and interpersonal skills, cognitive restructuring, creative problem solving, well-balanced nutrition, regular physical activity, art and music therapy, journal writing, creative writing, humor, and role play.

15.3 Application of Research Question

This section addresses the question, "How can parents, school personnel, and community members play roles in the prevention of eating disorders among children?" Each of these groups can positively influence children and adolescents by promoting self-esteem, teaching coping skills, and staying alert to behavior that may indicate disordered eating patterns. Prevention of eating disorders in a society that exerts so many pressures on children requires the participation by all groups who are in a position to positively influence them.

15.4 Tips for Primary Prevention of Eating Disorders in Children

Education is considered one of the principal vehicles for primary prevention. Educational programs and activities can be implemented in a variety of settings, including homes, schools, health-care facilities, community centers, and churches; and they are most effective when they target families, schools, and communities simultaneously. These strategies need to be multifaceted and emphasize a wide range of components, including: (a) the development of positive self-esteem, self-efficacy, and a healthy body image; (b) development of important life skills, including personal and social skills and coping skills; (c) promotion of experiences that encourage self-confidence and independence; (d) education about the importance of balanced nutrition and physical activity to health and wellness; (e) opportunities to challenge sociocultural myths and attitudes regarding body shape and size and gender roles; and (f) activities that promote change of unhealthy beliefs and practices regarding body weight regulation within the social milieu.[12,13]

15.4.1 Parents and Other Caregivers

As primary caregivers in the early years of life, parents are considered the fundamental socializing agents and overseers for a child's interaction with the larger environment.[26] In addition, children's fear of fatness begins early and is strongly influenced by parental attitudes, thereby creating a strong motivation to involve parents in the education process.[13,16,24] According to Smolak and Levine,[16] parental involvement in the prevention process is so crucial for several reasons. First, research with adolescents and college women points to possible links between maternal attitudes and behaviors and daughters' eating and dieting behaviors. Second, adolescent eating attitudes seem to be affected by family members' teasing, and teasing is thought to play a role in prepubertal anorexia nervosa. Third, parents are in charge of what food is in the home and what foods a child can eat, and are likely to exert even more control over eating behaviors of younger children. Therefore, it is possible that parents encourage dieting behaviors in children. Such diet promotion is more likely to occur if a parent is struggling with her/his own personal issues regarding body weight, body image, and dieting. Also, if children are overweight, parents may encourage dieting as a means for losing body fat.

Studies have shown a link between body-image disturbances and problematic eating.[27-30] Kelly[31] presents evidence of a possible connection between negative body image and risky sexual behaviors. Another reason why parents and caregivers play such a critical role is that children develop feelings and attitudes about their bodies at an early age, and these affective factors are largely dependent upon the care they receive. Costin[20] explains that during the early years, a child develops a sense of "body self" that can have lasting impact. A healthy body image involves a healthy sense of body boundaries — feeling separate from but equal to others. However, when a child is abused or neglected by a caregiver, the child develops poor body boundaries, poorly defined self, and thus a negative body image.

Because parents and other caregivers are instrumental in promoting the healthy development of children, including the development of a healthy body image, the following guidelines may be beneficial in the prevention of eating problems in children.

- Be loving and nurturing; NEVER abuse or neglect a child.

- Be a vigilant role model who practices healthful behaviors, such as effective communication, sensible eating and exercise habits, and effective stress-management and coping techniques.

- Avoid labeling foods "good" or "bad," and do not use food as a form of reward or punishment.

- Talk with your children about cultural messages regarding body shape and size. Discuss magazine ads, television commercials and shows, and movies that convey subtle and overt messages that "thin is in."

- Read your children stories and poems that deal with eating disorders as well as related topics, such as body image, self-esteem, individual uniqueness, growth and development, emotions and feelings, friendship, and communication. Children's literature is an effective medium for teaching about sensitive health-related topics. Talking with children about what they read helps them to verbalize their comprehension by paraphrasing messages they learn from reading and expressing their thoughts about what characters are feeling and experiencing.

- Help children develop competence and independence by mastering challenges. According to Seligman,[32] focusing on the "doing well" side of self-esteem helps children become more self-confident and optimistic. When children successfully overcome frustration and achieve goals, their self-esteem is bolstered and their self-efficacy increases, which sparks further success.

- Help girls build feelings of self-value that are not dependent on others' approval, particularly approval from males.[33]

- Be watchful for behavior that may indicate unhealthy attitudes toward the body, eating, and exercise. A remark that, "I can't eat a piece of birthday cake because it will make me fat," is indicative of distorted thinking and needs to be challenged. Teach children how to change negative thought patterns by providing concrete examples and regular opportunities to practice cognitive restructuring.

- Encourage the development of the four conditions of self-esteem. Children need to be given ongoing opportunities to develop a sense of uniqueness, sense of connectedness (belonging), sense of power (competence), and the sense of role models (people they feel are worthy of emulation, who have values and beliefs that guide their actions in various situations and exhibit a strong sense of purpose in life).[34]

15.4.2   School Personnel

Eating disorders can produce long-lasting, negative effects on academic performance, interpersonal relationships, and overall health and wellness.[33] Because children and youth spend a great deal of time in school, school personnel can play significant roles in the primary prevention of eating disorders via classroom instruction, enhanced detection and referral, and the ongoing professional development of school employees.[33] According to Neumark-Sztainer,[35] prevention should be directed to children and young people of all ages (preschool through college) through learning opportunities that promote healthy eating and exercise; encouragement related to body acceptance; and teaching of key social and personal skills, including those necessary for building healthy relationships and for developing critical thinking and problem-solving skills. In addition, she asserts that opportunities should be provided to promote gender equality and empowerment.

15.4.2.1   Teachers and Coaches

The following tips are designed to help teachers and coaches be proactive in the prevention of problematic eating.

- Consistently strive to help children develop self-esteem and self-efficacy (see Appendix 15-A). Focus on what children do well, and continually offer them opportunities to achieve realistic goals and experience success.
- Practice health-enhancing behaviors such as sound nutrition, regular physical activity, and effective stress management and coping strategies. Model and teach these life skills to students.
- Topics such as mental and emotional health (including self-esteem and depression), body image, dieting, and gender stereotypes are often sensitive and difficult to discuss. Examine your own attitudes and beliefs about these issues, and educate yourself about eating disorders.[33]
- Monitor students for initial signs of problems. Be concerned when a child shows signs of possessing low self-esteem and distorted body image; communicates dissatisfaction regarding body weight, shape, or size; and/or displays unhealthful eating and exercise behaviors.
- Know your limits, and understand the correct procedure for referrals. Be knowledgeable about community services that can help students and their families.[33]
- Health education teachers and physical education teachers possess rich opportunities to incorporate instruction about nutrition, physical activity, and stress management and relaxation techniques into their programs.
- Health education teachers, physical education teachers, and coaches should promote lifelong physical activity to enhance health and wellness, and not advocate exercise as a method to lose weight and/or alter body shape.
- Coaches and physical education teachers should correct misconceptions such as "no pain, no gain"[36] and "more is better." In addition, they should offer students opportunities to engage in a variety of non-competitive physical activities.
- Many athletes are at high risk for developing eating disorders, particularly those involved in gymnastics, dance, cheerleading, fitness classes, track, and wrestling. Coaches and instructors should talk to athletes about eating disorders and look for warning signs of potential problems.

- Classroom teachers can incorporate prevention lessons into language arts, mathematics, science, and social studies. Eating Disorders Awareness and Prevention (EDAP), a non-profit organization, has a variety of materials that promote self-esteem, body image, and healthy eating. One prime example is the EDAP Puppet Prevention Program (kindergarten through fifth grade), which encourages healthy eating habits and acceptance of body-size diversity. In addition, EDAP has recently partnered with Kathy Kater, LICSW, psychotherapist and eating-disorder therapist, to publish *Healthy Body Image: Teaching Kids to Eat and Love Their Bodies Too!*[37] which is a curriculum for grades 4 to 6 that promotes healthy eating and body image. The resource manual cites objectives and concepts that can be adapted for use at any age. (See Appendix 15-A.)

- Incorporate family involvement activities for class assignments and projects that target the prevention of eating disturbances. Birch[38] suggests a family involvement calendar as a creative way to involve the family in the health education process.

- Other ideas include using workbooks that students and parents complete together, inviting parents to the school to view activities and projects created by the students, and having students put on plays or prepare meals for their parents.[16]

- Give students and parents a copy of Basic Assertive Rights. (See Figure 19.2 in Chapter 19.) Use the list as a focal point for a family involvement activity, and encourage student-parent dialogues about these rights and how they relate to the prevention of eating disturbances and related problems.

15.4.2.2 School Nurses

School nurses are in a unique position to prevent eating disorders because of their focus on child health promotion and their routine contacts with many students.[36] School nurses can be more proactive in the prevention of eating disorders by implementing the following suggestions.

- Observe children's behavior for warning signs that they may have eating disturbances.

- Understand the correct referral process, and be knowledgeable about community resources.

- Conduct in-service workshops for teachers, coaches, and other school personnel regarding the prevention of eating disorders. Include information about risk factors, signs and symptoms, health consequences, complications, and community resources.

- Educate children about health. Help them learn the importance of eating well, exercising regularly, getting adequate sleep and rest, and practicing stress management and relaxation techniques.

- Educate students regarding the prevention of eating disturbances.

- Be a positive role model regarding personal health behaviors.

- Be an advocate for the health rights of children by correcting misconceptions about eating problems and involving parents in the prevention process.

- In the absence of a school counselor or psychologist, the school nurse may play the role of health counselor by increasing school and community awareness and educating and counseling students and families about eating disorders.

15.4.2.3 *School Counselors and Psychologists*

Because of their expertise in mental and emotional health, school counselors and psychologists play prominent roles in the prevention of eating disorders among children.[39,40] In talking with and listening to students, these professionals may be the first to detect signs of distorted thinking and body dissatisfaction that can lead to problematic eating. They can help children develop cognitive restructuring skills and learn to be more accepting of self and others. Other suggestions for school counselors and psychologists include:

- Conduct in-service and staff development programs concerning the prevention of eating disorders.
- Collaborate with school nurses, teachers, and coaches to develop and implement prevention programs.
- Conduct behavioral health interventions with individuals and groups of students.[41] Talk with children about the importance of health-promoting behaviors; teach them behavioral self-management skills, such as relaxation and other stress management skills, impulse control, and anger management.
- Distribute family newsletters that provide information about the prevention of eating disorders and include ideas for prevention activities.
- Conduct evaluations to assess the outcomes of the prevention programs and related activities.
- Act as a liaison in the coordination of school and community services.[41]
- Serve on community coalitions, and speak to community groups about the prevention of eating disorders.

15.4.2.4 *School Food Service Personnel*

Those who work in school food service often have unique opportunities to observe students' eating behaviors and should report any warning signs that may indicate eating disturbances. However, as Benson[42] notes, school food service personnel should use caution and discuss concerns with a school counselor or other reliable professional after considerable observations. In addition to the detection of possible eating problems, school food service personnel should consider these suggestions:

- Be knowledgeable about nutrition; know the types and amounts of dietary fats that are recommended for proper growth and development.[42]
- Provide menus that offer a healthful variety of tasty foods and reinforce important nutrition concepts that children learn in the classroom.
- Establish a committee of teachers and students to provide feedback on menus.[42]
- Let each classroom plan a menu that reflects sound nutrition, based on the principles outlined in the Food Guide Pyramid and the Dietary Guidelines for Americans.
- Provide opportunities for students, teachers, and parents to plan special food events that encourage healthful eating. For example, ethnic groups can prepare healthful versions of their favorite foods for a special evening of festive ethnic food sampling.
- Talk with children about being healthy and energetic—not about calories, body weight, or dieting.[42]

TABLE 15.3

Schools and Communities: Activity Ideas for the Awareness and Prevention of Eating Disorders in Children

- Sponsor health fairs at schools and other central points centered around themes that educate children, families, and other community members about health and wellness, healthy lifestyles and healthful choices, and available school and community resources and services. Health fairs can specifically target the prevention of eating disorders.
- Hold poster contests for students that promote the awareness of eating-disorders prevention. Ask local businesses to display the posters.
- Sponsor speech and debate contests that focus on the theme of eating-disorder prevention.
- Have students create songs and public service announcements (PSAs) that deal with themes surrounding the prevention of eating disturbances. Ask local radio and television stations to air the songs and PSAs.
- Hold special school activities in the evenings or on the weekends, for example wellness clubs, family fitness nights, or fitness walks. Activities can be tailored to target prevention of eating disturbances.
- Sponsor open educational forums in the schools on important issues related to the prevention of eating disorders, such as parent-child communication, media awareness/literacy, and bolstering self-esteem.
- Use the local school as a site for events, meetings, and screenings that promote the prevention of eating disorders.
- Provide eating disorder prevention facts and tips to local newspapers to use as sidebars for related stories.[43]
- Use eating disorder prevention facts and tips to spark discussion at community meetings, or in response to the question, "What can I do to help prevent eating disorders in children and youth?"[43]
- Share the facts and tips in other formats, such as bookmarks, cards, mail inserts, church bulletin inserts, magnets, flyers, bus and subway signs, and shopping bag panels.[43]
- Involve the religious community, and encourage it to play a proactive role in promoting awareness and prevention of eating disorders.
- Support well-known non-profit organizations such as Eating Disorders Awareness and Prevention (EDAP), and help disseminate their prevention and awareness information and programs.
- Engage health care providers (physicians, nurses, dentists, dieticians, and mental health professionals) to distribute information and provide programs to the community.

All school personnel can be advocates for organizational change, particularly if the school climate is not conducive to the prevention of eating disturbances and related issues. For example, school staff can help develop health-enhancing policies at the district level by requiring health education to be incorporated in the entire curriculum.

15.4.2.5 *The Community Connection*

The West Virginia Healthy Schools Program (WVHSP) is a prime example of how schools and communities can work together to promote health and wellness by implementing child nutrition and safe and drug-free school programs.[43] One of the salient results of having schools and communities work together to foster healthy children is explained by Valentine:[43] "Students who see the community interested in their health, have positive role models to follow, and are provided opportunities to reinforce knowledge about health through community-sponsored activities will be much more likely to take their health education lessons seriously." Schools and communities can work as partners to plan and implement activities that target the prevention of eating disturbances. (See Table 15.3.)

Additional suggestions include the following:

- Health-care providers (e.g., pediatricians, nurses, dieticians, dentists) can instruct parents about sound nutrition via one-on-one meetings, parent education classes, videos, books, and tip sheets. Information about nutrition and physical activity, developmental stages of growth, and body image/satisfaction can help parents to be more proactive in helping their children avoid problematic eating behaviors.

- Health-care providers need to address more sensitive issues such as prevention of child abuse and neglect and the promotion of mental and emotional health. Programs can cover important topics such as effective parenting, anger management, stress management and coping skills, effective communication, interpersonal skills, and relationships.

- Other significant points of contact within the community include child-care centers, community recreation centers, gyms and health clubs, discount stores, malls, hair and nail salons, barber shops, and neighborhood associations. Prevention information and programs that are provided through these channels can be particularly effective for reaching disadvantaged populations who often are isolated from the prevention-services loop.

- Coalitions can work to change the socio-cultural environment of the community so that the community is more supportive of gender equality and more accepting of diversity in body weight, shape, and size.

- Local radio/television stations and newspapers can periodically run articles and public service announcements that target prevention of eating disorders. National associations such as Eating Disorders and Prevention (EDAP) can provide quality education materials at minimal cost.

15.5 Summary

Parents, school personnel, and entire communities can be effective change agents for the prevention of eating disorders. Health-promotion efforts need to be multifaceted and encompass the whole child through the development of physical, mental and emotional, social, spiritual, and environmental health. Furthermore, prevention efforts should target skills and challenges that are distinctive for each stage of development.[24]

Neumark-Sztainer[35] has developed a model for a comprehensive school-based program on the prevention of eating disorders that links the school and community. In addition, she takes a proactive stance regarding sweeping socio-cultural change when she asserts:

> School-based programs should serve as catalysts for broader societal changes if eating disturbances are to be prevented. Such changes should include the way in which women are portrayed in the media; expectations regarding roles of both genders; acceptance of a wider range of body weights and shapes; and increased opportunities for healthy eating and exercise, in particular in low-income areas where exercise facilities are not available.

No individual should underestimate his or her ability to make a positive difference in the prevention of eating disorders among children. Even small changes have the capacity to produce a powerful ripple effect that can transform society. When parents, school personnel, and entire communities unite and engage in proactive endeavors to enhance the health and well-being of children, they create a legacy of tremendous impact and enduring value.

References

1. Pransky, J., *Prevention: The Critical Need*, Burrell Foundation, Springfield, MO, 1991, chap. 1, p. 14.
2. Bloom, M., *Primary Prevention Practices*, Sage Publications, Thousand Oaks, CA, 1996, 6.
3. Koff, E. and Rierdan, J., Perceptions of weight and attitudes toward eating in early adolescent girls, *Journal of Adolescent Health*, 12, 307, 1991.
4. Hill, A. J., Preadolescent dieting: implications for eating disorders, *International Review of Psychiatry*, 5, 87, 1993.
5. Hill, A. J., Oliver, S., and Rogers, P. J., Eating in the adult world: the rise of dieting in childhood and adolescence, *British Journal of Clinical Psychology*, 31, 95, 1992.
6. Maloney, M. J., McGuire, J., Daniels, S. R., and Specker, B., Dieting behavior and eating attitudes in children, *Pediatrics*, 84, 482, 1989.
7. Thelen, M. H., Lawrence, C. M., Powell, A. L., Body image, weight control, and eating disorders among children, in *The Etiology of Bulimia Nervosa: The Individual and Familial Context*, Crowther, J. H., Tennenbaum, D. L., Hobfoll, S. E., and Parris Stephens, M. A., Eds., Hemisphere, WA, 1992, chap. 5.
8. Collins, M. E., Body figure perceptions and preferences among preadolescent children, *International Journal of Eating Disorders*, 10, 199, 1991.
9. Childress, A. C., Brewerton, T. D., Hodges, E. L, and Jarrell, M. P., The Kids' Eating Disorder Survey (KEDS): a study of middle school students, *Journal of the American Academy of Child and Adolescent Psychiatry*, 32, 843, 1993.
10. Brodie, D. A., Bagley, K., and Slade, P. D., Body-image perception in pre- and post-adolescent females, *Perceptual and Motor Skills*, 78, 147, 1994.
11. Casper, R. C., Fear of fatness and anorexia nervosa in children, in *Child Health, Nutrition, and Physical Activity*, Cheung, L. W. Y. and Richmond, J. B., Eds., Human Kinetics, Champaign, IL, 1995, chap. 4.
12. Cheung, L. W. Y., Current views and future perspectives, in *Child Health, Nutrition, and Physical Activity*, Cheung, L. W. Y. and Richmond, J. B., Eds., Human Kinetics, Champaign, IL, 1995, chap. 6.
13. Halmi, K. A., Commentary 2: prevention strategies for eating disorders, in *Child Health, Nutrition, and Physical Activity*, Cheung, L. W. Y. and Richmond, J. B., Eds., Human Kinetics, Champaign, IL, 1995, 243.
14. Connolly, C. and Corbett-Dick, P., Eating disorders: a framework for school nursing initiatives, *Journal of School Health*, 60, 401, 1990.
15. Griffiths, R. A. and Farnill, D., Primary prevention of dieting disorders: an update, *Journal of Family Studies*, 2, 179, 1996.
16. Smolak, L. and Levine, M. P., Toward an empirical basis for primary prevention of eating problems with elementary school children, *Eating Disorders*, 2, 293, 1994.
17. Piran, N., Prevention: can early lessons lead to a delineation of an alternative model? A critical look at prevention with schoolchildren, *Eating Disorders*, 3, 28, 1995.
18. Worell, J., Todd, J., Development of the gendered self, in *The Developmental Psychopathology of Eating Disorders: Implications for Research, Prevention, and Treatment*, Smolak, L., Levine, M.P., and Striegel-Moore, R., Eds., Lawrence Erlbaum Associates, Mahwah, NJ, 1996, chap. 6.
19. O'Halloran, M. S., *Focus on Eating Disorders*, ABC-CLIO, Santa Barbara, CA, 1993, chap. 8.
20. Costin, C., Body image disturbance in eating disorders and sexual abuse, in *Sexual Abuse and Eating Disorders*, Schwartz, M. F., and Cohn, L., Eds., Brunner/Mazel, New York, 1996, chap. 8.
21. Page, R. M. and Page, T. S., *Fostering Emotional Well-Being in the Classroom*, Jones and Bartlett, Boston, 1993, chap. 4.
22. Attie, I. and Brooks-Gunn, J., The development of eating regulation across the life span, in *Developmental Psychopathology*, Dante, C. and Cohen, D. J., Eds., John Wiley & Sons, New York, 1995, chap. 10.

23. Connors, M. E., Developmental vulnerabilities for eating disorders, in *The Developmental Psychopathology of Eating Disorders: Implications for Research, Prevention, and Treatment*, Smolak, L., Levine, M. P., and Striegel-Moore, R., Eds., Lawrence Erlbaum Associates, Mahwah, NJ, 1996.

24. Graber, J. A. and Brooks-Gunn, J., Prevention of eating problems and disorders: including parents, *Eating Disorders*, 4, 348, 1996.

25. Benson, H., *The Relaxation Response*, William Morrow, New York, 1975.

26. Graber, J. A. and Brooks-Gunn, J., Prevention of eating problems and disorders: including parents, *Eating Disorders*, 4, 357, 1996.

27. Sands, R., Tricker, J., Sherman, C., Armatas, C., and Maschette, W., Disordered eating patterns, body image, self-esteem, and physical activity in preadolescent school children, *International Journal of Eating Disorders*, 21, 159, 1997.

28. Phelps, L., Augustyniak, K., Nelson, L. D., and Nathanson, D. S., Adolescent eating disorders, chronic dieting, and body dissatisfaction, in *Children's Needs II: Development, Problems, and Alternatives*, Bear, G. G., Minke, K. M., and Thomas, A., Eds., National Association of School Psychologists, Bethesda, MD, 1997.

29. Richards, M. H., Casper, R. C., and Larson, R., Weight and eating concerns among pre- and young adolescent boys and girls, *Journal of Adolescent Health Care*, 11, 203, 1990.

30. Striegel-Moore, R. and Smolak, L., The role of race in the development of eating disorders, in *The Developmental Psychopathology of Eating Disorders: Implications for Research, Prevention, and Treatment*, Smolak, L., Levine, M. P., and Striegel-Moore, R., Eds., Lawrence Erlbaum Associates, Mahwah, NJ, 1996.

31. Kelly, M., *My Body, My Rules: The Body Esteem, Sexual Esteem Connection*, Planned Parenthood of Tompkins County, Ithaca, NY, 1996, 22.

32. Seligman, M. E. P., *The Optimistic Child: A Revolutionary Program that Safeguards Children against Depression and Builds Resilience*, Houghton Mifflin, Boston, 1995.

33. Levine, M., *How Schools Can Help Combat Student Eating Disorders: Anorexia Nervosa and Bulimia*, National Education Association, Washington, D.C., 1987.

34. Bean, R., *The Four Conditions of Self-Esteem: A New Approach for Elementary and Middle Schools*, ETR Associates, Santa Cruz, CA, 1992.

35. Neumark-Sztainer, D., School-based programs for preventing eating disturbances, *Journal of School Health*, 66, 64, 69, 1996.

36. Connolly, C. and Corbett-Dick, P., Eating disorders: a framework for school nursing initiatives, *Journal of School Health*, 60, 401, 1990.

37. Kater, K. J., *Healthy Body Image: Teaching Kids to Eat and Love Their Bodies Too!* Eating Disorders Awareness and Prevention, Inc., Seattle, WA, 1998.

38. Birch, D. A., Involving families in school health education: implications for professional preparation, *Journal of School Health*, 64, 296, 1994.

39. Fetro, J. V., *Personal and Social Skills: Understanding and Integrating Competencies across Health Content*, ETR Associates, Santa Cruz, CA, 1992.

40. The Joint Committee on Health Education Standards, *The National Health Education Standards: Achieving Health Literacy*, 1995, The American Cancer Society, Atlanta.

41. Zins, J. E. and Wagner, D. I., Health promotion, in *Children's Needs II: Development, Problems and Alternatives*, Bear, G. C., Minke, K. M., and Thomas, A., Eds., National Association of School Psychologists, Bethesda, MD, 1997.

42. Benson, K., School children, eating disorders, and you, *School Food Service Journal*, 44, May 1993.

43. Valentine, J., Schools and communities work together for healthy children, *Wellness Management*, 11, 11, 1997.

44. O'Donnell, N. S., *Early Childhood Action Tips*, Families and Work Institute, 1998.

Appendix 15-A: Sample Educational Activities for the Prevention of Eating Disorders in Children

Activity 1: Feelings*

My Feelings and Yours Unit Goal — Feelings Grab Bag

Purpose: Identifying feelings and perceiving other's feelings.

Materials: Magazine pictures of people showing a variety of feelings; grocery or other large bag.

Activity: Have the children take turns selecting pictures from the grab bag. Ask the children to describe situations as they perceive them and to discuss the feelings that the people pictured might have. Encourage them to use as many different feeling words as they can. For pictures that suggest several emotions or explanations, talk about how different people can have different feelings about the same situation.

In the Science and Discover Center — Sounds of Laughter

Purpose: Comparing and identifying voices and laughter.

Materials: Blank tape; an audiocassette recorder.

Preparation: Tape-record each child's laugh or age-appropriate jokes and riddles. If you tape children laughing, leave a pause after each entry and then identify the child who just laughed. Tape different types of laughter (giggling, high, low, booming, staccato).

Activity: Children can identify their classmates' laughter, enjoy the jokes or riddles, or imitate different types of laughter. At the end of the tape or after this activity is completed, ask children how they feel when they laugh — physically (stomach, chest, and shoulders move; mouth smiles or opens; eyes may close) and emotionally (happy, cheerful, silly, relaxed).

Follow-up: When the children have listened to the tape at least once, ask whether they know any stories, jokes, or riddles, can imitate any stories, jokes, or riddles, or imitate any funny cartoon characters. You also can collect age-appropriate jokes or anecdotes, write them on index cards, and store them in a shoebox labeled "Funny Box." Children can choose cards whenever they like, and an adult can read them.

* From Breighner, K. and Rohe, D., *I Am Amazing*, American Guidance Service, 1989. With permission.

Activity 2: Stress Management/Relaxation Techniques

1. Enhance Personal Health
   a. Proper nutrition, regular exercise, and adequate rest and sleep
   b. Adopt a positive mindset, and put problems in perspective.
   c. Nourish spiritual health (e.g., prayer, praise and worship, etc.)
   d. Practice altruism. Giving to others is very healing!
   e. Implement humor into your life — smile and laugh more!
2. Nourish Interpersonal Relationships
   a. Build a strong support network, and foster a sense of connectedness with others.
   b. Talk with a trusted confidante about what is bothering you.
3. Practice Relation Techniques
   a. Slow, deep breathing — Breathe in deeply and silently count to three; hold your breath and count to three to yourself again. Then slowly exhale as you slowly count to five to yourself. Repeat several times until your body reaches a relaxed state.
   b. Progressive relaxation — Systematically tense and relax each muscle group in the body. Start at the top of the body and work all the way down to the feet. When tensing the muscle, hold for four seconds and then relax.
   c. Visualization — Imagine a place where you are calm and relaxed and visually "go there." For example, imagine you are walking along a beach; you can feel the breeze in your face, hear the gentle rolling of the waves, and hear the birds above you. You feel the stress of life leave your body as you become calm and relaxed.
4. Cognitive Restructuring

   Learn how to consciously reframe your negative thoughts into positive ones. For example, when faced with a difficult situation/circumstance, tell yourself that the trial will make you stronger and that "this, too, shall pass."

Activity 3: Self-Efficacy*

I Can Do This

Have children think of some activity they really like to do or that they think they do well. Ask the children to draw, demonstrate, or talk about what they like to do. They can display their pictures for the group to see, show the group something they do well, teach the class how to do something, or talk to the group about something they can do. Encourage the group to show appreciation and acceptance of each thing a child contributes.

Materials

Markers, crayons, poster board, paper, props children need for their demonstrations.

Other Ideas

> Make sharing special things, skills, and ideas with one another a regular classroom activity.
>
> Invite family members to visit and talk about something they do or their child does well.
>
> Read *I Like Me!* by Nancy L. Carlson (New York: Viking, 1988)
>
> Read *I Make Music*, by Eloise Greenfield (New York: Black Butterfly, 1991).
>
> Play "I'm Never Afraid," by Bonnie Raitt (*Free To Be … A Family*. A&M, 5196).

Talent Show

Have each child choose one special skill or talent to present in a show for parents, another class, or other groups. Help children identify a wide range of skills they may have, including drawing, running, using a computer, building with blocks, making up songs or stories, and using a hammer. Allow children to arrange space, make invitations, practice their talents, make props, or design costumes for the show. Invite local media to attend.

Materials

Props and costumes, music, space for staging the show, paper, markers, paint, signs.

Other Ideas

> Divide the class into small groups and let each group stage a talent show, with the other children serving as the audience.
>
> Invite school and community leaders to visit and show their talents.
>
> Invite family members to visit and perform for the class.
>
> Read *Gina*, by Bernard Waber (Boston: Houghton Mifflin, 1995).

"About Me" Display

Designate a space in the classroom for the children to set up a display. It might include their favorite things, drawings or pictures of themselves, pictures of their homes and families, and things that are important to them. Allow the children to add to the display for several days. At the end of that time, each child could make an invitation for someone to come and view his or her "About Me" display.

---

* From Smith, C.J., Hendricks, C.M., and Bennett, B.S., *Growing, Growing Strong: A Whole Health Curriculum*, 1997. With permission.

Materials
Markers, poster board, favorite items, designated space for each child.

Other Ideas

Collect boxes of similar size to let children make "About Me" boxes.

Videotape the children talking about or explaining items in their "About Me" display or boxes and let them invite people to see the video.

Do research and make a class display about a famous person.

Visit a museum to see displays about people.

Read *All About You*, by Catherine and Laurence Anholt (New York: Viking, 1992).

Play "Yourself Belongs to You," by The Fat Boys (*Free To Be … A Family*. A&M, 5196).

Activity 4: Body-Esteem*

Media Scavenger Hunt

Purpose: To examine media representations of bodies and discuss potential effects on self-esteem.

Preparation: Provide a variety of magazines for the group or have participants bring in magazines they don't mind cutting up. Have scissors, glue, or tape available for sharing, and large poster boards or sheets of newsprint on which to display the cutout images.

Procedure: Break the children into smaller groups of four to six. Ask them to look through the magazines for: (a) pictures or words that tell people how to look or what to be like, and (b) people that look like themselves, their friends and family members. Have them affix the images they cut out onto large paper and give the large group time to look at them. Allow time for each small group to talk about their posters and any thoughts they had about media messages while putting the display together. With the larger papers prominently displayed, move to a guided large group discussion.

Discussion Questions:

1. Is there one message about people that comes across more frequently than any others?
2. What images were the easiest to find?
3. What messages do those images give the magazine reader?
4. What images were difficult to find?
5. Were any images consistently negatively represented?
6. Do you think the messages sent out by the pictures seen here have any effect on people? If so, what?
7. What do you think the media could do differently to provide more diverse images of people?

Body Collage

Purpose: To explore the differences between how we look and feel and how we think we should look and feel.

Preparation: Have a variety of artistic materials available for each participant — large pieces of paper, colors, pencils, markers, magazines to cut pictures from, fabrics, glue, paint, glitter … whatever you have. Full-length mirrors are a great addition to this activity for any participant who has a difficult time envisioning herself/himself.

Procedure: Have the materials available for each participant to create two pictures on a paper. One is the *What I Am* picture, and the other, the *What I Should Be* picture. Before beginning, have all participants think about themselves. Provide a few questions/thoughts to get the process going:

---

* From Kelly, M., My Body, My Rules: *The Body Esteem, Sexual Esteem Connection*, Planned Parenthood of Tompkins County, Ithaca, NY, 1996. With permission.

1. Close your eyes and picture yourself, your *whole* self.
2. When you see yourself, do you focus on any particular area? Do you avoid looking at any part of yourself?
3. Can you think of any messages you've received from outside sources about the way you look?

Keeping those thoughts in mind, move on to the collages. Have people work on their own or in self-selected small groups. As they finish, give them the options of displaying their artwork and giving a brief description to the group.

Follow-Up Questions:

1. Look at your artwork: are there things that your ideal body could do that your real body cannot?
2. How much of your *should be* body's representation comes from external messages?
3. What is your favorite thing about your body as it is?

Your Favorite Tree

Purpose: To explore the variety of natural shapes and sizes that exist — especially useful for younger audiences.

Preparation: Have paper and coloring materials available for each participant.

Procedure: Ask the group if anyone has ever seen a tree. Explain that although most of us have seen a tree, there were probably different things about it that made it special. Have each participant think about her/his tree and try to remember how it looked, how tall it stood, what its branches looked like, how many leaves it had, what colors made it beautiful, etc. Ask everyone to think of one word that describes her/his tree, and, one at a time, share that word with the group. Give a piece of paper to each person and make coloring materials available. Have each person draw her/his tree and be sure to draw those features that make it unique. Once the group has finished, display the pictures for everyone to see.

Follow-Up Questions:

1. When you look at the trees, what is the first thing you notice?
2. What things are the same? What things are different?
3. Do all the trees look alike?
4. What makes *all* the trees special?

Discussion Point:

People are like trees in a forest. As you look around in a forest, whether it is real or imaginary, you can see trees, plants, flowers, and bushes that live in the same environment and look different. Likewise, people have curly red hair, small noses, or long brown legs.

Part V

Developing Healthy Attitudes and Behaviors to Manage the Stress Associated with an Eating Disorder

16

Behavior Modification

Anna Tacón and Yvonne Caldera

CONTENTS

16.1 Learning Objectives

After reading this chapter you should be able to:

- Know what behavior and behavior modification are;
- Understand research bases of behavior modification;
- Acquire basic principles used in behavior modification;
- Recognize basic procedures used in modifying behavior;
- Apply basic modification principles and procedures to eating disorders.

16.2 Research Background

Knowing that a problem exists is the first step toward change leading to the next step in the process of change and self-direction: acceptance. The most basic component of this process is behavior, and transition to healthy behaviors needs to be a gradual process in which they are incorporated into a person's repertoire of responses. Behaviors are grounded in the concrete, tangible world of the physical — small units of behavior link to form new patterns of response — and provide short-term anchors in long-term goal management.

16.2.1   Definitions, Characteristics of Behavior, and Behavior Modification

Behavior modification is a psychological approach that focuses on the alteration of behaviors that are not intrinsic characteristics of an individual. When dealing with individuals with eating disorders, for example, behavior modification is not used to treat anorexia, but to change the eating behaviors of individuals with anorexia. The roots of this approach are originally derived from experimental research with laboratory animals.[1] Overt behavior is considered to play a major role in clinical dysfunction; therefore, this approach emphasizes the primacy of behavior in the development of adaptive functioning strategies in everyday life.[2]

Human behavior has several characteristics: behaviors can be defined as actions; they can be observed and described by others; and behavior and environment have reciprocal impacts on each other.[3] Above all, behavior is simply what people do and say. Since behavior involves actions not characteristics or traits, one may observe, label, measure, identify, or describe a behavior, but not a person — actions do not correspond to static aspects of an individual's personality. This approach is helpful when dealing with eating disorders, because the focus is on adjusting behaviors to improve and maintain healthy living patterns, rather than addressing an invisibly assumed personality flaw or character weakness.

Characteristics of behavior modification work in conjunction with basic attributes of behavior.[3] The first characteristic of any behavior modification regime is to focus on behavior and associated principles derived from over 40 years of research in applied behavior analysis.[1] The scientific study itself is called experimental analysis of behavior or behavior analysis;[4] the scientific study of human behavior is termed experimental analysis of human behavior or, more commonly, applied behavior analysis.[5] In behavior modification, the behavior to be modified is called the target behavior, which can be a behavioral excess or deficit. Behavioral excess is an undesirable target behavior that needs to decrease in frequency, duration, or intensity, whereas a behavioral deficit is one that needs to increase in frequency, duration, or intensity. Binging and purging behaviors are examples of behavioral excesses; retaining a meal after eating is an example of a behavioral deficit that should increase in frequency.

Another characteristic of behavior modification is the emphasis on current events as they relate to the target behavior, de-emphasizing the past and other hypothetical or underlying factors as its cause. The goal of behavior modification is to identify and modify the synergy between the immediate environment and the behavior. Although past experiences could have contributed to the development of the behavior in question. The focus is on current experiences, as these can be changed. Past experiences cannot. For example, we must identify the environmental factors that are contributing to an individual's purging behaviors. Common environmental factors could be photographs and images of very thin models in magazines the individual frequently purchases. Once those environmental events or controlling variables have been identified, a modification plan can be designed and implemented, part of which would be to remove these intrusive images from the individual's immediate environment.

Similarly, a basic aspect of behavior modification is specificity which precisely describes the procedure or technique to be implemented to insure that desired environment-behavior changes occur each time. The effectiveness of a modification program is assessed by measuring behavior before and after intervention, obviously to determine the behavior change resulting from a given modification technique. Lastly, after a precise description and implementation of a behavior modification strategy have been determined, the treatment is frequently applied by a lay person rather than a professional.[6] An adolescent's parents, for example, could help ensure that their child is not continually exposed to these images.

16.2.2   Operant Conditioning, Basic Principles, and Procedures

In his laboratory experiments with animals, Skinner explored the impacts of various consequences on behavior, and concluded that many behaviors are influenced primarily by their consequences.[1,4,7,8] Skinner termed the consequences operants to indicate that they were responses that operated on the environment. An example is the operant of purging. Skinner's operant conditioning, also known as instrumental conditioning, is based on the principle that such behaviors are instrumental in determining consequences or outcomes. Thus, operants are distinguished by being controlled, motivated, or influenced in advance by their presumed outcomes. "ABC" components of operant conditioning are antecedent events (A), behaviors (B), and consequences or contingent outcomes (C). Basic principles include positive and negative reinforcement, extinction, punishment, and stimulus control (discrimination and generalization). Basic procedures of behavior modification include shaping and chaining, prompting and fading, contingency contracts, self-management, alternate response training, and systematic desensitization.

16.2.3   Basic Principles in Behavior Modification

16.2.3.1   *Reinforcement*

Reinforcement is the major tenet of operant conditioning, and therefore requires special attention. Basically, the principle of reinforcement refers to an increase in the frequency or likelihood of a behavior when that behavior is immediately followed by a certain consequence. The consequence contingent upon a given behavior strengthens the probability that the behavior will occur again, and the consequence that increases the frequency of an operant behavior is known as a reinforcer. For example, every time an individual purges, she feels less full; feeling less full is reinforcing. Another example of reinforcement is the constant negative attention the anorexic receives when she does not eat during mealtime. Even though the parent may reprimand the adolescent in an effort to entice the adolescent to eat, that disapproval actually increases the fasting behavior. A reinforcer is not an inherently "good" or "bad" event; it is only the process by which a response is strengthened and becomes more likely to occur in the future.

Positive reinforcement occurs when a behavior is followed by a stimulus or event immediately afterward. Such stimuli are commonly known as rewards. However, the defining feature of a reinforcer is its ability to increase the frequency of a behavior; hence, not all rewards fit that criterion. An example of a positive reinforcer in a behavior modification plan for a child or adolescent exhibiting anorexia would be taking the child to the movies after he or she eats a balanced meal.

Negative reinforcement is an increase in the frequency of a response by removing, withdrawing, or subtracting a stimulus immediately after a behavior. This permits escape or avoidance of an aversive stimulus, which results in strengthening the behavior. Avoidance and escape, however, are not synonymous. In escape behavior, the aversive stimulus or event is already present; in avoidant behavior, the organism avoids the aversive stimulus before its occurrence, usually due to the recognition of a signal or warning before the aversive event. For example, a reprimand by an adolescent's parents, if removed, could serve as a negative reinforcer for her to begin eating.

Reinforcement effectiveness is influenced according to the schedule by which the reinforcer is administered. The schedule of reinforcement specifies whether a reinforcer will be given every time a desired response is exhibited (continuous reinforcement) or only after a certain number (intermittent reinforcement) of responses are given. For example, at the beginning of a behavior modification program, the patient is praised every time a meal is completed. Once eating regularly has been accomplished, praise is administered once in a while.

16.2.3.2 *Extinction*

Extinction is a principle of behavior modification which means the withholding or cessation of a previously experienced reinforcer will gradually reduce and ultimately cause the behavior to cease. Thus, if a behavior no longer produces the reinforcing consequences, it will stop. Numerous studies have demonstrated the effectiveness of gradual extinction for decreasing problem behaviors.[6,13–15] In a bulimic, for example, the behavior to be extinguished is purging. Often, groups of adolescent girls will reinforce a bulimic for her courage in vomiting. The praises serve as an incentive to the bulimic to maintain the practice of purging. A behavior modification plan should include educating friends so that they do not continue to reinforce the bulimic behavior, or not to allow the bulimic to associate with such friends in order to eliminate their reinforcement. The purpose of these two techniques is to eliminate purging.

One behavior modification procedure that combines reinforcement and extinction is differential reinforcement. Specifically, this procedure is intended to increase the frequency of a desired behavior via reinforcement, while also decreasing the frequency via extinction of an undesired behavior that may interfere with the desired behavior. Several behavior modification studies have supported the use of differential reinforcement for various behaviors in various contexts.[16–18] The behavior modification plan should include positive reinforcers when an anorexic eats a balanced meal, and the elimination of praise when she loses weight.

16.2.3.3 *Punishment*

The principle of punishment has negative connotations, probably due to misconceptions and misapplications. It should be emphasized, however, that most proponents of behavior modification typically avoid the use of punishment, primarily due to the availability of a wide range of positive reinforcers, and also because of the undesirable associations that may result from its the use.[2] In behavior modification, the application of punishment is a technical term that refers to a process in which the consequence of a behavior likely results in the decreased performance of the specific behavior in the future Thus, in line with the ABC components of operant conditioning, punishment is simply one type of a contingent consequence of behavior. Two procedural formats are positive and negative punishment.

Just as positive and negative reinforcements deal with the presentation or removal of a consequent stimulus, positive and negative punishments operate on the identical principle. Positive punishment is the presentation of a stimulus considered aversive or unpleasant by an individual following the occurrence of the specified behavior, so as to decrease the probability of a recurrence of that behavior in the future. After an episode of purging, a child or adolescent may receive positive punishment through added chores, duties, or assignments for a week. Negative punishment, on the other hand, is the removal of a considered positive reinforcer following a behavior, the intended result again being to decrease the likelihood of recurrence of that behavior. An example would be a parental refusal to allow an adolescent anorexic daughter the privilege of going to the gym to exercise after refusal-to-eat behaviors.

16.2.3.4 Stimulus Control: Discrimination and Generalization

A behavior is under stimulus control when the probability of its occurrence increases in the presence of a specific stimulus. This occurs because reinforcement was administered only when that specific stimulus was present. This principle specifies that responses will vary, depending upon the presence of different stimuli; when an individual responds one way in the presence of one stimulus and another way in the presence of another, that individual has made a discrimination.[2] Specifically, an antecedent stimulus that is present when a behavior is reinforced is termed a discriminative stimulus, and when a behavior is differentially controlled by such antecedent stimuli, the behavior is said to be under stimulus control. Generalization, on the other hand, takes place when a behavior occurs in the presence of stimuli that are similar to the discriminative stimulus.

Principles of stimulus control are important for behavior modification because the goal is to change target behaviors by altering the existing relationship between the conditions prior to the behavior (antecedent context), the behavior, and the consequences. In a behavior modification plan for an adolescent with anorexia, eating is reinforced when she sits down at her parents' dining room table. Eventually, eating will be under stimulus control of the setting. Whenever the adolescent enters her parents' dining room, she expects to be rewarded and therefore eats her meal. Later, when she is invited by a friend's parents to eat in their dining room, she is likely to generalize her behavior and thus eat her meal.

16.2.4 Basic Procedures in Behavior Modification

16.2.4.1 Shaping and Chaining

Frequently, the development of a new behavior cannot be achieved by response reinforcement because the behavior may be so complex that its components do not exist in an individual's repertoire. To establish a new aspect of a behavioral response, shaping is used. Shaping is a procedure by which successive approximations of a target behavior are reinforced; thus, the final goal behavior is achieved by reinforcing the small units or approximations toward the final response, rather than reinforcing the final response alone.[2] Shaping has been applied in medical settings[19] and in studies to modify existing behavior.[20,21] For example, getting an anorexic to eat a full meal may be a difficult task at the beginning of the program. Instead of withholding reinforcement until she completes a full meal, her eating behavior may be shaped gradually. In the beginning, she should receive reinforcement for eating any amount of food. After that, she should receive reinforcement only when she eats a bit more, until she is able to eat a full meal.

Most behaviors consist of a sequence of several responses. A complex behavior consisting of many component behaviors occurring in a certain sequence is thus called a behavioral chain.[3] Chaining procedures teach an individual to incorporate a chain of behaviors into a repertoire of behavioral responses. An example of chaining for an anorexic would be sitting at the table, placing a napkin on her lap, holding utensils, bringing food to her mouth, chewing, swallowing, and repeating the last three behaviors until her plate is empty. Reinforcement initially would come when a chain is completed; gradually, reinforcement would follow only after all the chain units of behavior have been completed and the plate is empty.

Another helpful strategy is known as written task analysis. This objective, documented format helps to guide appropriate performance and sequence of component behaviors in a desired behavioral chain. The analysis clearly and specifically lists every instruction (component) in the chain in proper sequence; this detailed list of instructions helps an individual to perform a task correctly.[3] Both shaping and chaining demonstrate the significance of small steps or components in behavior modification programs which are concurrent with the accomplishment of small or short-term goals as parts of any long-term goal achievement.

16.2.4.2 Prompting and Fading

The behavior modification procedure of prompting is a method used to develop appropriate stimulus control for a specific behavior; prompts or cues are used during discrimination training, so that the subject will produce the desired behavior in the presence of the discriminative stimulus. Basically, prompting is use of stimuli that help to initiate a response (instructions, gestures, providing direction or guidance during a behavioral action, or modeling of a behavior).[2] When a prompt produces the desired response, the behavior can be reinforced. As behavioral training progresses and the need for prompting decreases, fading or gradual removal of the prompt occurs. Fading, moreover, is a way to transfer stimulus control from facilitating prompts to discriminative stimuli.[3]

As stated above, a behavior modification program for an anorexic should include reinforcement whenever the anorexic eats at her parents' dining room table. While eating in this setting, the anorexic should be given a prompt such as a statement like "bon appetit" or "nourishment for the body." Every time the anorexic eats in the dining room after being prompted with that phrase, she is reinforced. Later, she can go to a restaurant and be prompted to eat. Eventually, no prompting will be needed and fading can be initiated. Other methods of facilitating new behaviors include behavioral rehearsal and the use of models to enhance behavioral induction.

16.2.4.3 Contingency Contracts

Often reinforcement contingencies are designed in the form of behavioral or contingency contracts between individuals who design behavior change (professionals) and the individuals (clients) whose target behaviors are goals for change. The procedure precisely specifies the consequences for certain behaviors; that is, contracts specify reinforcers as determined by contingent behaviors.[2] Contracts have been used in studies of a variety of target behaviors, including adult weight loss, weight maintenance, and academic performance in children, adolescents, and college students.[9–12]

Contingency contracts have five basic components.[3]

First, the target behaviors are clearly defined in objective operational terms; target behaviors may include desirable behaviors to be increased, undesirable behaviors to be decreased, or both. Second, specific statements as to when a target behavior must be performed are required; this provides a deadline and enables the professional to determine implementation of the contracted contingencies. Third, the target behaviors must be observable in order to be objectively measured. Fourth, the contract specifies reinforcement (positive or negative) for the target behaviors, as well as sanctions for failure to meet the agreed-upon terms (positive and negative punishment). Finally, the contract clearly identifies the roles of all parties involved, including who will be responsible for implementing the contingencies relevant, for example, in the case of an adolescent, a parent. Probably the greatest advantage of such contracts is the participation of the individual with the targeted behaviors. Taking an active role in negotiation and creation of the contract may increase the individual's performance and sense of control, rather than having her feel the program was imposed on her without her input.

16.2.4.4 Self-Management

Self-management occurs when an individual engages in one behavior to control the occurrence of another behavior — the target behavior — at a later time.[22,23] Self-management strategies ultimately permit application of self-control, as people do in everyday life situations, and the goal of behavior modification is to train individuals to control their behaviors and achieve self-selected goals.[2] To avoid the eternal debate of associated free will versus determinism, self-control or management procedures in behavior modification will include techniques in which the client plays an active role, and occasionally the sole role, in administering treatment and applying the appropriate behavior modification strategies.[2]

Self-management strategies include a variety of controlling behaviors to increase the future occurrence of a controlled behavior (target behavior). Examples of strategies include appropriate goal setting, self-monitoring, self-reinforcement and self-punishment, positive self-talk such as self-praise, self-instruction involving cues to desired behavior, arranging social support, and developing a behavioral contract.[2,3] Of the above, perhaps the most crucial techniques are appropriate goal setting and self-monitoring.

The most self-defeating goals are unrealistic, inappropriate, or unachievable. Such goals set an individual up for failure. Appropriate goal setting, therefore, identifies a desirable level of target behavior to be achieved. The goal should be objectified by being written. The target behavior should be precisely described, and a reasonable time frame determined for achieving this goal. Intermediate or short-term goals within the main goal should be specified. Intermediate goals build upon a baseline level of behavior and indicate progress toward the final goal.[3]

Goal setting is usually intertwined with self-monitoring techniques. Appropriate goal setting is best implemented in conjunction with accurate monitoring of behaviors; this provides a record of effectiveness with which to evaluate progress. Self-monitoring consists of a person's systematic observation of his or her own behavior. Since many behaviors are automatic, they usually go unrecognized and, accordingly, uncensored or open to revision. Self-monitoring devices such as daily log sheets for recording behaviors can increase awareness and bring home the reality of the behavior. Variations of self-monitoring in conjunction with behavioral recording in a diary journal may also provide motivation and take on reinforcing properties. Although self-monitoring strategies alone do not alter behavior, such techniques may initiate behaviors that do, such as self-reinforcement or self-punishment.

16.2.4.5 Alternate Response Training

A form of self-control is interference or replacement of an undesired behavior with another behavior.[2] Obviously, an individual needs an alternate response to replace the undesired response. Examples here could include various forms of relaxation or anxiety reduction strategies, such as progressive relaxation, meditation, exercise, biofeedback, yoga, positive thoughts, etc. Forms of relaxation have been widely used as alternates because of their incompatibility with and mediation of anxiety.[2] The goal is for the behavior to serve as an acceptable option to interfere with or replace the undesired behavior. Relaxation training is particularly important if systematic desensitization is to be applied.

16.2.4.6 Systematic Desensitization

Systematic desensitization is one of the most widely employed procedures in behavioral approaches to treatment. The basic assumption for using this technique is that anxiety is a learned/conditioned response that can be inhibited by a response incompatible with anxiety. Basically, anxiety-producing stimuli are repeatedly paired with relaxation training until the connection between those stimuli and the anxious response is eliminated.[24] This technique involves three basic steps: relaxation training, development of an anxiety hierarchy, and desensitization.[25] The client is taught how to progressively relax and follows a regimen of daily practice outside of sessions. Following this phase, an agreed upon anxiety hierarchy is created, involving anxious/aversive stimuli of varying intensity. After these two phases are completed, the pairing of anxious stimuli with relaxation is begun. In a relaxed state, the client is exposed to the lowest-level arousing stimuli in the hierarchy and proceeds up the anxiety ladder; when the client experiences anxiety, the experience is halted and relaxation is induced. After a relaxed state is again achieved movement up the anxiety hierarchy continues, with relaxation inducement as needed, and the original pairing of stimulus and anxiety response is eventually replaced with stimulus and associated relaxation.

16.3 Application of Research Question

How can behavior modification principles and procedures be applied to eating disorders? Behavior disorders typically have two major foci. First, because inappropriate or harmful behaviors are assumed to be reinforced, their reinforcers need to be identified and eliminated where possible, or the context in which they occur is modified. Second, maladaptive behaviors need to be replaced with health-enhancing behaviors. An appropriate modification plan can be formulated and implemented only after an intense behavioral assessment is made. The assessment should be based on observing the frequency, intensity, and duration of client behavior. Antecedent events, the contexts in which the undesired behaviors occur, and, most importantly, the determination of contingent reinforcers must also be considered in formulating the plan.

The assessment phase involves obtaining reports from the client and gathering information from spouse, family members, and other people close to the client about their observations of the client's behavior. The assessment phase is a good time to encourage the client to use a journal or diary as a self-monitoring device. This allows the professional to establish a baseline and helps increase the client's self-awareness of behavioral responses. It also helps him or her identify associations involving feelings, moods, behaviors, stimuli impacts, and antecedent/contextual factors associated with the problem behavior. The self-monitoring mechanisms will become more specific and detailed as a modification plan is designed and implemented to assess effectiveness.

Once a behavior modification program is designed and agreed upon with client input, a contingency contract should concretely specify the terms of the plan aimed at achieving the target behavior, the contingent consequences (reinforcement or punishment), and time frame. Self-management procedures should include detailed behavioral record-keeping and use of self-monitoring techniques. Reinforcement strategies and discrimination training should be applied with regard to positive consequences contingent upon target behavior and sanctions or punishments when target behavior is not achieved. Alternate response training, especially training in relaxation techniques should be implemented as a means to provide behavior replacement options and enhance overall benefits of the program. This will also serve as an important component, particularly if the decision is made to apply systematic desensitization during the modification program. Finally, if behaviors need to be developed within a client's repertoire, modeling, rehearsal, shaping and chaining, and prompting and fading techniques can be utilized.

References

1. Skinner, B., *The Behavior of Organisms: An Experimental Analysis*, Appleton-Century-Crofts, New York, 1938.
2. Kasdin, A., *Behavior Modification in Applied Settings*, 4th ed., Brooks-Cole Publishing, Pacific Grove, CA, 1989.
3. Miltenberger, R., *Behavior Modification*, Brooks-Cole Publishing, Pacific Grove, CA, 1997.
4. Skinner, B., What is the experimental analysis of behavior? *Journal of Experimental Analysis of Behavior*, 9, 213, 1966.
5. Baer, D., Wolf, M., and Risley, T., Some current dimensions of applied behavior analysis, *Journal of Applied Behavior Analysis*, 1, 91, 1968.
6. Kasdin, A., *Behavior Modification in Applied Settings*, 5th ed., Brooks-Cole Publishing, Pacific Grove, CA, 1994.
7. Skinner, B., *Contingencies of Reinforcement: A Theoretical Analysis*, Appleton-Century-Crofts, New York, 1969.
8. Skinner, B., *About Behaviorism*, Alfred A. Knopf, New York, 1974.
9. Jeffery, R., Bjornson-Benson, W. Rosenthal, B. Kurth, C., and Dunn, M., The effectiveness of monetary contracts with two repayment schedules on weight reduction in men and women from self-referred and population samples, *Behavior Therapy*, 15, 273, 1984.
10. Kramer, F., Jeffrey, R., Snell, M., and Forster, J., Maintenance of successful weight loss over one year: effects of contracts for weight maintenance or participation in skills training, *Behavior Therapy*, 17, 295, 1986.
11. Kelly, M. and Stokes, T., Student-teacher contracting with goal setting for maintenance, *Behavior Modification*, 8, 223, 1984.
12. Miller, D. and Kelly, M., The use of goal setting and contingency contracting for improving children's homework, *Journal of Applied Behavior Analysis*, 27, 73, 1994.
13. Lerman, D. and Iwata, B., Prevalence of the extinction burst and its attenuation during treatment, *Journal of Applied Behavior Analysis*, 28, 93, 1995.
14. Mazaleski, J., Iwata, B., Vollmer, T., Zarcone, J., and Smith, R., Analysis of the reinforcement and extinction components in contingencies with self-injury, *Journal of Applied Behavior Analysis*, 26, 143, 1993.
15. Rincover, A., Sensory extinction: A procedure for eliminating self-stimulatory behavior in psychotic children, *Journal of Abnormal Psychology*, 6, 299, 1978.

16. Goetz, E. and Baer, D., Social control of form diversity and the emergence of new forms in children's block-building, *Journal of Applied Behavior Analysis*, 6, 209, 1973.

17. Sulzer-Azaroff, B., Drabman, R., Greer, R., Hall, R., Iwaata, B., and O'Leary, S., *Behavior Analysis in Education 1967-1987: Reprint Series*, Vol. 3, Society for the Experimental Analysis of Behavior, Lawrence, KS, 1988.

18. Reid, D., Parsons, M., and Green, C. *Staff-Management in Human Services: Behavioral Research and Application*, Charles C Thomas, Springfield, IL, 1989.

19. O'Neill, G. and Gardner, R., *Behavioral Principles in Medical Rehabilitation: A Practical Guide*, Charles C Thomas, Springfield, IL, 1983.

20. Howie, P. and Woods, C., Token reinforcement during the instatement and shaping of fluency in the treatment of stuttering, *Journal of Applied Behavior Analysis*, 15, 55, 1982.

21. Jackson, D. and Wallace, R., The modification and generalization of voice loudness in a fifteen-year-old retarded girl, *Journal of Applied Behavior Analysis*, 7, 461, 1974.

22. Watson, D. and Tharp, R, *Self-Directed Behavior: Self-Modification for Personal Adjustment*, 6th ed., Brooks-Cole Publishing, Pacific Grove, CA, 1993.

23. Yates, B., *Applications in Self-Management*, Wadsworth, Belmont, CA, 1986.

24. Wolpe, J., *The Practice of Behavior Therapy*, 4th ed., Pergamon Press, Elmsford, New York, 1990.

25. Morris, R., Fear reduction methods, in *Helping People Change: A Textbook of Methods*, 3rd ed., Kanfer, F. H. and Goldstein, A.P., Eds., Pergamon Press, New York, 1986.

17

Restructuring Cognitive Distortions

Marcia Abbott

CONTENTS

17.1 Learning Objectives

After completing this chapter, you should be able to:

- Understand the definition of a cognitive distortion and list common ones associated with eating disorders;
- Explain the cognitive view of the maintenance of bulimia nervosa (BN) and anorexia nervosa (AN);
- Identify cognitive distortions in the verbalizations of eating disorder patients;
- Understand methods to help change distorted thought patterns;
- Know when and how to refer patients for more intensive help.

0-8493-2027-5/01/$0.00+$.50
© 2001 by CRC Press, Inc.

17.2 Research Background

17.2.1 Cognitive Behavioral Model

In his now classic *Cognitive Therapy of Depression*,[1] Aaron Beck, M.D. explained that irrational and distorted patterns of thinking lead to negative emotions and self-defeating behaviors. He theorized that learning how to recognize specific thoughts and beliefs that precede negative emotional reactions and behaviors could provide the chance to change unhealthy thinking patterns. Many irrational patterns are acquired from early childhood and lead to emotions and behaviors that are almost automatic and spontaneous. In patients with eating disorders, cognitive distortions lead to feelings of low self-esteem; mistaken attributions of problems in life to weight, shape, and appearance; and maintenance of eating disorders as ways to manage weight and emotions. For example, a person with anorexia believes that she controls her environment as long as she maintains a low weight. She may believe that she cannot be successful or liked by others unless she is thin. The thinner she becomes, the more weight she wants to lose because her perception of perfection becomes distorted as does her image of her body. The patient with bulimia nervosa commonly believes that she cannot lose weight without binge/purge episodes, laxatives, diuretics, or over-exercising. This belief is maintained even though the patient may remain at an average weight for her height. The mechanism of binging and purging causes swelling which contributes to the body image distortion and serves to provide proof to the patient that she is, indeed, fat.

In clinical practice it is often observed that a patient's concern with her body shape and weight frequently has become a preoccupation by the time she enters puberty. She may recall criticism of her size or weight by a parent, teacher, or other authority figure. She incorporates what she hears as a part of her self-esteem and body image and develops distorted cognitive beliefs at a preconscious level. Her irrational and self-defeating behaviors with food stem from these irrational beliefs. The fears and tensions that are dealt with through the use of these behaviors reflect deficient coping abilities in several areas including developmental transition (from childhood to puberty), maturity fears, autonomy (separating from parents and going away from home), sexuality, and dysfunctional family relationships. The preoccupation with food and weight becomes consuming and the patient is distracted from overwhelming feelings of anxiety, fear, and depression triggered by developmental or family events. She, therefore, mistakenly feels in control of herself and those around her although her eating behaviors are out of control. As she becomes more and more ill, her perception of negative comments about her thinness is distorted and she sees them as compliments.

Garner, et al.[3] point out that our culture has a strong influence on beliefs and expectations. The media constantly glorify the virtues of dieting and thinness. Eating disorders are considered culture-bound disorders since they rarely occur outside the Western world where the ideal body is very thin.[5] Young girls are bombarded by images of ultra-thin models, actresses, and entertainers, and incorporate these images into their beliefs about their own body images. Even when a celebrity comes forward to reveal problems with an eating disorder, little impact is made on an adolescent's distorted body image. A young person begins to develop the irrational belief from these media examples that being thin equals happiness and success. These values are reinforced in some cases by a family member who gives praise for weight loss, particularly from a mother whose self-image is also culture-bound.

Irrational eating behaviors become habit patterns that persist independently of emotional situations that occur. What starts as desire to lose a few pounds becomes an obsession. The more the patient loses, the more she restricts her diet, and the more fearful she becomes of food. She begins to limit food choices based on irrational beliefs. For example, she may believe that any fat intake will result in an instant weight gain, so she will cut out fat entirely, or she may believe that white foods have fewer calories than other foods.

Cognitive distortions occur in the areas of personality functioning, self-esteem, self-efficacy, and competence. They color the patient's perception of food and what effects particular foods and eating patterns have on weight loss. Therefore, the use of the cognitive behavioral model is best used in the context of a multidisciplinary setting in which cognitive distortions are addressed by both a psychotherapist and a registered dietitian.

17.2.2   Common Cognitive Distortions of Eating Disorder Patients

Based on Beck's[6] taxonomy of thinking errors, Garner et al.[3] have linked various types of cognitive distortions to faulty distortions that are peculiar to eating disorder patients.

17.2.2.1   *Dichotomous Reasoning*

Dichotomous reasoning involves thinking in extreme and absolutiste terms — all-or-nothing thinking. A patient may tend to divide food into "good" and "bad" categories. For example, she may say that fat is "all bad" and vegetables are "all good," not realizing that some fat is essential to good nutrition and that potatoes, although considered vegetables, are carbohydrates. This type of thinking also extends to personality functioning and personal relationships. She expects perfection in grades, sports, acceptance from others, happiness, and self-control. If she finds herself lacking in one area, she feels she is a total failure. Examples of dichotomous thinking are as follows:

- If I eat one thing that's not on my diet, I've blown the whole thing and might as well binge.
- If I miss exercising for one day, I might as well not exercise at all.
- If I have any sexual contact, I will be totally promiscuous.
- If I express anger at all, I'll explode in rage.
- If I'm not in total control, I'll lose control of everything.

17.2.2.2   *Overgeneralization*

A patient's pattern of drawing a general conclusion about her ability, performance, and worth on the basis of a single incident is called overgeneralization.[1] Examples common to eating disorder patients include:

- If I make a B on this test, I'm a total failure.
- If my boyfriend breaks up with me, I'll never have another relationship.
- If I gain one pound, I am totally fat.
- If I disagree with my mom, she'll never love me again.

17.2.2.3   *Catastrophizing*

Catastrophizing is magnification of the negative consequences of a particular event. The following are examples of this distortion.

- I must be thin in order to be happy. If I gain weight, I'll always be fat.
- All my problems in life are a result of the way I look. If I don't look perfect, my life is miserable.
- If my mother gets mad at me, she'll hate me forever.

17.3   Application of Research Question

The value of the research knowledge contained in this chapter is in helping a patient recognize and reform cognitive distortions. Modifications of Beck's model of cognitive-behavioral therapy have been researched and the procedures have been recommended for use when counseling eating disordered patients. Fairburn,[2] Garner and Garfinkel,[3] and Halmi[4] recommend that treatment take about 20 weeks. It should be semi-structural, problem-oriented, and mainly concerned with the patient's present and future rather than the past. The process can be summarized by the following discussion points.

1. Because eating disorder patients are, in general, resistant to treatment and secretive about their thoughts and behaviors, plenty of time should be taken to establish a therapeutic and trusting relationships with them.

2. The patient is taught to monitor her own thoughts and discover irrational perceptions or beliefs. Education on body weight regulation, the adverse effects of dieting, and the physical consequences of anorexia and bulimia are introduced to help deal with the common cognitive distortion that these behaviors do not have negative or long-term consequences. A journal and homework assignments are recommended.

3. The patient should learn to recognize the connection between distorted perceptions and irrational behaviors. For example, through the use of a daily journal, the patient may notice that her hours of exercise increase as she contemplates going to the senior prom. This connection might indicate an increase of anxiety based on her irrational belief that she must be thin to get a date. As her fear of failure increases, her level of exercising, incidence of binge and purge episodes, and restriction of food intake will also increase.

4. The patient and the therapist should examine the validity of the patient's beliefs. The therapist should question the beliefs in a kind and nonthreatening manner, and let the patient know she is accepted no matter what her beliefs are. The therapist asks questions to confront the irrational beliefs, for example:

   How do you know you can't get a date for the prom if you weigh what you *do now*?

   How do you know that people think you're fat and don't like you?

   How many calories per week do you have to overeat to gain one pound?

   Does it mean you're a total failure in life if you don't go to the prom?

5. The patient is taught to substitute healthy and positive thoughts which are more realistic and logical for her earlier irrational beliefs. She should be encouraged to verbalize these thoughts to trusted friends so that she can gain a more reality-based view. She should confront her irrational thoughts by writing down pros and cons on the issues. She should ask herself what objective data support her thoughts. Are there data that cast doubt on her thoughts? She should also ask herself what other people would think under similar circumstances.

6. After learning to use the information she has gathered to change her beliefs and substitute healthy and positive thoughts, she should practice by verbalizing the new thoughts with her therapist.

7. The new thoughts should be used to guide behavior even if the patient does not fully believe them. For example, if she is studying for a test and her anxiety level is increasing, she may find herself obsessing about carbohydrates and constantly wanting to eat. If she has changed her belief that she is hungry to a belief that she is anxious, she can use a relaxation technique such as deep breathing to calm herself instead of rushing off to binge. That will give her time to analyze her thoughts. A common problem for an anorexic is the irrational belief that if she eats anything, she will gain weight. She practices new beliefs by forcing herself to stay on her meal plan even though she is afraid to do so. To accomplish this monumental change, she needs to trust her therapist and to get positive support from those around her.

Some patients are very resistant to the cognitive behavioral process. They feel that exploring their thoughts and attitudes is too intrusive, especially since some of their thoughts and attitudes are learned from their families. They often feel guilty revealing family histories to therapists because they feel they are betraying family secrets. This is almost always the case if a family history includes serious problems with abuse or addiction. Other patients are unable to engage in cognitive restructuring because of limited intelligence or a tendency to be concrete thinkers. These patients can sometimes benefit from a group approach. This allows them to relate to other eating disorder patients who share their problems. Appendix 17-A lists resources that may be helpful.

If eating disordered behavior accompanies another diagnosis, (addiction, depression, anxiety, borderline personality disorder, or obsessive-compulsive disorder), the patient should be referred for therapy to a well-trained expert and a physician should evaluate the patient for prescription of medication. This is particularly important if suicidal or homicidal ideation or tendency to self-injure is present.[1]

17.4 Case Studies

Two case studies are presented for demonstration purposes. The first involves an 18-year-old college sophomore who developed bulimia nervosa. The second study is a patient with anorexia nervosa. The histories of the illnesses are presented and examples of common cognitive distortions are included. The names of patients and details of the cases are disguised to protect confidentiality.

17.4.1 Becky: A Case Study of Bulimia Nervosa

Becky was an 18-year-old college sophomore who was presented by her parents for evaluation and treatment of binging and self-induced vomiting. The behavior continued daily for nine months. Becky said, "I'm out of control. I've tried so hard, but I can't stop the binging and purging." Her binging and purging episodes increased steadily to a rate of two to three times per day. In addition, she did an hour of aerobics exercises and an hour of weight lifting every day. She denied the use of laxative, diuretics, or other purgatives. Her height is 5 feet 5 inches tall, and her weight was 110 pounds. She was very concerned about her body weight and felt that her hips were too big and her thighs were too fat. She was obsessed with weight and weighed herself three times a day. If her weight was up even a pound she had a bad day because she believed that people could tell she gained weight. She also reported difficulty with sleeping, nightmares, and dysphoric moods. She isolated herself in a college dorm room, and dropped out of social groups. Because she was so obsessed with her weight and felt so hopeless, she developed some passive suicidal ideation. Her attention and concentration were impaired. She was formerly an A student whose grades dropped to Cs. Her anxiety level increased dramatically as she became sicker with more frequent binging and purging episodes. She denied the use of alcohol and drugs.

Her physical symptoms included palpitations, sensitivity to cold, dry skin, brittle hair, bitten fingernails, swollen parotid glands, dizziness, and dental erosion. She recalled fainting twice in the recent past. Her menstrual periods were irregular, and lab work indicated an electrolyte imbalance. Her EKG was normal.

17.4.1.1 Family History

A review of Becky's family history reveals some of the causes for the development of her cognitive distortions. Becky's father, an alcoholic, is a successful farmer and businessman. Her mother, a homemaker, has been treated for depression and is very passive. She makes excuses for her husband's abusive and strict behavior. Becky's sister is 2 years younger, and drinks and uses cocaine. Becky has been embarrassed about her sister's behavior since they were in grade school together. She describes her sister as rebellious, passive-aggressive, and angry most of the time. Becky describes her relationship with her mother as very close. She and her mother shared personal problems and Becky describes their relationship as "best friends." Becky felt pressure to succeed and not disappoint her depressed mother.

Her mother was also overweight and always on a diet. She complained to her daughter about problems with their father, saying that maybe he would love her more and not drink so much if she lost weight.

Becky believes that if she is perfect in every way, her family life will improve. Becky was student body president and a cheerleader in high school. She developed a competitive spirit with the other cheerleaders, and at times they competed to see who could be the thinnest or lose the most weight. She also participated in a church youth group. She made As in school and feared that a B would prevent her from getting into a good college.

Becky had one boyfriend throughout high school and had been sexually active with him, but she had never been pregnant. When Becky went to college, her boyfriend stayed in their small town to work because he was unable to afford college. He became very jealous, demanded that she come home every weekend, and did not want her to participate in social activities at school. He became especially angry when she joined a sorority. He began to comment about her figure and weight, and called her a social climber. He broke up with her after the second month of school.

Becky became very depressed and described herself as a total failure. She said "I'm a little fish in a big pond." She was lonely and upset and went on a fasting diet and lost 20 pounds because she thought the reason her boyfriend broke up with her was because she had gained the "freshman ten." It was then that the binging and purging began. Even though she had lost almost 15% of her average body weight, she viewed herself as fat and had a severely distorted body image. Since she continued to feel severely depressed, she believed that she had not lost enough weight. She began to weigh herself more frequently and believed that if she gained 1 pound she was totally fat and out of control. She believed that all her problems were due to her weight and appearance. When her grades began to fall due to her depression and inability to concentrate, she began to make self-statements about her lack of intelligence. This caused her self-esteem to fall even further as she compared herself to others who made good grades. She felt totally unable to function in college, and when she went home for a holiday, she revealed her problem to her parents who sought help.

17.4.1.2 *Treatment Recommendations and Resolution*

The psychologist who evaluated Becky recommended cognitive behavioral therapy to help restructure her irrational beliefs and cognitive distortions. Becky was also seen by a registered dietitian to help her with her irrational beliefs about food. In addition, she participated in assertiveness training and communication skill training to help raise her self-esteem. Antidepressant medication was prescribed by her family physician and a close watch was kept on her physical condition. She limited her exercise to one hour per day in order to balance her food intake and number of calories expended. The family met with her for several sessions so they could learn how to be supportive of her and her efforts to change her beliefs about food and herself. She learned in family therapy that she was not the cause of or the cure for the family's problems.

17.4.2 Sally: A Battle with Anorexia Nervosa

Sally is attractive and has a figure that others admire. Some girls envy Sally for her good grades, her success at everything she tries, her helpful attitude, and her closeness with her parents. However, when Sally was brought to the attention of her physician, she weighed 90 pounds and was 5 feet 5 inches tall. She told her physician that she saw herself as fat and that she only needed to lose a little more weight. She was sure that her parents were overreacting by saying that she was too thin, and they were trying to control her behavior. Sally's preoccupation with weight began in an effort to lose a few pounds. She had wanted to try out for the high school drill team and thought if she lost a few pounds she would have a better chance. She began to diet. At first she drew praise for her appearance. Other girls wished that they could drop a few pounds and have the will power Sally had.

She enjoyed exercising that will power and felt superior to her friends. Soon she dropped below the weight goal she had set but still thought that she looked a little fat, specifically in the hips and thighs. She increased her exercising and began to avoid eating with others because they always seemed to force food on her and make remarks about her weight. Eventually, breakfast at home became a battle because she refused to eat anything. As Sally's anorexia worsened, she began to lose perspective. She believed that she would never lose enough weight, and no matter how low her weight was on the scale, she would always be fat. Even though she was gradually starving herself to death, she would say, "Just 5 more pounds and my life will be perfect." Family members watched her weight go down and watched her sit for hours at the dinner table unable to force herself to eat even the smallest amount of food.

She developed a habit of eating with a very small plate and a baby fork to make the food look smaller on the plate. She also limited her diet to foods that were white because she believed white foods contained fewer calories and would make her gain less weight than colored foods. She believed that certain foods made her gain weight in particular places. For example, she said that she could see the size of her thighs increase if she ate bread. She constantly weighed herself and continued to compare herself unfavorably with other people. She began to hide her exercising from her family by running in place for hours in her room after everyone had gone to sleep. She also became obsessed with computing the number of calories in any food offered to her. She worried whether she should risk the calories in a stick of gum, toothpaste, and cough drops. She would not lick postage stamps for fear that they had calories. She also became obsessed with the preparation of food. She believed that her mother hid extra calories in her food and wanted to make her fat. She took over the family's menu planning, grocery shopping, cooking, and clean up. She took pride in cooking gourmet dishes that her family enjoyed and, at the same time, refused to taste them. She also limited her fluid intake because liquids made her stomach feel full and that meant she was fat. Her thinking was so obsessive and her brain so starved for nutrition that she lost her ability to concentrate. Her grades and performance declined, and she seemed depressed. The menstrual periods stopped and she felt weak and dizzy.

17.4.2.1 Development of the Disease

Sally came from a family that appeared picture perfect. Her parents were older and her father placed great emphasis on her intellectual and athletic achievements, but ignored her budding womanhood. She was given everything material that she wanted, based on her parents' desires, not her own. Her mother was obsessed with weight and provided a role model for Sally's weight loss. Sally tried to please her mother; she repressed her anger and any thoughts that were contrary to what was expected of her. She was very submissive to her parents, and they recognized that she was "a people pleaser." She could never be good enough and feared making her parents angry if she should fail. She was seeking impossible perfection. She denied her feelings of hopelessness and helplessness and was willing to lose her health to be thin.

The more weight Sally lost, the more she felt in control of her life. In reality, her thinking and eating were totally out of control, and the distortions in her perception were causing a vicious circle of weight loss. She wanted to make herself attractive and at the same time feared her own sexuality. It is possible that her desire to be abnormally thin was a way of denying her needs for male attention. She also identified strongly with female role models on television who seemed to be happy and successful and had abnormally thin bodies.

17.4.2.2 Treatment and Progress

By the time Sally arrived for treatment, her weight was so low that she was in danger. She was hospitalized, regained some physical strength and weighed about 100 pounds. After that, she participated in cognitive behavioral therapy to help raise her self-esteem and change her distorted image of herself and of her body. She began to notice that whenever she became unsure of herself or insecure, she would restrict her food. She was able to separate the way she handled her emotions from her behaviors with food. Her obsessive-compulsive nature was actually a help in establishing new eating patterns that were very strict. Although she had difficulty gaining weight, she was able to maintain a weight that allowed her to think and concentrate and do a limited amount of exercise. Her physical health improved and her menstrual cycle began again. She had more energy. She continued to, at times, be compelled to restrict her food, but she used cognitive restructuring to talk herself out of it. She had frequent sessions with her therapist when she felt herself getting out of control.

17.4.3 Questions

1. What were the cognitive distortions that Becky experienced?
2. What were the cognitive distortions that Sally experienced?

17.4.4 Answers

Question 1

1. Others can tell if I gain 1 pound.
2. I am responsible for my sister's behavior. If she looks bad, so do I.
3. If my mother is overweight, then I must be also.
4. My father will love me more and won't drink so much if I'm thin.
5. I have to be the thinnest to be the best cheerleader.
6. If I make a B, I won't get into college.
7. If I don't have a boyfriend, I'm a total failure.
8. My boyfriend broke up with me because I'm fat.
9. The thinner I am, the happier I'll be.
10. My grades are falling because I'm stupid.

Question 2

1. If I lose 5 pounds I'll make the drill team.
2. I'm better than my friends because I can lose weight.
3. My life will be perfect when I lose 5 more pounds.
4. White foods have less calories.
5. If I eat bread, my thighs will be fatter.
6. My mother wants me to be fat.
7. If I have food or water in my stomach, I am fatter.
8. I have to be perfect to please my family.
9. I can't have angry feelings because it would mean I'm a bad person.
10. When I'm thin, I'm in control.

References

1. Beck, A.T., Rush, J., Shaw, B., and Emery, G., *Cognitive Therapy of Depression*, Guilford Press, New York, 1979.
2. Fairburn, C.G. and Wilson, G.T., *Binge Eating: Nature, Assessment, and Treatment*, Guilford Press, New York, 1993.
3. Garner, D.M. and Garfinkel, P.E., *Handbook of Psychotherapy for Anorexia Nervosa and Bulimia*, Guilford Press, New York, 1985, 365.
4. Halmi, K.A., *Psychobiology and Treatment of Anorexia Nervosa and Bulimia Nervosa*, American Psychiatric Press, Washington, D.C., 1992.
5. Nicola, V.F., Anorexia multiforms: self-starvation in historical and cultural context. Part 1. Self-starvation as a historical chameleon, *Transcultural Psychiatry Research Review*, 27, 245, 1990.
6. Beck, A.T., *Cognitive Therapy and the Emotional Disorders*, International Press, New York, 1976.

Appendix 17-A: Resources for Eating Disorder Information and Treatment

American Anorexia/Bulimia Association, Inc.
165-W 46th St., Suite 1108
New York, NY 10036
(212) 575-6200
http://www.AmAnBu@aol.com
AOL members-aol.com/amanbu

Anorexia Nervosa and Related Eating Disorders, Inc.
P.O. Box 5102
Eugene, OR 97405
(541) 344-1144
http://www.anred.com

Center for the Study of Anorexia and Bulimia
1841 Broadway, 4th Floor
New York, NY 10023
(212) 595-3449

National Association of Anorexia Nervosa and Associated Disorders
P.O. Box 7
Highland Park, IL 60035
(847) 831-3438

Overeaters Anonymous Headquarters
World Services Office
2190 W. 190th Street
Torrance, CA 90504

Remuda Ranch
Center for Anorexia and Bulimia, Inc.
1 East Apache
Wickenburg, AZ 85390
1-800-445-1900
http://www.remuda-ranch.com

The Renfrew Center of Florida
7700 Renfrew Lane
Coconut Creek, FL 33073
1-800-RENFREW

American Anorexia/Bulimia Association, Inc.
133 Cedar Lane
Teaneck, NJ 07666
(201) 836-1800

Canyon Lakes Residential Treatment Center
2402 Canyon Lakes Drive
Lubbock, TX 79415
(806) 762-5782

National Eating Disorders Association
6655 South Yale Avenue
Tulsa, OK 74136
(918) 481-4044
Fax (918) 481-4076
E-mail – www.laurcate.com

Remuda Ranch Center for Anorexia and Bulimia
10000 N 31st Avenue
Suite D400
Phoenix, AZ 85051
1-800-445-1900

The Center for the Study of Anorexia Nervosa and Associated Disorders
Box 271
Highland Park, IL 60035

Eating Disorders Awareness and Prevention
603 Stewart Street, Suite 803
Seattle, Washington 98101
(206) 382-3587 phone
(206) 829-8501 fax

18

Kudos for Me: Self-Esteem

Michelle Pettus

CONTENTS

18.1 Learning Objectives

After reading this chapter you should be able to:

- Define self-esteem;
- Understand how low self-esteem affects each dimension of wellness;
- Recognize behaviors that reflect high and low self-esteem;
- Utilize activities to boost self-esteem.

18.2 Research Background

"All of the significant battles are waged within the self."[1] One of the most crippling health concerns in society today is not a deadly disease or a threatening social disaster but rather, a gradual, consuming internal battle — low self-esteem. The dynamic may bleed into other areas of life including mental, physical, spiritual, social, occupational, and emotional well-being. Self-esteem has been defined as the difference between the real self and the ideal self. The real self reflects the person as he or she truly is, while the ideal self is who the person wishes to be. The greater the difference between the two, the more a person's self-esteem is lowered. Other terms describing self-esteem include self-acceptance, self-concept, and self-efficacy. Self-esteem is reflected through self-talk, countenance, and outlook on life. It is based on a lifetime of experiences and relationships. The keys to self-esteem are connectiveness, uniqueness, power, values, and role models.[2]

Connectiveness provides satisfaction in knowing that one's relationships are significant, nurturing, and affirmed by others. Uniqueness represents an individual's feeling of possessing qualities that make him or her special and different. These qualities are also respected and admired by others. Power gives one the sense of having the ability to access and use inner resources to influence circumstances in life. This may also be described as having an internal locus of control, a concept developed in the 1960s by psychologist Julian Rotter. An individual who has an internal locus of control feels responsible for his or her actions and draws upon internal resources of self-confidence, faith, intuition, and will power. An internal locus of control can be seen in people who seek information, are goal-directed and are able to cope with problems. Power empowers. Unlike an internal locus of control, an external locus of control means an individual is at the mercy of outside influences and it is often the cause of apathy and complacency. Examples of external factors include other people, luck, the weather, chance, or the zodiac.

The last key to self-esteem means having role models and a sense of values. This key stresses the importance of knowing people we feel are worth emulating and having the confidence to distinguish right from wrong and good from bad. Having values and beliefs can provide constant guidance and direction, encourages an individual to know more or less where life is headed, and enables him or her to make sense out of what is going on internally and externally.

Self-esteem is high in those who accept their strengths and weaknesses, recognize themselves as unique and valuable, trust themselves to maintain a steady disposition through life's storms and changes, and have the confidence that they can reach their deepest personal goals and aspirations.[3]

Self-esteem may also be influenced by gender. Dr. John Gray, author of *Men are from Mars; Women are from Venus*, suggests that men receive their sense of self from personal accomplishments while women are esteemed by others. He goes on to say that a woman's self-esteem rises and falls like a wave. When a woman's wave rises, she feels she has an abundance of love to give, and when it falls, she feels an inner emptiness and needs to be filled with love.[4]

If a woman's self-esteem comes from others, she may give so much and make so many sacrifices to please others that she finds herself in a tangled web with no more resources to draw upon. This phenomenon ties back to the keys of self-esteem mentioned earlier and is in direct contrast to the sense of power and internal locus of control needed for self-esteem. The toll of low self-esteem on an individual's intellectual, occupational, social, emotional, spiritual, and physical dimensions of wellness will be explored.

Intellectually, low self-esteem hampers a person's potential to expand his or her knowledge. Students may be apprehensive about raising their hands in class to ask questions for fear of looking stupid or drawing attention to themselves. Procrastination can set in as individuals feel overwhelmed and perhaps incompetent to tackle difficult assignments and meet pending deadlines. Poor time management ties in closely with procrastination. Another factor in poor time management is inability assert a need for personal time — time alone, time to work, think, rest, plan, dream, and do whatever is of interest.

Occupationally, low self-esteem may attribute to the mediocrity seen in society. Individuals resist setting life-building goals for fear of failure rather than adopting Benjamin Franklin's outlook: "I haven't failed, I've only had about ten thousand tries." Apathy may set in as persons find themselves meeting only minimum job requirements rather than taking ownership of their work and seeking ways to improve.

Socially, a person suffering from low self-esteem may either immerse herself into another person, work, food, or family, or withdraw completely. Behavior that includes bitterness, belittling, and constant comparisons can be attributed to low self-

Anorexia Nervosa–Bulimia
A Multi-Dimensional Profile

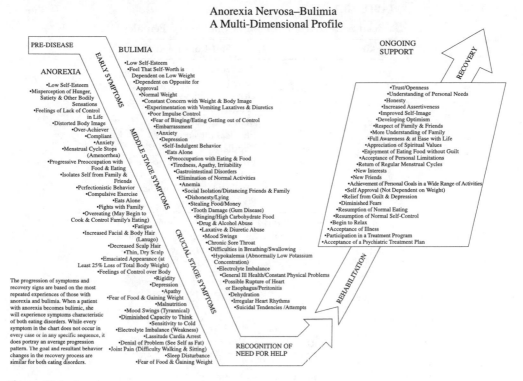

Figure 18.1

Anorexia nervosa and bulimia: a multi-dimensional profile.

esteem. Disassociation might occur when a person gives up his or her identity to please others.

The downward spiral of low self-esteem continues. People become depressed, defensive (extremely sensitive to criticism), frustrated with their lack of ability to validate problems, or stressed out. Interestingly, high self-esteem is considered the best defense against stress.[2] A person may become very self-centered as he or she tries to make sense of events. This affects his or her spiritual well-being by robbing him or her of peace and stability.

Physical consequences can accompany low self-esteem as well. Irresponsible drinking, drug abuse, casual sex, and eating disorders maybe linked to low self-esteem. Figure 18.1 shows the progression of symptoms and recovery signs of victims of anorexia and bulimia. The first item on the list of pre-disease/early symptoms of anorexia *and* bulimia is low self-esteem.

Peggy Fogle and Teresa Pangan of the University of North Texas presented research on eating disorders at the Southwest College Health Association Conference in South Padre Island, TX in 1997. Table 18.1 shows their findings on the ten most valued self-concept traits in college-age females. Table 18.2 lists seven triggers of eating disorders, and the two main predisposing factors of eating disorders. The influence of self-esteem is clearly apparent.

Self-esteem is a central element in overall well-being. Therefore, it is important to discuss several ways to boost self-esteem:[2]

1. Disarm the negative critic inside. Forgive yourself or your mistakes and be conscious of your self-talk. Positive self-talk enhances performance; negative self-talk decreases performance and confidence and can lead to depression. Techniques for controlling negative self-talk include thought-stopping,

TABLE 18.1

Valued Self-Concept Traits in College-Age Females

Ranking	Self-Concept Trait
1	Academic ability
2	Assertiveness
3	Drive to achieve
4	Leadership
5	Mathematical ability
6	Physical attractiveness
7	Popularity
8	Popularity with opposite sex
9	Public speaking
10	Intellectual self-confidence
11	Social self-confidence

Source: From Fogle, P. and Pangan, T., Development of a multidisciplinary approach for treating college students suffering from eating disorders, presented at Southwest College Health Association Conference, South Padre Island, TX, November, 1997.

TABLE 18.2

Triggers That May Lead to the Development of an Eating Disorder

A single traumatic event
A 2- to 3-year period of unusual stress or pain
Onset of a mood disorder
Having been a very sensitive child
A controlling environment
Lack of validation of feelings
Predisposing factors
Inability to accept one's own complexity
One or more significant relationship disruptions

Source: From Fogle, P. and Pangan, T., Development of a multidisciplinary approach for treating college students suffering from eating disorders, presented at Southwest College Health Association Conference, South Padre Island, TX, November, 1997.

changing negative and irrational thoughts to positive thoughts, countering, and having a positive attitude.[5] Thought-stopping may be the use of a trigger word (e.g., Stop!) or physical action (e.g., clapping).

2. The negative and irrational thoughts that should change are as follows:

   (a) perfection is essential;

   (b) catastrophizing — making the situation worse than it is in actuality;

   (c) worth depends upon achievement;

   (d) one-trial generalizations — one failed attempt discourages any others.

3. Several strategies can be used to divert the mind from negative self-talk. Avoiding people who are negative or put people down can also safeguard self-esteem. Avoid self-blame for everything that goes wrong. The countering strategy uses facts and reason to refute negative thinking.

4. Give yourself positive reinforcement. When constructing affirmative statements, the affirmations should be believable. Positive self-talk may be used for acquiring skill, changing bad habits, initiating action, and motivating. By accentuating the positive, a person can focus on his or her good qualities and become more genuine. A person can set herself up for success by doing activities she is good at, not expecting perfectionism, resisting comparisons to others, and setting realistic goals.

5. Avoid "I should have" thinking.

6. Focus on who you really are.

7. Avoid comparisons with others.

8. Diversify your interests. For example, if an individual's self-identity centered upon his or her athletic talent and an injury or accident destroyed the ability to participate in athletics, it would be detrimental to his or her self-esteem if he or she had no other interests.

9. Improve your "connectedness." A person should spend time with those who make him or her feel better about himself or herself. Those who are envious and use that envy to chip away self-esteem should be avoided as should those who are negative or put others down.

10. Reassert yourself and your value before and during a stressful event.

11. Use SMART (specific, measurable, action-oriented, realistic, and time-specific) goals.[5]

18.3 Application of Research Question

How does one measure self-esteem and what activities can be used to raise self-esteem, if self-esteem is low? Several assessment tools can be found in the literature on the measurement of self-esteem. A sample assessment instrument can be found in Appendix 18-A. Sample activities are described in Appendix 18-B.[6]

References

1. Canfield, J., Hansen, M. V., Rogerson, H., Rutle, M., and Clauss, T., *Chicken Soup for the Soul at Work*, Health Communications, Deerfield Beach, FL, 1996, 242.
2. Seaward, B., Stress-prone and stress-resistant personalities, in *Managing Stress*, Jones and Bartlett Publishers, Boston, 1994, chap. 6.
3. Henderson, J., personal communication, 1998.
4. Gray, J., *Men are from Mars; Women are from Venus*, HarperCollins, Glenview, IL, 1992, 112.
5. Weinberg, R.S. and Gould, D., *Foundations of Sport and Exercise Psychology*, Human Kinetics, Champaign, IL, 1995, 344.
6. Mrosla, H., Lessons to remember, *Guideposts*, September, 15, 1999.

Appendix 18-A: Self-Acceptance Scale

The following self-assessment scale provides individuals the opportunity to evaluate attitudes toward themselves and find a measure of self-acceptance. Please answer the following questions about yourself. There is no right or wrong answer for any statement. The best answer is what you feel most reflects yourself. Please respond to each item on the scale according to the following scheme:

1 (not true at all)   2 (slightly true)   3 (about half true)   4 (mostly true)   5 (true)

Place the number for the best response on the line *before* the statement number. Remember that the best answer is the one that applies to you.

*____ 1. I wish someone would tell me what to do when problems arise.   ____

____ 2. No matter what others may think, I'm a worthwhile person.   ____

*____ 3. I don't take compliments very well because I think the person isn't being truthful.   ____

*____ 4. I find it hard to accept criticism or others' negative remarks.   ____

*____ 5. I'm never quite satisfied even when I think I should be.   ____

*____ 6. I wish I was more like other people – I feel so different.   ____

*____ 7. If I were to show my true self, I'm scared people would be let down.   ____

*____ 8. I often feel inferior to others.   ____

*____ 9. I behave the way others expect me to so they'll like me.   ____

____10. I trust myself and feel strong enough to handle things.   ____

*____11. I often don't go out of my way to make friends – they wouldn't like me.   ____

*____12. Though a person may not mean it, I'm very sensitive to his or her words and easily feel criticized or insulted.   ____

____13. I can face tomorrow's trouble.   ____

*____14. I know I'm not the person I make other people believe I am.   ____

____15. I am not worried if judged by others.   ____

*____16. Around people I don't say much – that way I won't stick my foot in my mouth.   ____

____17. I think I'm on an even keel with others and can develop positive relationships.   ____

*____18. I let other people set the standards for my life.   ____

Total   ____

Scoring:
For all items without an asterisk (*), transfer your score from the left of the question to the space at the end of the statement on the right-hand side. For all items marked with an asterisk (*), reverse the scores you have given and write them in the space given at the end of each statement on the right-hand side. Thus, for an item/statement

marked with an asterisk, if you have given yourself a score of 1, it will change to a 5, and a score of a 2 will become a 4. A score of a 4 becomes a 2, and a score of a 5 becomes a 1. A 3 score remains a 3. Once you have transferred all the scores, sum them up and determine your total score. Note it on the space provided at the end of the scale on the right-hand side.

Interpretation:
18 – 50   Indicates a low level of self-acceptance
51 – 75   Indicates a moderate level of self-acceptance
76 – 90   Indicates a high level of self-acceptance

Modified from Self-Acceptance Scale, *Self-Esteem and Positive Performance*, American Institute for Preventive Medicine, 1990.

Appendix 18-B: Activities to Increase Self-Esteem

Activity #1

Distribute index cards and ask an individual or group to make a list of five positive personal attributes and five negative personal attributes. Discuss which list took the most time to complete. Individuals may find it easier to criticize than praise themselves.

Activity #2

Distribute index cards and ask an individual or group to jot down the things he or she does well, his or her personal accomplishments, and the reasons he or she is cared for by others. This list may be saved as a reminder and as a self-esteem boost.

Activity #3

Distribute index cards with this saying written on them:

> *Grant me the serenity to accept the things I cannot change*
> *The courage to change the things I can*
> *And the wisdom to know the difference*
>
> [Author unknown]

Ask the group or individual to reflect on this prayer and answer the following questions.

Are there negatives in my life that can be changed?

Are there circumstances that need to be accepted because change is not possible?

Are there self-criticisms that aren't really true?

Activity #4

This activity is geared for groups and is most beneficial in team, organizational, resident hall floors, and other close-knit settings. Sister Helen Mrosla who shared her experience in *Guideposts Magazine* (September, 1999), inspired the idea. The activity allows individuals to mill around the room and take an active role in the exercise. Each member of the group needs a pencil and blank piece of paper taped to the back of his or her shirt. The paper may be heart-shaped to symbolize love or a hand cutout signifying a "pat on the back." Individuals are instructed to anonymously write something positive (not a compliment on a physical attribute) about the person on each person's back. At the end of the activity, participants remove the pieces of paper and read the positive comments. Each person is encouraged to save the list as a reminder of the positive qualities others recognize.

19

Communication, Expressing Feelings, and Creative Problem Solving

Marilyn Massey-Stokes

CONTENTS

19.1 Learning Objectives

After completing this chapter, the reader will be able to:

- Discuss how weak communication skills may contribute to eating difficulties;

- Discuss how the inability to healthfully express emotions may contribute to eating problems;
- Discuss the skills essential for effective communication;
- Explain how a practitioner can help a female with eating problems learn to communicate more effectually;
- Explain how a practitioner can help a female with eating problems learn to express her emotions in appropriate, health-promoting ways;
- Discuss the significance of creative problem solving as a life skill;
- Discuss strategies a practitioner can use to help a female with eating problems learn to creatively solve problems;
- Discuss how emotional toughness can help buffer a person from experiencing eating problems or developing eating disorders;
- Explain the strategies an individual can implement to develop emotional toughness;
- Explain the concepts of "four rooms" and "sharpen the saw," and discuss how they relate to wellness and the prevention of eating disorders.

19.2 Research Background

19.2.1 Emotional Vulnerabilities

Studies suggest that emotional vulnerabilities are salient predictors of eating difficulties,[1] and researchers have investigated psychological variables that may play roles in the development of eating disturbances and clinical eating disorders. Several authors have found negative body image and body dissatisfaction to be associated with more eating disorder symptoms in adolescence.[1-3] Negative body image and body dissatisfaction are often linked to emotional distress. For example, Levine[3] explains that misconceptions of external body shape constitute a distorted body image, of which there are two types — perceptual and emotional. He adds that anorexics who experience emotional body image distortion "can see that they are too thin, but they either rejoice in this 'achievement' or they cling to slenderness as protection against a body that they loathe in its normal form." Furthermore, negative body image and body dissatisfaction often are linked with other psychological variables such as shame;[4] depression;[1,3-6] low self-esteem;[1,4,6,7] low self-efficacy;[2] perfectionistic tendencies;[1,6,8] fear;[4] anxiety;[1,3,5,7] impulsivity;[1,2] lack of boundaries and control;[4] lack of self-confidence and feelings of insecurity;[1,2,7,9] and lack of interoceptive awareness.[1,3,5,7]

19.2.2 Barriers to Effective Communication and Expressing Feelings

The National Mental Health Association[10] describes emotionally well people as possessing three basic characteristics: (1) They feel comfortable about themselves and are not overwhelmed by their feelings and emotions; (2) They interact positively with others and enjoy satisfying and lasting relationships; and (3) They are able to meet the demands of life. In terms of mental and emotional wellness, it is important for individuals to learn how to identify their feelings, acknowledge their feelings, and express them appropriately. When emotions are blocked and not acknowledged, negative emotional energy can lead to a sense of helplessness, hopelessness, and overall distress. To try to cope with negative emotions, young people may engage in self-destructive behaviors, including harmful dietary practices.[11] Schafe and Parsons[4] assert that individuals with eating disorders seem to be self-medicating their negative feelings through misuse of food.

Various factors that erect roadblocks to the healthy expression of feelings have been linked to eating anomalies. For example, anorexics generally are out of touch with their emotions and frequently do not know what they feel or how to express their feelings.[3,9] In addition, young women who suffer with anorexia tend to exhibit denial of negative feelings and denial of the disorder.[6] They attempt to please others by being "good little girls"[12] and may deny feelings of anger and frustration, thereby avoiding conflict.[6]

Bulimics also suffer from low self-esteem and self-confidence. In addition, they have trouble setting limits and boundaries because they do not want to disappoint others and be disliked. Like anorexics, bulimics are perfectionistic and often are afraid to express anger. If others are angry or upset, the bulimic often accepts the blame and tries to amend the situation. Because it is impossible to control other people's moods and actions, bulimics feel a great deal of frustration and are likely to suffer from guilt and depression due to what they see as personal failure.[5] Impulsivity and emotional instability are two other characteristics commonly associated with bulimics. Impulsivity may partially explain why bulimics are two to four times as likely as the general population to abuse alcohol and drugs. With regard to emotional instability, bulimics have low tolerance for frustration and experience great difficulties controlling their feelings, especially anger.[3]

Chatoor[5] asserts that an eating-disordered individual controls eating with emotions and external cues instead of internal physiological signals. Moreover, research reveals an intriguing difference in the ways anorexics and bulimics deal with emotions through food. Anorexic, restricting individuals generally are unable to eat when they are emotionally upset, whereas bulimic individuals are likely to binge in response to the same feelings.[5]

The psychological traits of compulsive overeaters are similar to those of anorexics and bulimics. Compulsive overeaters usually experience dysphoria, anxiety, perfectionism, and low self-esteem. Despite their outward appearance of contentment, many of them say they are sad, lonely, and frustrated. They lack the security of knowing that others love and accept them. Finally, they are unable to set limits on the demands that others place upon them, and they have great difficulty in expressing anger and frustration.[6]

One factor associated with the complexity of eating disorders is family dynamics, discussed in Chapter 9. The way a family handles communication and conflict are two dynamics that are linked to the development of eating disorders. Minuchin, Rosman, and Baker[13] explain that within families of anorexics, direct communication often is blocked, and conflict is avoided. As a result, problems are left unresolved and continue to resurface. Conflict often is heightened when a family member does not communicate effectively. This may be due to lack of coping skills (including stress management and anger management), lack of assertiveness, passivity or aggressiveness, poor listening skills, and (or as well as) underdeveloped critical thinking and creative problem solving skills.

What happens in a family has powerful and long-lasting impact. In a healthy family system, individual growth and expression of boundaries, feelings, and needs are encouraged. In contrast, within a dysfunctional family system, rules are rigid, communication is closed, and individual growth is stifled.[4] Those who study and write about family of origin explain that communication patterns learned and practiced within the family are carried forward into other relationships.[13,14] For example, if a girl lives in a home where the family suppresses conflict and represses angry feelings, she is very likely to continue those behavior patterns. Certain familial characteristics in the area of communication may contribute to eating problems, such as avoidance of open conflict[5,9] and lack of conflict resolution.[5,9,13]

Additionally, studies reveal that within families of eating-disordered women, parental support, empathy, and nurturance often are lacking, and expression of feelings is not encouraged.[1,4,13] Chatoor[5] asserts that individuals who fail to express their needs and feelings remain unaware of their inner feelings and consequently fail to develop strong senses of self. In her work with adolescent anorexic girls, Chatoor noticed that the girls "have perfected the art of focusing on others and reading their cues while remaining unaware of their own needs and emotions."

19.2.3   Communication

19.2.3.1   Communication Basics

Strong communication skills are vital to health and wellness. Effective communication improves self-esteem, increases self-efficacy, reduces stress, and helps a person develop and experience quality interpersonal relationships. Communication is a dynamic process that involves the transmission of information and meaning from one individual to another. Communication is a learned skill — a process by which one develops the ability to clearly express thoughts, feelings, beliefs, opinion, reactions, values, hopes, and dreams.

A basic axiom of communication is that *one cannot not communicate*. Therefore, silence, withdrawal, and other forms of denial are types of communication.[15] To paraphrase a common saying, "The three most important words for a successful relationship are communication, communication, and communication." Strong communication skills are requisite to overall health and wellness and essential for interpersonal relationship growth. Effective communication encompasses a variety of skills, including critical thinking, problem solving, assertiveness, empathic listening, the ability to interpret nonverbal signals, and the ability to effectively manage conflict.

Barriers to communication interfere with the transference of a message and, as a result, can greatly hinder communication and even damage interpersonal relationships. Typical roadblocks to effective communication include the following.[16,17]

- Speaker and listener have different "languages."
- Listener's personal biases affect response to the speaker.
- Speaker and listener are resistant to change.
- Insufficient time is set aside for discussing an issue.
- Listener is not actively listening.
- One or both parties overgeneralize ("You always..." or "You never...").
- Blaming and belittling lead to negative responses through the use of "you" statements, such as "You are always late" or "You never listen to me."
- Listener redefines a speaker's message by adding his or her own thoughts to the message.
- One or both parties have tunnel vision (viewing life as black or white rather than seeing gray areas).

TABLE 19.1

Interpreting Nonverbal Communication

Nonverbal Signals	Interpretations
Eye Contact	
Steady, warm	I'm listening (or, I like you)
Staring	You're weird (or, I don't like you)
None or fleeting	I'm bored (or, I'm anxious/resistant)
Peering over glasses	I'm skeptical
One eyebrow raised	I disapprove (or, I don't believe you)
Hand Gestures	
Drumming, tapping pencil	Hurry, I'm impatient (or, you bother me)
Clenched fists	I'm angry (or, I'm tense)
Relaxed	I'm open to you (or, I feel relaxed)
Firm handshake or touch	I care about you (or, I feel you're important)
No physical contact	I want to keep my distance
Pointing finger	I'm blaming you (or, now, understand this)
Body Postures	
Facing	I like you (or, I'm straightforward with you)
Turned away	I want to avoid you
Slouched	I'm relaxed (or, I'm not taking this seriously)
Erect	I'm on edge (or, I'm taking this seriously)
Forward lean	I'm interested
Backward lean	Who cares?
Open arms or legs	I like you (or, I'm relaxed)
Closed arms or legs	I don't like you (or, I'm feeling defensive)
Physical Distancing	
Close	I feel warm or friendly (or, I'm trying to intimidate you)
Far away	I feel distant (or, I feel superior)
Above the other	I am superior
Below the other	I am beneath you
At the same level	We are equals
Head Movements	
Nodding	I agree (or, I understand)
Head shaking	I disagree (or, I'm confused)
Cocking head to one side	I doubt it (or, I'm amused, or I'm listening)
Facial Expressions	
Smile	I like you (or, I want your approval)
Frown	I'm confused (or, I don't like this or I don't like you)
Clenched teeth	I'm tense (or, I'm feeling threatened)
Open mouth	I'm relaxed (or, I'm surprised or in wonder)
Curled lip	I'm disgusted (or, I'm mocking you)

Another barrier to effective communication occurs when the speaker's body language contradicts the verbal communication, and the listener receives a mixed message. This type of mixed message interrupts the two-way flow of thoughts and feelings and can cause frustration, resentment, and conflict. It is helpful for both the speaker and listener to understand the meanings conveyed through forms of nonverbal communication such as eye contact, hand gestures, and body postures. Table 19.1 explains how to interpret nonverbal signals.

19.2.3.2 Assertiveness

One of the key characteristics of an effective communicator is assertiveness. Assertiveness is the ability to express oneself without violating the rights of others. Assertiveness is characterized by open, honest communication that is self-enhancing and expressive. Before a person can clearly state her needs, however, she needs to believe she has a legitimate right to have these needs. Table 19.2 lists basic assertive rights.

TABLE 19.2

Basic Assertive Rights

1. The right to act in ways that promote your dignity and self-respect as long as others' rights are not violated.
2. The right to be treated with respect.
3. The right to say "no" and not feel guilty.
4. The right to experience and express your feelings.
5. The right to slow down and think.
6. The right to change your mind.
7. The right to ask for what you want.
8. The right to do less than you are humanly capable of.
9. The right to ask for more information.
10. The right to make mistakes.

Source: From Rogers, M. A., Gonzalez, J., Mullen, R., and Montgomery, M., *Talking and Listening to the Children: A Family Based Program for Children, Teens, Single Parents and Blended Families*, Talking and Listening to the Children, Inc., Lubbock, TX.

When a female does not believe she has these basic assertive rights (or is not aware of them), she may react very passively to circumstances in her life. When a person allows the needs, opinions, and judgments of others to become more important than her own, she is likely to feel frustrated, hurt, anxious, and even angry. Because females often are socialized to be passive communicators and people pleasers in our society, it is imperative to offer them opportunities to learn and practice assertiveness so they can be more effective communicators. Girls and women who are not accustomed to communicating assertively may initially and incorrectly view this form of communication as selfish. Selfishness is aggressive and involves expressing rights at the expense, degradation, or humiliation of another. Assertiveness is a positive trait that does not violate the rights of others.

19.2.3.3   *Self-Disclosure*

Self-disclosure is the highest level of communication that is reserved for intimate relationships; it requires openness, honesty and trust.[16] Self-disclosure is characterized by mutual sharing of happiness, sadness, fears, and aspirations. Being intimate requires one to open up and take risks by sharing innermost thoughts and feelings with another person. However, individuals with disordered eating tend to avoid intimacy and self-disclosure because they fear rejection. They are afraid that others will not like or love them for who they really are. Furthermore, it is difficult to self-disclose when one suffers from low self-esteem and is not in tune with inner needs.

Another facet of self-disclosure involves a practitioner's self-disclosure to a client. As a recovered anorexic who works with clients suffering from eating disorders, Goldkopf-Woodtke[18] provides insight into this controversial issue. She explains that one of the disadvantages of using self-disclosure with clients is that therapy can become more difficult if a client develops hostility and feelings of competitiveness. Clients also may expect quick results from a therapist who has "been there." Self-disclosure has advantages in that clients have less difficulty in opening up to someone who has experienced similar trials, and they feel more comfortable with a therapist who, through personal experience, possesses a clearer understanding of the complex issues that are involved. In addition, a therapist can be a positive role model to her clients and others by conveying the message that, "You *can* conquer this — I'm living proof that it can be done!"

19.2.3.4 Empathic Listening

In Stephen Covey's bestseller *The Seven Habits of Highly Effective People*,[19] Habit 5 concerns the "single most important principle" of effective interpersonal communication: "Seek first to understand, then to be understood." Covey describes a paradigm for listening different from what most people practice. He explains that most of us listen at one of four levels: (1) we may *ignore* the person and not listen at all; (2) we may *pretend* to listen; (3) we may engage in *selective listening* by hearing only certain parts of the conversation; or (4) we may practice *attentive listening* and pay attention to what is said. Few people practice the fifth level, the highest form of listening, called *empathic listening*. Covey explains:

> Empathic (from *empathy*) listening gets inside another person's frame of reference. You look out through it, you see the world the way they see the world, you understand their paradigm, you understand how they feel…. The essence of empathic listening is not that you agree with someone; it's that you fully, deeply, understand that person, emotionally as well as intellectually.

Next to physiological survival, the greatest need of a human being is psychological survival — to be understood, to be affirmed, to be validated, to be appreciated. When a person listens with empathy to another person, she gives that person "psychological air." The need for "psychological air" strongly impacts communication,[19] particularly in the areas of problem solving and conflict resolution.

19.2.3.5 Conflict Resolution

Conflict is natural in human relationships because people have their own needs, desires, past experiences, and world views. Conflict is not necessarily harmful to a relationship; it may indicate that the relationship is growing and reaching a deeper level of intimacy. However, if conflict is not handled in a constructive way, it will damage — and ultimately demolish — the relationship.[20] Therefore, a fundamental communication skill that is critical to overall success and positive interaction with others is the ability to resolve conflict in a peaceful, constructive manner. The desired outcome for conflict resolution is negotiation that produces a win-win situation in which both individuals or groups succeed in having their needs met. Effective conflict resolution requires a panoply of skills, including effective communication, empathy (including empathic listening), anger management, problem solving, and decision making. Becvar and Becvar[21] assert that "direct expression of feelings, including the components of description, prescription, and negotiation, plus the skill of paraphrasing feelings, are fundamental to constructive resolution." Several approaches to resolving conflict exist. The section on improving communication skills in this chapter outlines basic steps for successful conflict resolution.

In summary, "problem solving and conflict resolution are therefore enhanced to the degree that we can admit others' perceptions as valid for them, can clearly express our feelings and reactions when we experience conflict, can provide opportunities for discussion, and can allow the other person to respond in a way that is comfortable for him or her."[21]

19.2.4 Expressing Feelings

One of the basic tenets for learning to effectively cope with feelings is to understand that feelings are not facts. A person may feel a certain way. That does not mean that the feeling is reality. For example, girls and women often make the statement, "I feel fat." The feeling does not necessarily equate with actual body weight. Females "feel fat" to displace uncomfortable feelings that they are generally encouraged to stifle — anger, fear, anxiety, loneliness, etc. — or to represent situations that are unsafe for them to describe.[22] Furthermore, Becvar and Becvar[21] suggest that feelings are intimately related to the "way it's supposed to be" and the "way it is not supposed to be." They also suggest that "our maps of the way things are 'supposed to be' are learned, are relative, and thus are subject to review, revision, and perhaps expansion to include a wider range of acceptable behavior." This concept has wide application for helping girls and women move toward greater self-acceptance and helping them resolve conflicts in their relationships.

Goldkopf-Wootke[18] contends that we send our children mixed messages about expressing feelings: "Today we tell our children that it is okay to have feelings — it is okay to be angry. But do we really give them the freedom to express that anger as they move through stages of growth and assertion that are filled with frustration and confusion?"

Another significant point of discussion is the problematic tendency to label feelings as "good" or "bad." Children quickly learn that good feelings — happiness, joy, love, and gratitude — are acceptable, while bad feelings — anger, fear, anxiety, frustration, and sadness — are not acceptable. Consequently, children often internalize these messages and begin to believe that if they experience bad feelings, they must be bad people, which, in turn, can lead to feelings of guilt and shame. Becvar and Becvar[21] contend, "The basic social message is that we are to be happy all of the time. But, feelings do not work that way. More often than not, the harder we try to get rid of a feeling we are not 'supposed to have,' the more we tend to experience that feeling."

The following guidelines can be used by practitioners to help themselves as well as others learn to resolve this dilemma.[21]

- There are no good feelings and no bad feelings. We need all our feelings to be complete, whole human beings.
- Whatever you are feeling, it is appropriate to feel as you do, given your experience and your interpretation of this event. You have a right to feel as you do, and you do not need to apologize, explain, or defend your feelings.
- Feelings can and do change if your interpretation of events changes.
- Although your feelings are not subject to conscious control and you have no choice except to feel what you feel, you have a choice about what you do with those feelings.

A critical point to keep in mind is that behavior change precedes feeling change.[21] On occasion, a person needs to be emotionally tough and act as if she feels a certain way, even if she has to "fake it." For example, even if an individual feels anxious about performing or speaking in front of a group of people, she needs to consciously focus on acting the way she wants to feel — relaxed and self-confident. When a person follows through with an action in spite of trepidation, she adds a deposit to her "emotional bank account" and experiences more elevated self-esteem and increased self-assurance as a result.

Feelings are useful because they help us better understand ourselves and our connections with others. Negative feelings often are suppressed because a person does not want to face the problems they signify. Negative feelings and emotions signal unmet needs. Ignoring or blocking negative feelings prevents needs from being met, which can lead to unhappiness, unsatisfying relationships, and health-related problems, such as depression, eating difficulties, and substance abuse. Many people are ill at ease expressing their uncomfortable feelings, and those battling eating problems generally stifle their true feelings to the detriment of health and well-being. Anger is a particularly difficult emotion with which to deal because many females have been taught to suppress their anger because it is unladylike. If anger is not appropriately and outwardly expressed, it is directed inward and can attribute to low self-esteem and depression and lead to unhealthy behaviors such as eating problems.

Identifying (or naming) feelings is very difficult for some individuals, particularly when they have buried their feelings for a long time. A person may experience negative emotions, but she is unable to pinpoint precisely what she feels. Identifying feelings is requisite for being able to appropriately express them. In learning to tune into feelings, Loehr[23] employs an interesting telephone analogy. To illustrate this concept, suppose a person is experiencing negative emotions (e.g., anxiety, frustration, sadness). These emotions mean that her inner "telephone" is ringing. She needs to answer it to find out what is bothering her. Perhaps her emotional discomfort is due to insufficient sleep and relaxation or lack of regular exercise or a nutritious diet. Perhaps she is inadequately coping with stress or not directly facing a problem. When she pays attention to her feelings and "answers the phone," she is then free to hang up and return to a positive emotional state. She must: (1) hear the phone announcing the negative feeling; (2) take the message concerning physical or psychological pain; and (3) fulfill the need, or the phone will start ringing again, more loudly, carrying more pain. The causes of troubling feelings must be identified so that a person can take proactive measures to alleviate the situation. If internal signals are ignored, the problem festers, increasing the likelihood that the individual will react in harmful ways (e.g., through unhealthy eating and/or exercise behaviors).

Finally, Kinoy[24] cites a follow-up study conducted after 26 years that revealed four salient factors contributing to the recovery of six anorexics: *personality strength, self-confidence, being ready,* and *being understood.* In order for individuals suffering with disordered eating to be understood, they must learn to be assertive, and they need to feel safe to express their feelings. The following comments are from women in treatment/recovery from eating disorders.[18] Notice the connection to feelings and emotions.

- My feelings are similar to the ones I felt in 1983 when I was bulimic. However, this time I didn't eat away my problems. I went back into therapy as quick as I could.
- I learned to like myself and deal with issues that bothered me by talking about them — not eating my way around them.
- I always basically knew food was not as much the problem as it was a lack of love, feeling alone, and hating myself.
- I am much better but much worse, because I am feeling now.

19.2.5 Creative Problem Solving

Females who battle eating problems and disorders often are dealing with problems that affect the entire being — mind, body, and spirit. If problems are not directly confronted and successfully resolved, negative stress (or distress) is likely to occur. When an individual experiences continuous distress with little or no relief, she is at higher risk for succumbing to illness. She also is at greater risk for engaging in harmful behaviors such as unhealthy dieting, substance abuse, and risky sexual behaviors.

A female with eating problems generally possesses an external locus of control. Instead of possessing an internal locus of control characterized by self-confidence and self-efficacy, she tends to exhibit vulnerability to external influences (other people and life situations). Girls and women who suffer from eating disorders generally feel out of control in certain aspects of their lives. In the attempt to exert some control, many engage in harmful self-restricting diets and/or unhealthy, strict exercise regimens that often lead to health problems, including full-blown eating disorders. Eating disorders wreak havoc on life by disrupting the balance of mind, body, and spirit and feeding an ever-spiraling loss of control.

Seaward[25] notes that change is inevitable, and people generally meet change with a certain degree of resistance. Furthermore, change often is equated with chaos, and chaos spells stress. Nevertheless, creativity can help bring order to the chaos and to help us embrace change. A crucial skill for coping and gaining control over life is the ability to creatively solve problems. Because problems, changes, and stressors are ingredients of daily life, the ability to creatively solve problems is imperative for high-level health and wellness. For many people, creativity is a foreign concept because they are quick to say, "I'm not creative." However, Seaward infers that everyone is creative and that creativity takes time and effort.

19.3 Application of Research Question

19.3.1 Enhancing Life Skills

Health promotion and prevention programs call for emphasis on the development and enhancement of life skills rather than on pathology.[26] Health promotion encompasses development of the whole individual, which includes the interrelated dimensions of physical, mental and emotional, social, and spiritual health. For that reason, effective health promotion and prevention programs (as well as intervention programs) must address individual interests and needs within each of these four dimensions. Strong communication and problem solving skills, healthful expression of feelings, and mental toughness are essential for total health and wellness and requisite for health-enhancing behaviors such as healthful eating and exercising. Programs can include strategies for building these crucial life skills in order to empower the individual and augment self-confidence, self-esteem, and self-efficacy.

19.3.2 Improving Communication Skills

A crucial dimension of assertive communication is the use of "I" statements to communicate thoughts and feelings openly and honestly. "I" statements allow a person to express feelings directly while still respecting another person's point of view. They allow a speaker to take responsibility for her own thoughts, feelings, and needs without blaming others. A sample outline for communicating with "I" statements is:

> I feel _____ (state a feeling) when _____ (state an exact behavior) because _____ (state the need related to that feeling and any thought or belief connected to it). What I want is _____ (describe the exact behavior that would meet the need).

Assertiveness increases self-confidence and self-efficacy. Assertive communication also improves key life skills such as decision making, problem solving, and conflict resolution. Assertiveness leads to self-empowerment, and it is an essential skill in learning to navigate through life's twists and turns. Assertive communication does not solve all problems, nor does it ensure happiness. However, lack of assertiveness can be linked to the inability to openly and honestly express feelings, which, in turn, can lead to great inner turmoil and difficulties with interpersonal relationships. Appendix 19-A describes techniques for building assertiveness.

Seaward[25] posits that effective communication includes listening, attending, and responding skills. The following steps[25] can be rehearsed through role play to develop more effective communication skills, particularly empathic listening. One person takes the role of the speaker while the other becomes the listener; then they reverse their roles.

- Assume the role of the listener.
- Maintain eye contact.
- Avoid word prejudice (liberal, feminist, right-wing radical, or other prejudicial statements).
- Use "minimal encouragers" to indicate that you are on the same wavelength as the person speaking. Use short-word questions and repeat key words.
- Paraphrase the speaker to ensure understanding.
- Ask questions to improve the clarity of the message.
- Use empathy to reflect and share feelings.
- Provide feedback. Summarize the content of the message so that the speaker's thoughts and feelings are fully understood.

These eight steps also are useful in helping resolve conflicts because they require a person to listen with the intent to understand the other person's point of view. Other basic strategies can be implemented to further increase the likelihood of successful conflict resolution.[20,27]

- Remain calm and set the tone.
- Take responsibility for personal actions.
- Clarify the issue.
- Determine what each person wants.
- Use "I" statements to express needs and feelings.
- Listen empathically to the needs and feelings expressed.
- Identify and evaluate possible solutions.
- Agree on a solution and solidify the agreement.
- Implement the agreement.
- Evaluate the agreement and renegotiate if necessary.

The speaker-listener technique as described by Markman, Stanley, and Blumberg[28] (Appendix 19-B) offers an alternative mode of communication when issues are hot or sensitive. This technique can be useful for conversations that focus on resolving conflict. For additional exercises to help an individual develop more effective conflict resolution skills, refer to Becvar and Becvar's book titled *Pragmatics of Human Relationships*.[21]

TABLE 19.3

Anger Management Strategies

- Talk it out with an objective person (friend, parent, teacher, clergy, therapist) who is an active listener and will give you feedback that may help you to deal with or understand your anger better.
- Close your eyes and breathe deeply as you become better aware of your feelings. You may find it helpful to count your breaths; try to stay with your feelings until they gradually begin to subside.
- Use visual imagery — close your eyes and imagine a calm, peaceful place. Breathe deeply, and stay in your special place until you feel calmer.
- Use writing as an outlet for your feelings. You can use writing as a mode of catharsis. For example, write poems or stories, or keep a personal journal in which you record your feelings. Give yourself the freedom to express yourself freely. Another idea is to write a letter to the person with whom you are angry. You can choose to tear it up or mail it. If you decide to mail it, it is wise to wait a few days and reread it to make sure that you really want to mail it. Seeing words on paper helps clarify feelings and provides a clearer mindset about the situation.
- Release your anger in nonviolent ways that do not hurt you or others (e.g., punch a boxing bag, hit a pillow, play angry notes on a piano or drum, go to a private place to scream and yell, cry, etc.).
- Exercise! The physical release can be helpful; exercise produces endorphins, which are naturally occurring chemicals in the brain that produce a feeling of well-being.
- Listen to music that calms you.
- Watch something calming — a beautiful sunset, the moon and stars, a body of water, etc.
- Hold and/or play with a favorite pet.
- Read books that soothe you (e.g., the Bible, poetry, etc.).
- When you have calmed down, talk with the person with whom you are angry.

Source: Adapted in part from Kramer, P., *The Dynamics of Relationships: A Guide for Developing Self-Esteem and Coping Skills for Teens and Young Adults*, Equal Partners, Silver Spring, MD, 1994, 111–112. With permission.

19.3.3   Learning How to Healthfully Express Feelings

It is vital for practitioners to help females with problematic eating behaviors or disorders learn to recognize and accept the entire range of human emotions — including the difficult, negative emotions such as fear, anger, frustration, guilt, and anxiety — and encourage healthful expression of feelings and emotions. This is not a simple one-step solution. The process takes time, patience, and nurturing guidance. Geneen Roth contends that, "Feelings cannot be skipped; you get out of them by going through them."[9] Appendix 19-C covers exercises that can help a person accept feelings, express feelings directly and appropriately, and deal effectively with feelings expressed by others.[21] Appendix 19-D includes an activity for learning to communicate empathically. These exercises can build communication skills and help an individual identify and express "feeling" words. These exercises may be uncomfortable at first; nevertheless, if a person resolves to practice, she has the opportunity to experience the personal victory of taking a positive step toward self-growth.

Another beneficial skill is anger management, which includes the ability to constructively express anger. Anger can be a helpful emotion in that it can motivate one to take action to correct a situation or take a strong stand against injustice and inequality.[17] Anger becomes damaging when it is repressed, ignored, or inappropriately expressed. Angry feelings must be appropriately expressed so that an individual does not experience the negative repercussions of harboring pent-up anger. Numerous constructive strategies can be employed to appropriately express anger (see Table 19.3).

Feelings also can be addressed as an integral component of nutritional education and counseling for people with eating disorders. Not only does the nutritionist work with the client on establishing a well-balanced eating plan, but she/he also talks with the client about the emotions that underlie the eating patterns. Marx[29] explains that compulsive eaters must learn to take charge of their physical, emotional, and mental needs. In doing so, they must learn to develop healthy responses to the following questions.

- Who am I?
- What are my *own* thoughts, values, ideas, and feelings?
- What are my *own* wants and needs?
- What frightens me, angers me, pleases me, saddens me?
- What can I do besides eat when I feel fear, anger, joy, or sorrow?
- How can I eliminate obsessive thoughts and compulsions that lead me to eat?
- What stresses me and makes me tense?
- What can I do besides eat when I feel tense and stressed?
- How can I ask for what I need and want?
- How can I learn to accept my right to ask for what I need and want?
- How can I learn not to abandon myself for the sake of others?
- How can I learn to love and accept myself and be patient with myself while I heal?
- How can I learn to forgive myself?

These are painful questions to answer, and it takes time and diligence to work through them. However, in time, this self-work becomes freeing and fulfilling. "It is like coming home."[29] Kahm[30] suggests that a practitioner working with a bulimic client can ask a patient: (1) What is going on? (2) How does that make you feel? (3) Does eating help? (4) Does it solve problems? and (5) What can you do instead? The practitioner can alter the questions so that they are more relevant to anorexic clients. For example, the practitioner can substitute, "Does it help you to severely restrict your daily food intake?" for the third question. The fourth question can be phrased, "What can you do to express your feelings in a way that promotes your health and wellness?"

A brainstorming session can yield ideas for what a client can do beyond "eating away her problems" or starving herself to deny her problems. Various expressive and experiential techniques can serve as valuable tools to help uncover buried feelings and emotions.[31] Examples of these strategies include journaling;[31] creative writing;[11] story-telling;[22] using analogies;[31] art;[4,22,31] massage;[31] role play;[22] and movement/dance. In learning to express feelings through creative and expressive activities, a person struggling with an eating disorder gains a sense of competence and control, which bolsters self-esteem and strengthens self-efficacy. Other ideas for avoiding emotional eating include engaging in deep breathing, prayer, and meditation; visual imagery; yoga; and other relaxation techniques. Exercising (in moderation and for the right reasons), talking to a trusted confidante, listening to music, and working on an important project can also be beneficial.

For additional ideas, Appendices 19-C and 19-D include "feelings" vocabulary lists that can help a person find words that express her feelings. Appendix 19-E lists activities that can help a person examine the connection between feelings and body attitude, body image, and body messages.

19.3.4 Increasing Problem-Solving Skills

A primary component of eating disorder prevention and early intervention programs is building personal competence by developing an internal locus of control and cultivating adaptive coping skills.[2] Numerous personal and social skills can help empower an individual, such as communication (including conflict resolution), decision making, goal setting, and creative problem solving. Likewise, adaptive coping strategies such as emotional toughness and stress management/relaxation techniques help buffer individuals from developing eating disorders.

Creative problem solving is crucial to personal happiness and success because to fully participate in life, one must frequently encounter challenges of varying degrees of perplexity. For effective problem solving to develop, an individual must possess solid communication skills, a positive mind-set, and a willingness to work on strengthening abilities to be creative. To stimulate the brain's creative "muscles," Seaward[32] recommends reading two books written by Roger von Oech: *A Whack on the Side of the Head* and *A Kick in the Seat of the Pants*. Although a problem can have multiple solutions, some basic steps can be taken to simplify and demystify the creative problem-solving process. Seaward[25] submits the following strategies as a "map" for creative problem-solving skills: (1) describe the problem; (2) generate ideas; (3) select and refine an idea; (4) implement the idea; and (5) evaluate and analyze actions.

McGaffey[33] offers these thoughts about problem solving and listening: "Problem solving starts with how you listen. There is a way to listen that produces action and determination not only to solve the problem, but to build character and self-esteem." Some questions a person can ask include: What were the actions or inactions that produced the problem? What resources are missing? What needs to be learned? What assistance is needed and from whom? These questions can help avoid communication roadblocks, such as blaming or wallowing in self-pity and complaint, and reduce the chance for negative attitudes, resentment, or hopelessness to set in. These questions allow a person to keep trying, keep learning, and keep moving toward fulfillment of personal goals and visions.[33] As a result of facing problems with courage and honesty, a person experiences a sense of competence that positively fuels self-respect.

Another way a person can bolster problem solving skills is to create a personal mission statement or "personal constitution" that guides and supports her through life. According to Covey,[19] a personal mission statement focuses on what one wants to be (character) and do (contributions and achievements), and it encompasses personal values and principles. Furthermore, a personal mission statement brings centering to an individual's life, thereby helping her experience a sense of clarity, a sense of organization and commitment, and a sense of exhilaration and freedom.

A person can begin to develop a personal mission statement by setting short-term and long-term goals. Some salient factors should be considered in the goal-setting process.[19] First, goals are based upon values and aspirations, and require self-awareness and personal vision. Second, they reflect the way people envision their different roles (individual, daughter, sister, girlfriend, student, employee, etc.). Third, they represent what a person wants to accomplish in each role during a specified period of time. Well-written goals possess certain characteristics. They are clear, specific, and measurable; realistic and manageable; positively focused (on what a person *will* do as opposed to what she *will not* do); and written.[16,34] It is important for an individual to set both types of goals because short-term goals are essential "baby steps" for achieving long-term goals. Viewed another way, short-term goals are the *strategies*, whereas long-term goals serve as the *destination*.[34] According to Robert Riley, "You can eat an elephant if you do it one bite at a time." After a client becomes more comfortable with the goal-setting process, she can then work on creating a personal mission statement. Two valuable resources that offer excellent ideas for building skills for setting goals and creating personal mission statements are *The Wellness Book*[34] and *First Things First*.[35]

19.3.5 Developing Emotional Toughness

According to Loehr,[23] "maximum health, happiness, and productivity occur when sufficient physical and emotional toughness are acquired to effectively manage the volume of stress in one's life." Individuals become physically and emotionally tough by experiencing balanced cycles of stress and recovery in various areas of their lives. Being emotionally tough means "being able to deal with life in flexible, responsive, strong, and resilient ways. It means you control your emotions rather than the other way around. It means you can weather life's storms and seize life's opportunities. It means that when the going gets tough, you're tougher." Dr. Loehr proposes the following strategies for staying mentally tough and protecting oneself from the damaging effects of negative stress.

- Acknowledge that what you think has a significant impact on how you feel.
- Take full responsibility for what and how you think. While you may not always be able to prevent negative thoughts, you can choose not to entertain them.
- Think more flexibly. Use cognitive restructuring to reframe the situation in a more positive light.
- Think more responsively. Be responsive to the ringing phone of negative feelings.
- Think more energetically. Think *fun*, and positive energy will begin to flow.
- Think more resiliently because "This, too, shall pass."
- Think more humorously. Being able to laugh puts you in emotional control.
- Be more disciplined in the way you review your mistakes. What can I learn from them?

These emotional toughness strategies are advantageous to all individuals as they strive to develop inner strength and resilience. Furthermore, they can be particularly efficacious in helping females with eating problems to develop essential emotional skills to productively cope with life's challenges and demands.

19.4 Summary

An Indian proverb states, "Everyone is a house with four rooms—a physical, a mental, an emotional, and a spiritual room. Most of us tend to live in one room most of the time; but unless we go into every room every day, even if only to keep it aired, we are not a complete person." For an individual to develop high-level wellness and achieve her best in life, she must take the time to regularly visit and nourish each of her "rooms." This practice parallels Stephen Covey's Habit 7 — *Sharpen the Saw* by renewing the four dimensions. When we proactively take time to "sharpen the saw," we preserve and enhance the greatest asset we have — ourselves.[19] By developing communication and problem solving skills and learning how to be emotionally tough and healthfully express emotions, we begin the journey to excellence and success. As Covey states, "This is the single most powerful investment we can ever make in life — investment in ourselves, in the only instrument we have with which to deal with life and to contribute. We are the instruments of our own performance, and to be effective, we need to recognize the importance of taking time regularly to sharpen the saw in all four ways."

References

1. Connors, M. E., Developmental vulnerabilities for eating disorders, in *The Developmental Psychopathology of Eating Disorders: Implications for Research, Prevention, and Treatment*, Smolak, L., Levine, M. P., and Striegel-Moore, R., Eds., Lawrence Erlbaum Associates, Mahwah, NJ, 1996, chap. 12.
2. Phelps, L., Augustyniak, K., Nelson, L. D., and Nathanson, D. S., Adolescent eating disorders, chronic dieting, and body dissatisfaction, in *Children's Needs II: Development, Problems, and Alternatives*, Bear, G. G., Minke, K. M., and Thomas, A., Eds., National Association of School Psychologists, Bethesda, MD, 1997, chap. 81.
3. Levine, M. P., How Schools Can Help Combat Student Eating Disorders: Anorexia Nervosa and Bulimia, National Education Association, Washington, D. C., 1987, 43, 93.
4. Schafe, M. C. and Parsons, J. M., Eating disorders: A holistic approach to treatment, in *Controlling Eating Disorders with Facts, Advice, and Resources*, Lemberg, R., Ed., Oryx Press, Phoenix, AZ, 1992, 139.
5. Chatoor, I., Child development as it relates to anorexia nervosa and bulimia nervosa, in *Controlling Eating Disorders with Facts, Advice, and Resources*, Lemberg, R., Ed., Oryx Press, Phoenix, AZ, 1992, 10, 12.
6. Thurstin, A. H., Symptoms of eating disorders: behaviorial, physical, and psychological, in *Controlling Eating Disorders with Facts, Advice, and Resources*, Lemberg, R., Ed., Oryx Press, Phoenix, AZ, 1992, 15.
7. Attie, I. and Brooks-Gunn, J., The development of eating regulation across the life span, in *Developmental Psychopathology*, Dante, C. and Cohen, D. J. Eds., Wiley, New York, 1995, chap. 10.
8. Slade, P., Prospects for prevention, in *Handbook of Eating Disorders: Theory, Treatment and Research*, Szmukler, G., Dare, C., and Treasure, J., Eds., Wiley, New York, 1995, chap. 21.
9. O'Halloran, M. S., *Focus on Eating Disorders: A Reference Handbook*, ABC-CLIO, Santa Barbara, CA, 1993, 78.
10. National Mental Health Association, *Mental Health 1-2-3*, Alexandria, VA, 1992.
11. Massey, M. S., Promoting emotional health through haiku, a form of Japanese poetry, *Journal of School Health*, 68, 73, 1998.
12. Casper, R. C., Fear of fatness and anorexia nervosa in children, in *Child Health, Nutrition, and Physical Activity*, Cheung, L. W. Y. and Richmond, J. B., Eds., Human Kinetics, Champaign, IL, 1995, 211.
13. Minuchin, S., Rosman, B. L., and Baker, L., *Psychosomatic Families: Anorexia Nervosa in Context*, Harvard University Press, Cambridge, MA, 1978, chap. 2.
14. Becvar, D. and Becvar, R., *Hot Chocolate for a Cold Winter Night: Exercises for Relationship Enhancement*, Love, Denver, CO, 1994, chap. 14.
15. Watzlawick, P., Beavin, J. H., and Jackson, D. D, *Pragmatics of Human Communication: A Study of Interactional Patterns, Pathologies, and Paradoxes*, W. W. Norton, New York, 1967, chap. 2.
16. Fetro, J. V., *Personal and Social Skills: Understanding and Integrating Competencies across Health Content*, ETR Associates, Santa Cruz, CA, 1992, 158.
17. Kramer, P., *The Dynamics of Relationships: A Guide for Developing Self-Esteem and Coping Skills for Teens and Young Adults*, Equal Partners, Silver Spring, MD, 1994, 89.
18. Goldkopf-Woodtke, M., Recovery, in *Eating Disorders: New Directions in Treatment and Recovery*, Kinoy, B. P., Ed., Columbia University Press, New York, 1994, chap. 10.
19. Covey, S. R., *The Seven Habits of Highly Effective People: Restoring the Character Ethic*, Simon & Schuster, New York, 1989, 129, 240, 241, 289.
20. Insel, P. M., Roth, W. T., Rollins, L. M., and Petersen, R. A., *Core Concepts in Health*, 8th ed., Mayfield, Mountain View, CA, 1998, chap. 4.
21. Becvar, D. J. and Becvar, R. S., *Pragmatics of Human Relationships*, Geist & Russell, Galena, IL, 1997, chap. 6–7, 65, 121, 123–126, 169, 187.

22. Friedman, S. S., Girls in the 90's, *Eating Disorders*, 4, 240, 1996.

23. Loehr, J. E., *Toughness Training for Life*, Penguin Group, New York, 1993, chap. 7, 35, 120.

24. Kinoy, B. P., Preface, in *Eating Disorders: New Directions in Treatment and Recovery*, Kinoy, B. P., Ed., Columbia University Press, New York, 1994, xi.

25. Seaward, B. L., *Managing Stress: Principles and Strategies for Health and Well Being*, 2nd ed., Jones and Bartlett, Sudbury, MA, 1999, chap. 13.

26. Graber, J. A. and Brooks-Gunn, J. B., Prevention of eating problems and disorders: including parents, *Eating Disorders*, 4, 348, 1996.

27. Meeks, L., Heit, P., and Page, R., *Comprehensive School Health Education: Totally Awesome Strategies for Teaching Health*, 2nd ed., Meeks-Heit, Blacklick, OH, 1996, 172.

28. Markman, H., Stanley, S., and Blumberg, S. L., *Fighting for Your Marriage: Positive Steps for Preventing Divorce and Preserving a Lasting Love*, Jossey-Bass, San Francisco, 1994, chap. 3.

29. Marx, B. K., Out of balance, out of bounds: obesity from compulsive eating, in *Controlling Eating Disorders with Facts, Advice, and Resources*, Lemberg, R., Ed., Oryx Press, Phoenix, AZ, 1992, 45, 47–48.

30. Kahm, A, in *Eating Disorders: New Directions in Treatment and Recovery*, Kinoy, B. P., Ed., Columbia University Press, New York, 1994, chap. 2.

31. Costin, C., Body image disturbance in eating disorders and sexual abuse, in *Sexual Abuse and Eating Disorders*, Schwartz, M. F. and Cohn, L, Eds., Brunner/Mazel, New York, 1996, chap. 8.

32. Seaward, B. L., *Instructor's Resource Manual to Accompany Managing Stress: Principles and Strategies for Health and Well Being*, 2nd ed., Jones and Bartlett, Sudbury, MA, 1999, 77.

33. McGaffey, T. N., *The Courage to Lead: A Practical Way to Learn Leadership for Everyone*, 1994, 28, 29. Booklet available from Thomas N. McGaffey, 4732 Myerwood, Dallas, TX 75244; Tel: 214 980-7391, Fax: 214 233-3339.

34. Benson, H. and Stuart, E. M., *The Wellness Book: The Comprehensive Guide to Maintaining Health and Treating Stress-Related Illness*, Simon & Schuster, New York, 1992.

35. Covey, S. R., Merrill, A. R., and Merrill, R. R., *First Things First: To Live, to Love, to Learn, to Leave a Legacy*, Simon & Schuster, New York, 1994.

36. Wagner, S., Eating disorder treatment stories: four cases, in *Controlling Eating Disorders with Facts, Advice, and Resources*, Lemberg, R., Ed., Oryx Press, Phoenix, AZ, 1992, 57.

Appendix 19-A: Assertive Communication Techniques

1. Be specific, and clearly express what you want, need, think, and feel. Here are some examples:

   "I want to…"

   "I don't want you to…"

   "I need…"

   "Would you please…?"

   "I disagree. I think that…"

   "I have mixed reactions. I agree with these aspects for these reasons, but I am troubled about these aspects for these reasons."

2. Be direct. State your message to the person for whom it is intended rather than telling others.

3. "Own" your message. Acknowledge that your message comes from your frame of reference and your perceptions. You can reinforce this by using I-statements, such as:

   "I feel hurt when you say you'll call me and then you don't; it makes me feel I am not important to you."

   "I feel angry when you say that because I don't feel like you are cherishing and respecting me."

4. Ask for feedback from the listener. This gives the listener an opportunity to correct any misperceptions you may have and helps him/her to understand that you are expressing an opinion, feeling, or desire rather than a demand. Likewise, encourage others to be clear, direct, and specific in their feedback to you. Examples:

   "Am I being clear?"

   "Does this make sense to you?"

   "How do you view the situation?"

   "What do you suggest we do about the situation?"

5. Use nonverbal language that matches your verbal language. Eye contact, voice tone, facial expression, posture, and gestures should reinforce the assertive message, not detract from it.

6. Establish a proper climate to foster better communication. Practice these steps to establish a climate where open, honest communication can take place:

   Choose an appropriate time and place so that both parties can participate and listen without distraction.

   Keep an open mind.

   Listen empathically.

   Avoid judgmental statements.

   Avoid projecting superiority.

   Avoid people who tend to give negative feedback.

Appendix 19-B: The Speaker-Listener Technique*

The Speaker-Listener Technique is a valuable conflict resolution tool that offers people an alternative mode of communication when issues are hot or sensitive, or when they are likely to get that way. This simple, yet effective communication technique can benefit any conversation in which you want to enhance clarity and safety.[28]

Rules for Both:

1. The Speaker has the floor.

   Use a real object to designate the floor. You can use anything: a pen, a remote control, a paperback book, magazine, etc. If you do not have the floor, you are the Listener. Follow the rules for each role as designated below.
2. The Speaker keeps the floor while the Listener paraphrases.
3. Share the floor.

Rules for the Speaker:

1. Speak for yourself. Don't mind read!
2. Keep statements brief. Don't go on and on.
3. Stop to let the listener paraphrase.

Rules for the Listener:

1. Paraphrase what you hear.
2. Focus on the Speaker's message. Don't rebut.

* Adapted from Markman, H., Stanley, S., and Blumberg, S.L., *Fighting for Your Marriage*, Jossey-Bass, San Francisco, 1994, 63–69. With permission.

*Appendix 19-C: Expressing Feelings**

This exercise is designed to help you get in touch with your feelings. It may be uncomfortable to do at first, but try to override your feelings of discomfort to do the exercise so that you can experience the personal satisfaction of having taken a positive risk.

1. Turn your chairs so that you face each other directly. Decide which of you will keep time. Using no words, observe each other for one minute. During this minute just respond to each other, paying particular attention to your feelings. At the end of this minute, each of you will tell your partner (a) what feeling or feelings you experienced during the minute; and (b) how you felt about your feelings. Before beginning, paraphrase the instructions and check with each other to be sure you both understand the same thing.

2. Person A begins. Talk only about yourself and your feelings. No exceptions. Begin with, "I felt _____." Then reverse and let B have a turn. As your partner expresses his/her feelings, seek clarification when needed or allow your partner to elaborate by maintaining a respectful silence. Paraphrase his/her *feelings*, not agreeing or disagreeing, just understanding and helping her/him to feel understood.

3. Tell your partner what you experienced. What did you learn about yourself? About your partner? Paraphrase each other's feelings and thoughts.

We created a situation in which you might have felt a variety of feelings. The dilemma is that sometimes we feel feelings without knowing what to call them. Even when this is the case, we are not taught to report them directly. We are therefore going to ask you to do this exercise again. This time, however, we ask you first to scan the list of labels for feelings presented below. Some of the labels may make it easier for you to be more precise as you communicate, "I felt _____."

adorable	affectionate	agreeable	at ease
adequate	afflicted	awkward	afraid
apprehensive	afflicted	angry	annoyed
big-hearted	brilliant	bold	brave
blue	bewildered	caring	comforting
conscientious	considerate	cooperative	contented
confident	crushed	confused	constrained
censured	criticized	cowardly	combative
contrary	dedicated	determined	depressed
despairing	despondent	discouraged	disgusted
disliked	displeased	dissatisfied	disturbed
deflated	depreciated	diminished	demoralized
disagreeable	discontented	easy-going	elated
excited	excluded	embarrassed	exhausted
fair	faithful	friendly	firm
foolish	fearful	frightened	feeble
frail	furious	genuine	glad
gratified	grim	honorable	hopeless

* From Becvar, D. J. and Becvar, R. S., *Pragmatics of Human Relationships*, Geist & Russel, Galena, IL, 1997, 129–131. With permission.

hurt	helpless	hesitant	helpless
interested	inspired	important	intense
impaired	impatient	ill at ease	incapable
incompetent	inferior	insecure	inconsiderate
insensitive	intolerable	intolerant	joyful
kind-hearted	lovable	lone	laughed at
mellow	marvelous	neighborly	nice
nervous	neglected	obliging	open
offended	outraged	patient	peaceful
pleased	proud	powerful	pathetic
pained	puzzled	put down	reasonable
receptive	respectful	regretful	rejected
rebellious	sensitive	sweet	satisfied
superb	sharp	stable	sure
sad	silly	skeptical	scared
shaky	slighted	spiteful	tolerant
trustworthy	terrific	thrilled	terrified
unselfish	unhappy	unloved	unpopular
unsatisfied	unsure	uncomfortable	uneasy
useless	unruly	warm	wise
wonderful	worthless		

You may note after the second time through the exercise that you felt somewhat differently. Indeed we would predict that, for the context is now different. That is, your familiarity with the experience changes the context, its meaning to you, and thus your feelings. The first time you did the exercise you may have felt it to be very long. You may have felt frustrated that the instructions did not allow you to talk. You may have felt the urge to say something. When you could not do this, you may have changed your nonverbal behavior several times. The second time around, the experience may have been different in that you knew what to expect. You may have done it more playfully and had fewer of the negative feelings. In either case, we suspect that you had difficulty expressing your feelings. Probably it was also easier for one of you to do so. And it is always easier if you as listener can listen to the expression of feelings acceptingly and uncritically.

Appendix 19-D: Communication Dialogue and Feeling Words

1. Mirror what the other person is saying.
2. Validate that person's perception by saying, "I understand that because..." or "That makes sense to me because...."
3. Empathize: "I can imagine you might be feeling...."
4. Problem-solve: Ask partner for specific, concrete things you need from him/her to help solve the problem

FEELING WORDS FOR EMPATHIZING

abandoned	discouraged	inadequate	resentful
afraid	disgust	indifferent	sad
alienated	distant	insecure	shamed
angry	distrustful	invaded	smothered
animosity	dominated	invisible	sorrowful
annoyed	embarrassed	irritated	sorry
anxious	empty	isolated	suppressed
ashamed	excluded	left out	tense
bored	exhausted	lonely	terrified
cheated	fearful	mad	torn
cold	frustrated	neglected	trapped
controlled	guilty	nervous	unappreciated
cowardly	gutless	one down	uneasy
depressed	hated	ostracized	unimportant
despairing	helpless	put down	used
devalued	hopeless	rejected	violated
disappointed	humiliated	remorseful	withdrawn
disapproved of	hurt	repelled	
	ignored	repulsed	

Examples:

"I hear you saying that you are really upset that I'm always telling you what to do and not letting you make decisions on your own. That makes sense to me because I don't like it either when someone always tells me what to do, and I imagine you might be feeling controlled, dominated, and devalued."

"It sounds like you are angry with me for criticizing you, and you hate it when I make fun of you. I understand that because I don't like that happening to me, and I imagine you might be feeling put down, inadequate, insecure, and hurt."

"You're very tired from always doing all the work around here, especially when I come home and plop down in front of the TV. That makes sense to me because I don't do very much work around here, and I imagine you might be feeling resentful, exhausted, unappreciated, and lonely."

"I hear you saying you get angry when I keep asking you what is wrong, and I won't let it drop. That makes sense to me because I also get angry when someone keeps bugging me, and I imagine you might be feeling trapped, pressured, and anxious."

Appendix 19-E: Activities for Clarifying Feelings Related to Body Attitude, Body Image, and Body Messages*

Body Attitude Inventory

What's your first memory of a positive body message? A negative one?

What things (i.e., media, culture, family, peers) have most influenced your relationship with your body?

If you were to place the feelings you have about your body today on the continuum below, where would they fall? Do your feelings ever change?

Love ◄─────────────────────────────────────► Loathe

What do you think would be different in your life if your body matched the culturally ideal body?

As I See It

Purpose: To explore feelings and reactions participants have about certain body parts and identify the factors that played a significant role in the development of those feelings.

Procedure: Distribute the As I See It Worksheet to each participant. Ask them to take a moment to go down the list of body parts making a mark under the column that best describes their relationship to each listed part.

Discussion: Ask for comments on the experience of completing the worksheet. Be sure to discuss the following areas:

Was there one column that had more marks than the rest?

Thinking back through your life, can you recall a time when your responses would have been different? When and why do you think they would have been different?

What factors have played a significant role in the growth and change of your feelings about your body?

What things would need to change in order for your feelings to be different?

---

* Kelley, M., *My Body, My Rules: The Body Esteem, Sexual Esteem Connection — A Resource and Activity Guide*, Planned Parenthood of Tompkins County, Ithaca, NY, 1996, 31, 34–37. With permission.

As I See It Worksheet

Body Part	Very OK	Sort of OK	Definitely Not OK	Don't Think About It
Face				
Hair				
Eyes				
Ears				
Nose				
Teeth				
Belly				
Voice				
Hands				
Feet				
Waist				
Butt				
Legs				
Height				
Thighs				
Chest/Breasts				
Weight				
Smile				

Body Message Impact

Purpose: To examine the impact of learned body messages on feelings and behaviors and explore the potential influence of changing negative body messages to positive ones.

Preparation: Have one envelope prepared for each small group with each of the following topics written on individual index cards. Add more or change the topics if others are more applicable to your audience.

Television and music

Family

Magazines and newspapers

Friends

Religion

Procedure: Break the class into small groups, preferably no more than five people. Give each group an envelope. One person at a time will have a chance to address one of the topic areas while the group listens. Explain that this is not a time to debate issues, but to hear the participants' experiences with different people and the forms of media specifically related to their bodies. Have each person address the following questions in regard to the topic pulled from the envelope. Reconvene the large group and ask for anyone who is willing to briefly share her/his topic and its effect on self-perception.

What were the positive and negative message you learned about your body?

What effects did those messages have on the way you feel about and treat your body?

Have you taken any risks (for example, restrictive dieting, excessive exercise, risky sexual behavior) as a result of the body messages you learned?

What would you do differently if you were in control of your topic area (as a television executive, a parent, etc.) to allow the people your message touched to have more positive body views?

20

Spirituality

Leslie Lewis

CONTENTS

20.1 Learning Objectives

After completing this chapter you should be able to:

- Understand the spiritual aspect involved in eating disorders;
- Understand the spiritual quest of a person with an eating disorder;
- Recognize the need for time and room in the spiritual quest;
- Recognize the need for a spiritual or self-transformation in a person with an eating disorder.

20.2 Research Background

What is spirituality? The difficulty in answering this question has continually been a source of agony for many spiritual leaders. Kurtz and Ketcham[1] attest to this difficulty in their book, *The Spirituality of Imperfection*. They state, "To have the answer is to have misunderstood the question." This statement is proceeded by a story retold by Anthony de Mello.

> The disciples were absorbed in a discussion of Lao-tzu's dictum: *Those who know do not say; those who say do not know.* When the Master entered, they asked him what the words meant. Said the Master, "Which of you knows the fragrance of a rose?" All of them knew. Then he said, "Put it into words." All of them were silent.

0-8493-2027-5/01/$0.00+$.50
© 2001 by CRC Press, Inc.

"Spirit" is defined in the *Zondervan Pictorial Encyclopedia of the Bible* as "an incorporeal, sentient, intelligent being, or the element by virtue of which a being is sentient, intelligent, etc."[2] The human entity is evidenced by its mental, emotional, physical, and spiritual components. When a person is healthy, all parts function individually, but never to the exclusion of the others. When any part of the total person is excluded, the result is stress. Spirituality is the part of the person where centering takes place. Borysenko states that centering unites all parts of the human entity as one.[3]

Every individual is given a unique calling before birth. An image or pattern that the individual is to live out here on the earth has been selected. This calling, this "I am," is the individual's spiritual guide. In the process of living, however, the individual forgets all that took place before she was born and this leaves her deficient in relating to others, to her environment, and to God. The "I am" or "daimon," or calling remembers the original image and pattern chosen by the individual before birth and is therefore the carrier of the person's destiny. Greeks called this dynamic the daimon; Romans named it genius; Christians call it a guardian angel. Eskimos and other groups who follow shamanistic practices say the "I am" is the spirit of the individual, the free soul, the animal soul, or the breath soul. James Hillman's "acorn theory" holds that every person bears a uniqueness that asks to be lived and is already present before it can be lived.[4] The spiritual includes aspects of higher consciousness, awareness, transcendence, self-reliance, self-efficacy, self-actualization, love, faith, enlightenment, self-assertiveness, community, bonding, and a multitude of other virtues.[5]

R. M. Rilke wrote, "Spiritual pain is not so much a problem to be solved as a question to be lived."[6] The following sections allow the reader to understand the role spirituality plays in recovery from eating disorders. Furthermore, the reader is challenged to reflect on the continuum of spirituality ranging from the negative impact a sense of spirituality can play in recovery to the positive self-transformation that can result from true spiritual growth.

20.2.1   Spirituality and the Stress of Eating Disorders

In 1996, Catherine J. Garrett, a member of the faculty of Nursing and Health Studies of the University of Western Sydney, Australia, wrote an article entitled "Recovery from Anorexia Nervosa: a Durkheiman Interpretation."[7] In this publication, the author relies heavily on a book by Emile Durkheiman titled *The Elementary Forms of the Religious Life.* The article refers to a study of 32 people at different stages of the recovery process to reconceptualize the problem in sociological terms. The participants on many occasions referred to anorexia as a "spiritual quest." Recovery seemed to them to involve a rediscovery of their connections with their inner selves, with others, and with nature. These connections were for them the defining features of spirituality.

The paradox of spirituality is the sense of incompleteness, of being somehow unfinished, disconnected from others, the self, God, and nature. As humans we are imperfect and incomplete, and yet we yearn for completion, to be perfect, and have the answers to life's questions. All these yearnings remain basically unsatisfied. Healthy spirituality is the process of learning how to live daily with the tension between our desire for perfection and the reality of our imperfection. We are forever making mistakes, and yet those who judge us, including the voices of our environment, experiences, religions, and relationships call us to perfection. This is the essential paradox of living. The God of grace and ancient voices insists that this life is not a failed life, but rather it is the nature of *be-ing* human. It is the way we were created.[1]

Those with eating disorders seem to be involved in the struggle for spirituality. The struggle for them is a striving to find grace for themselves as they experience the discomfort that lies between expectations (which they accept as reality and life) on the one hand, and their perceptions of what they experience and their potential for failure on the other. This represents a struggle between life and death for them.

The ritual then becomes an act of *doing*. This doing grows out of the inability to trust *be-ing*. Spiritual pain and hunger for meaning are often spoken of as the real problems in the ritual. Anorexia and recovery are ritualistic attempts to construct the self. Each phase represents a distinct stage in the *rite of passage* to a new identity. To find meaning, purpose to life, and an acceptable identity seems to be the objective of the ritual. The attempt may be conscious or unconscious.

The negative phase of the ritual, or the need to do something about their perceived imperfection while living with the tension explained above, involves a confrontation with the inevitability of death. The negative phase sees death as a *condition* of the positive phase, in which participants intentionally choose to live.

Death seems to be the feared mysterious monster who stands in the shadows while each day the anorexic lives with the pressure of seeking perfection. In a society (even in a family) where only winners — smart, trim, sophisticated, healthy people who stand out in a crowd — are acceptable and where failure, a form of death, is not even acknowledged, the struggle serves as the basis for the need of the anorexic to *do* something. Every ounce of perceived "excess" is a reminder of his or her own earthiness. Every sign that his or her body is less than perfect is a reminder of mortality. In his or her value system, none of this is acceptable, especially in light of expectations imagined to be imposed by society, family, or peers.

The task is to achieve and maintain perfection while knowing that death could come at any time before a person has achieved the goal of a satisfactory identity. To face the struggle of being committed to the presence of death in order to live, while filled with doubts and fears, the anorexic commits to the ritual. Commitment has the most potential when it is in spite of doubt and not without doubt. The anorexic seems to know that to be totally alive she has to be closely related to her own death although she may be not want to articulate such a truth. The courage required to accommodate the ultimate paradox is the strength to live in the tension between life and death — the death of the old and the birth of the new.[8]

In summary, the recovery processes for persons with eating disorders are very similar to the processes of recovery from any form of human suffering in which the model of ritual is also applicable. For the 32 participants in Garrett's test,[7] the defining features of anorexia were those they believed had to be overcome. The eating disorders were only the symptoms of real problems such as self-loathing growing out of social expectations, dissatisfaction with their bodies, developmental stagnation, ongoing difficulties with eating, detachment from other people, and unresolved questions about death.

20.2.2   Spirituality and Recovery

However misguided their attempted spiritual transformations, the references to "spiritual pilgrimages" by those who described themselves as recovered, evidence the intention behind the ritual. Also, the hope of divine intervention seems to be present in the ritual. "You look for enlightenment … some sort of salvation to unravel your own tortured complexity of your self," was the testimony of Michael, a recovering anorexic. At the point of transformation, there is a reconnection described by phrases like "coming home." Jennifer expressed the need to return to where she was. "I want to go back to being cared for"[7] William James described the religious experience as frequently associated with some form of pathology. He described recovery as conversion. He called the spiritual experience a sensation of union, a direct connection with the

cosmos, with humanity, with nature, and with the divine energy.[9] Spirituality in healing (recovery) demands that the practitioner give time and room to the process. The
practitioner needs time for centering, for emptying, for grounding, and for connecting.

The centering process must include deep reflection of the real self. Answering questions such as, "Who am I?" and "What am I doing here?" is part of any healing process. For Native Americans, a spiritual quest ritual requires time devoted to
addressing questions like these that can only be answered in times of deep solitude.

The emptying process involves cleansing of consciousness. Many practitioners cite
the practices of meditation (clearing the mind of thoughts) and journal writing as
ways of emptying the spirit. Sustained centering by which old voices are cleared
away usually produces the emptiness that is desired.

Grounding is a process by which the spirit of the individual is filled with new
insights and knowledge which are made possible by the emptying step. In Eastern
cultures, the word *enlightenment* is used to refer to the grounding process. Grounding
comes from the connection that one begins to feel with his or her surroundings —
with the earth and as a part of nature.

The connecting process is the feeling of attachment to the community, to God or
a spiritual being greater than the individual, and to the world. As a result of connecting, the individual feels a sense of purpose and his or her connection with the
world happens.[3]

The more we are able to align ourselves with who we are and with the "dance of the
universe," the more we find our purpose in life. The measures by which we are
brought into harmony with ourselves determine the quality of healing and the speed
at which it takes place.[10]

"Give the disease a hearing!" is the attitude of psychotherapist Robert Sardello.[11]
His approach seems to be allowing the disease to find the person rather than seeing
the disease as something to be conquered because it is evil. Disease, whether in the
form of pain, negative emotion, confusion, or any other abnormality contains within
it a spiritual mystery or voice. This voice is speaking a truth about who the person
really is when he or she is allowed to experience life with its happy and sad times.
Allowing the disease the time and room necessary to make the meaning clear to the
person produces a sense of natural truth about the self.

When an authority figure, out of concern for an anorexic uses force to stop the ritual
by attempting to force-feed the hunger and constantly maintaining supervision over
the anorexic, the process of the ritual is interrupted. This action may even prove temporarily successful. However, the quest for meaning and understanding is not complete. The spiritual revelation is not yet part of the *experience* of the anorexic. The
seeming successful action may only delay the quest until the yearning of the anorexic
to find herself returns. That may happen very soon or after a year or several years. The
ritual may very well need to be carried out again in the same way or through some
other form of behavior that creates the life and death scenario. The hunger for meaning must find its substance, and it will. That is the objective of the ritual.

20.3 Application of Research Question

The sacred ritual or spiritual quest involved in eating disorders and recovery is a very
real process. It is very similar to the spiritual lesson that parallels the story in the New
Testament about Judas' final effort to control his friend Jesus. Judas is most commonly
remembered because of his betrayal of Jesus. The common belief of Judas' time

seemed to be that a king would come to the Jews, take up his earthly throne and thereby establish his rule. In doing, so he would rid the Hebrew nation of the oppression of Rome. This idea was generally accepted by Jesus' own disciples including Judas. They all seemed to grow impatient with Jesus' reluctance to move forward and return true meaning and identity to the chosen Jewish people. Judas' plan seemed to be to force Jesus to establish himself as the King and Savior of the Jewish nation calculating that Jesus would never submit to a trial as a common criminal, but rather be driven to defend himself and save the nation.

The anorexic attempts to hear from the spiritual part of her being by pushing the limits of her body, mind, and emotions. Her hope, whether conscious or unconscious, is that if her body is pushed to the limit, a transformation will come from the spiritual part of her being.

As a chaplain and as an individual, my experience is that the true self, that person each individual truly is, is the spiritual part of all of us. According to James Hillman, the spiritual being within us is born with a definite character, a calling, a fate, and an innate image. By *character*, he means we are born with definite bents and traits. The *calling* is the feeling that there is something that must be done in life. *Fate* to Hillman constitutes those pushes and pulls that gently move us in a certain direction. We all develop *innate images*. The innate image is the person the individual sees herself to be.

This self knows no fear, is not always rational, does not feel the need to impress anyone, does not judge anything as good or bad, is filled with joy and gratitude, and knows the self to be eternal. From birth, however, someone begins the process of telling us who they think we are. We get messages about our bodies from people and events around us. The body is told to be alive, pain-free, beautiful, healthy, trim, a winner, etc. The mind is told to be rational, smart, quick, humorous, serious, and so on. We are told that emotions are signs of weakness and should be avoided, ignored, and denied. After years of absorbing this kind of inaccurate information, the true self is buried under a sea of expectations, but the character, the calling, the fate, and the innate image do not die. However, for the anorexic, the agony of resolving the gap between the true self and the self that is perceived from external information seems insurmountable.

The anorexic longs to hear from the true or divine self. As in the case of Judas, it is determined that somewhere in the vise between life and death will be born the innate self that is the spirit of the individual. The ritual begins and continues, as the body screams, the confused mind calculates, and emotions fight over which one is the greatest. Healing will only come when the anorexic begins to feel a new sense of worth and purpose from within, rather than only from the external influences. The transformations may be slow, or in some cases, appear as revelations that are suddenly seen as truths. Healing can seem to be a miraculous event, or a natural process of losing trust in the old image and learning to trust the inherent image.

Allowing the spiritual quest to have "its hearing" gives meaning the opportunity to find the individual. To interfere and attempt to control the situation or force a solution may remove the spiritual aspect from the quest and reduce it to another overpowering event in which the seeker is proven inadequate again. Although forcing healthy action on an individual may temporarily stop the "bleeding," it is still a spiritual battle that must be engaged. When the battle is reignited, it may be fought with the same behavior or some other destructive behavior unless spirituality is also engaged in the battle.

Trained professionals must understand the spiritual process and trust it in order to build trust and respect for individuals they may be counseling. Spiritual guidance is as necessary a part of the recovery process as the expertise of medical and other professional practitioners.

20.4   Case Study

The dialogue which follows is taken from an interview with an attractive 25-year-old woman who spent almost 5 years engaging in the eating pattern of bulimia nervosa.

Monica:
I remember comparing myself to this other girl and I remember thinking I was fat. Those were the earliest thoughts I remember having that could in any way point to any patterns of troubled eating. Through high school, I hardly ate. I was never diagnosed as having an eating disorder, but I don't know why. Eating was an issue with my parents because my dad came from a family that was like, everyone sits down at the table and you finish everything on your plate, and I just would not do that. So that was a huge issue for him, and I don't know if I just chose to rebel or what, but in high school I never experimented with binging and purging but eating itself, well, I didn't eat much. I had counselors, groups, dietitians, and psychiatrists … it's ridiculous. I felt trapped … I had a boyfriend. We had plans and were going to get married but I broke it off. And I really didn't even do that well. I was a dietary major and I knew everything I was doing was not healthy. But I just never saw the need to concentrate on getting better. I didn't think it was that bad, ever. I mean, at some points I did because I always felt like really bad, but … then I met Eric, and after a while I ended up getting pregnant last January. And that changed … everything. It stopped. I chose to stop it. I was concerned about the baby.

L.L.:
How much had to do with how you looked?

Monica:
Oh, a shit load. I mean, I don't know how much … the weight, not so much the looks. The thing is I probably looked shittier than ever, because it's so hard on your body. You just get bloated, and you feel like … It just really takes a toll on your body. And you don't really lose that much weight either. I don't really think that anyone ever really helped me. Except me. I got pregnant and I wanted to be healthy, and even now, there's just no way. I just wonder why I spent so much time obsessing about food and throwing up … and I still don't know why I spent so much time doing that. It's like the focus is off me now. I mean, the focus for myself now is off me. I care way too much about him [the baby] to even think about it. I mean I don't even think about it actually.

L.L.:
So you don't see yourself ever going back to the old pattern of behavior?

Monica:
No, I don't … ever.

L.L.:
So, do you think of yourself as recovered?

Monica:
I guess so, but I didn't go through any program … I just hate the fact that I wasted so much time doing this. Everybody kept telling me, "Choose something else besides this" that I like. I just never did. But at this point in my life I don't see myself ever, ever doing that again.

L.L.:

It seems that the baby was a significant part of your story. So what if the pregnancy had never happened?

Monica:

I don't know. I'd probably be still doing the same thing. I don't know why though. It woke me up. I asked myself, what are you doing? You are, like, wasting your life away right now. I went from, like, going out, to doing nothing. I didn't want to do anything but concentrate on that [the baby], which is a good thing. I just wanted to focus on making sure that he had a good life. And I want to have a good life with him too. I don't want to be messed up or anything. This is the priority I have … just being a good mom and provider. And I don't think that's ever going to change.

L.L.:

Monica, what part does your spirituality play in all this? By that I mean your inner person who has the ability to communicate with the divine? Does this fit into the story?

Monica:

My parents are very religious. So we went to the Catholic church every Sunday, and after a while I just stopped. I hated it. For years I didn't go to church. I didn't pray. But still believed in God. When I became pregnant I started to think differently. I started thinking about God, and praying that everything will be okay. And I started going to church with my parents. I don't know if I'm going to church because he [baby] likes it or what. But It's nice, nicer than it's ever been. I feel good to go and I'm not sure why, yet.

L.L.:

All the time you were involved in the episode, did you think it was ever going to end?

Monica:

No! I never thought about dying. I knew I should have been taking it more seriously but I just didn't think about death. But I knew it does a lot of damage to your body. I thought girls that are really anorexic, if they are really bad they will go first. I thought they were more messed up than I was but … probably not.

L.L.:

When I talk about spirituality I am also talking about your connections with yourself, and with others, and the universe. Am I hearing you say that when you felt that connection, that is when things started to change and look differently to you?

Monica:

Yeah, there's more at stake than my little piddly … I mean, when I first became pregnant you have no idea. I had no idea the feeling that I had for him. I had these crazy thoughts about his dying or something happening to him. I was not exactly panicky about it but when you realize you only have one life on this earth, you have to make it the way you want to make it. That's why I get so pissed, when I think of how much of my life I wasted. I don't mean I need to live my life through my son but live a better life.

L.L.:

You have used the phrase, "a waste of time" often. Is that the way you feel about the bulimia?

Monica:

Oh! Absolutely! My God! Like a momentous waste of time. It doesn't accomplish anything. Bulimia sucks! Like a stupid vise. It doesn't do anything you think it will. It's just a tremendous waste of time. So why do it?

L.L.:

Monica, one last difficult question. What if something happened to the baby? Would you go back to the old life style?

Monica:

[Pause, with deep thought] No! No! The baby was just the trigger. But, no! I would not.

20.4.1   Questions

1. Is the individual on a spiritual quest?
2. Is there evidence of feeling disconnected?
3. What was the spiritual lesson learned from the bulimic process?
4. When was the spiritual lesson actually learned?
5. How much help was gained from outside sources?

References

1. Kurtz, E. and Ketchem, K., *The Spirituality of Imperfection*, Bantam Books, New York, 1992, 15, 19.
2. *The Zondervan Pictorial Encyclopedia of the Bible*, Spirit, Grand Rapids, MI, 1972, 503.
3. Borysenko, J., *Fire in the Soul: A New Psychology of Spiritual Optimism*, Warner Books, New York, 1993.
4. Hillman, J., *The Soul's Code*, Random House, New York, 1996, 6, 7.
5. Seaward, B. *Managing Stress*, Jones and Bartlett, Boston, 1994, 127–128.
6. Rilke, R.M., quote in Garrett, G.J., Recovery from anorexia nervosa: a Durkheimian interpretation, *Social Science Medical Journal*, 43, 1489, 1996.
7. Garrett, G.J., Recovery from anorexia nervosa: a Durkheimian interpretation, *Social Science Medical Journal*, 43, 1489, 1996.
8. May, R., *The Courage to Create*, Bantam Books, New York 1975, 3.
9. James, W., *The Varieties of Religious Experience*, Penguin/Mentor, New York, 1958.
10. Simonton, O.C., *The Harmony of Health: Healers on Healing*, Carlson, R. and Shield, B., Eds., Jeremy P. Tarcher, Inc., Los Angeles, 1989, 48.
11. Sardello, R., *Facing the World with Soul*, Lindisfarne Press, Hudson, NY, 1992, 65.

21

Exercise Prescription for Fitness and Health

Jacalyn J. Robert-McComb and Jeromi Kummell

CONTENTS

21.1 Learning Objectives

After reading this chapter you should:

- Understand the evaluation criteria for safe exercise participation;
- Understand the components of physical fitness;
- Recognize normative values for the components of physical fitness for girls and women;
- Be able to prescribe and assess a safe exercise program for physical fitness for girls and women;
- Understand the importance of a balanced exercise program.

21.2 Research Background

21.2.1 Evaluation Guidelines for Safe Exercise Participation

Initial screening for exercise program participation should include a health history questionnaire, basic lab reports (cholesterol, blood glucose, and triglycerides), and blood pressure assessment. A sample health history questionnaire is included in Appendix 21-A. The health history questionnaire should also include questions which address eating habits. For example, if an individual fasts all day, then binges and purges at night, it would be unwise to have her engage in a rigorous exercise program, such as aerobic dance, at 5:30 P.M. when her blood glucose levels would be unusually low. Acceptable values for cholesterol, blood glucose, and triglycerides can be found in Table 21.1. Cardiovascular risk factors (see Table 21.2) and major signs and symptoms suggestive of cardiovascular disease (see Table 21.3) should be identified from the health history questionnaire, lab reports, and blood pressure assessment.

Following this initial screening, individuals can be placed in one of three risk categories (see Table 21.4). Regardless of age, individuals who fall in the low risk category may begin moderate exercise programs without further medical evaluations. Moderate exercise is defined as 40 to 65% of heart rate reserve (see the sections on exercise prescriptions in this chapter). Individuals in the moderate risk category are males over 40 years of age and women over 50 years of age or who exhibit symptoms suggestive of cardiopulmonary disease. They should have medical examinations and clinical exercise tests prior to undertaking moderate exercise.

TABLE 21.1

Classification of Serum Cholesterol, Fasting Serum Triglycerides, and Resting Blood Pressure[a]

Variable	Value	Category
Systolic blood pressure (mm Hg)[a]	<130–139	Normal range
Diastolic blood pressure (mmHg)	<85–89	
	140–179	Mild-moderate hypertension
	90–109	
	>180	Severe hypertension
	>120	
Total cholesterol	<200 mg/dL (5.2 mmol/L)	Desirable cholesterol
	200–239 mg/dL (5.3–6.2 mmol/L)	
Borderline high cholesterol	>240 mg/dL (6.2 mmol/L)	High cholesterol
LDL cholesterol	<130 mg/dL (3.4 mmol/L)	Optimal LDL
	130–159 mg/dL (3.4–4.1 mmol/L)	Borderline high LDL
	>160 mg/dL (4.1 mmol/L)	High LDL
HDL cholesterol	<35 mg/dL (0.9 mmol/L)	Low HDL cholesterol
Serum triglycerides	<200 mg/dL (2.3 mmol/L)	Normal
	200–400 mg/dL (2.3–4.5 mmol/L)	Borderline high
	400–1,000 mg/dL (4.5–11.3 mmol/L)	High
	>1,000 mg/dL (11.3 mmol/L)	Very high

[a]Adapted in part from *JAMA*, 269, 3015–3023, 1993.

TABLE 21.2

Coronary Artery Disease Risk Factors[a]

Primary Modifiable Risk Factors	Defining Criteria
Diabetes mellitus	Persons with insulin dependent diabetes mellitus (IDDM) who are > 30 years of age, or have had IDDM for > 15 years, and persons with no insulin dependent diabetes mellitus (NIDDM) who are > 35 years of age should be classified as patients with disease
Current cigarette smoking	
Hypertension (or using prescribed antihypertensive medication)	Blood pressure > 140/90 mmHg
Hypercholesterolemia	Total serum cholesterol > 200 mg/dL
Sedentary lifestyle	Defined by the combination of a sedentary inactivity job involving sitting for a large part of the day and no regular exercise or active recreational pursuits

Secondary Nonmodifiable Risk Factors	Defining Criteria
Age	Men > 45 years; women > 55 or premature menopause without estrogen replacement therapy
Family history	MI or sudden death before 55 years of age in father or before 65 years of age in mother

Secondary Modifiable Risk Factors	
Obesity	Men above 20% body fat, women above 30% body fat
Chronic stress	Stress is defined as the inability to cope with a perceived or real threat. Chronic means that the event occurs on a regular basis. Physiological markers are elevated levels of catecholamines, cortisol, and other hormones associates with the stress response.

[a]Adapted in part from *JAMA*, 269, 3015–3023, 1993.

TABLE 21.3

Signs and Symptoms Suggestive of Cardiopulmonary Disease

1. Rapid or racing heart rate
2. Dizziness
3. Pain, tension, and weakness in the limbs while walking; relief from claudication during rest
4. Swelling of the ankles
5. Aches or discomfort in the chest, neck, jaw, and/or arms
6. Difficulty breathing with mild exertion
7. Shortness of breath at rest
8. Sudden difficulty in breathing while sleeping
9. Heart murmur
10. Exceptional fatigue with normal activities
11. Sudden dimness or loss of vision[a]
12. Sudden severe or unexplained headaches[a]
13. Sudden weakness or numbness of the face, arm, or leg on one side of the body[a]
14. Difficulty speaking[a]

[a]Symptoms have been noted as warning signs of a stroke. All symptoms must be interpreted in the clinical context in which they appear.

TABLE 21.4

Risk Stratification

Low risk	Individuals who are asymptomatic and apparently healthy with no more than one primary coronary risk factor either modifiable or nonmodifiable (see Table 21.2)
Moderate risk	Individuals who have signs or symptoms suggestive of possible cardiopulmonary disease or metabolic disease (see Table 21.3) and/or two or more primary or secondary coronary risk factors either modifiable or nonmodifiable (see Table 21.2)
High risk or have disease	Individuals with known cardiac, pulmonary, or metabolic disease

21.2.2   Components of Physical Fitness

21.2.2.1   *Cardiorespiratory Endurance*

Cardiorespiratory endurance is related to the development of the cardiovascular, respiratory, and muscular systems. The cardiovascular system supplies the body with oxygen and nutrients and is composed of the heart, blood vessels, and blood. The respiratory system function includes pulmonary ventilation, external respiration, and internal respiration. Cardiorespiratory endurance is an individual's capacity to take in, transport, and utilize oxygen for a sustained period during prolonged, rhythmical exercise. Cardiorespiratory endurance is a function of the ability of cardiovascular and respiratory systems to supply the needed oxygen for energy metabolism and the ability of muscles to uptake the supplied oxygen, hence the term *oxygen uptake*. It is best measured by a laboratory test to determine maximal oxygen consumption (VO_{2max}) or maximal oxygen uptake. Many factors exert effects on cardiorespiratory endurance including cumulative exercise training programs, heredity, sex, age, and body fat.

21.2.2.1.1   *Normative Values for Girls and Women*

Cardiorespiratory standards for girls are most easily calculated by a 1-mile walk/run test. To perform the test, a 1-mile course is marked off. A circular track is helpful and should be used if available. A girl is asked to complete the mile in the quickest time possible. She is allowed to walk or run at her discretion.

Standards for the 1-mile walk/run are set so that at the age of 5, girls should complete the course in 14 min. Time will then decrease 1 min per year for the next 2 years (age 6 — 13 min; age 7 — 12 min). After 8 years of age, however, the standard only decreases by 30 s (age 8 — 11:30). Girls ages 9 through 12 should be able to complete the course in 11:00. Girls aged 13 or more should complete the course in 10:30 or less.[1]

Other methods of determining cardiorespiratory fitness standards for girls include the .5 mile run, 1.5 mile run, and a 9-min run. As the name implies, the girls are asked to run rather than walk and run. This could be a disadvantage for field testing because of the wide range of fitness levels.

The .5-mile run is suggested for girls aged 5 through 9. Standards are as follows: (1) a 5-year-old girl should complete the course under 6:20, (2) a 6-year-old, under 5:40, (3) a 7-year-old, under 5:20, (4) an 8-year-old, under 5:00, and (5) a 9-year-old, under 4:45.[1]

Like the .5 mile, the 1.5-mile course is only suggested for a certain range of ages. The 1.5-mile run is suggested for girls aged 13 through 18. There are only two time standards in the 1.5-mile course. Girls 13 and 14 years old should complete the course under 17:00, whereas, any girl over the age of 14 should complete the course under 16:30.[1]

The timed run differs slightly from the distance runs. Time is fixed and yardage is calculated. Standards for girls are as follows: (1) age 5 — 1150 yards, (2) age 6 — 1250 yards, (3) age 7 — 1400 yards, (4) age 8 — 1500 yards, and (5) age 9 — 1520 yards. Girls 10 through 12 years of age should complete 1480 yards and girls over 12 should complete 1550 yards. The onset of puberty accounts for the decrease in expected yardage for girls aged 10 through 12.[1]

Cardiorespiratory standards for women are similarly assessed. Women can also run the 1.5-mile course for a time. However, women are assessed through a measurement called VO_{2max}. Women younger than 30 years of age should have a VO_{2max} of 38 or greater. After age 30, this figure will drop two points per decade, so a woman of 49 years should have a VO_{2max} of 34 or greater. After the age of 50, a woman's VO_{2max} will only decrease by one point per decade. For the 1.5-mile run, a time of 13:10 is equal to a VO_{2max} of about 38. After that, each additional 10 seconds subtracts 0.4 from the VO_{2max} score. This would mean that a time of 14 min would result in a VO_{2max} of 36 (0.4×5 intervals of 10 s each = 2; 38 − 2 = 36).[2]

If running is not your style and you prefer to walk, the 1-mile walk test is designed for you. Before you begin, you will need three items for your calculations. The first is your weight, the second is a stopwatch, and the last is a 1-mile walking course. A track is the preferred area for testing. Time yourself as you walk. Your walk should be at a brisk pace and should elevate your heart rate to over 120 beats per min. At the completion of your walk, check your pulse for 10 s. To convert that number into your pulse for a minute, multiply the value you obtained by 6. The next step is to convert the time from minutes and seconds into minutes. To do this, divide the seconds by 60 and the resulting figure will be a fraction of a minutes. The final step is to insert your information into an equation to find your VO_{2max}. The equation is:

$$VO_{2max} = 88.768 - (0.0957 \times \text{weight in pounds}) - (1.4537 \times \text{time in min}) - (0.1194 \times \text{heart rate}).$$

21.2.2.2 Muscular Strength and Endurance

Muscular strength is defined as the maximal force that can be exerted in a single voluntary contraction. Muscular endurance is defined as the repetition of submaxial contractions for a sustained period. Muscular strength and endurance are not necessarily related. Muscular strength and endurance depend on a variety of factors, some of which are the number of fibers contracting, types of muscle fibers contracting, sex, age, amount of body fat, diet, and types of exercises in training program. Strength and endurance gains are highly specific to the mode of training. Muscular strength and endurance can be developed through isotonic, isometric, or isokinetic training programs. During an isotonic (same tension) contraction, there is visible joint movement with a set amount of resistance or weight. Examples of isotonic contractions are those observed during weight lifting with machines or free weights. If there is no visible movement of the joint, or the resistance is immovable, the muscle contraction is isometric (same length). An example would be to hold a 5 s contraction at maximum intensity without moving the joint angle. An isokinetic contraction (same motion) is the movement of a muscle group at a constant speed throughout the full range of motion. The speed of contraction is controlled mechanically so that the limb moves through the full range at a set speed as on a Cybex machine.

21.2.2.2.1   Normative Values for Girls and Women

Commonly used methods to assess childhood muscular strength and endurance capabilities are sit-up and pull-up exercises. The maximum repetitions a child can perform in one minute are counted. Typically the standard is 20 sit-up repetitions for a 5-year-old girl. As a girl ages, the standard progresses by one sit-up per year. The standard for the pull-up exercise is one pull-up regardless of the age of the girl.[1]

The assessment for muscular strength and endurance for women is slightly more complex. Rather than performing only two exercises, the adult must perform five exercises. These exercises are: (1) latissimus dorsi pull-down, (2) leg extension, (3) bench press, (4) leg curl, and (5) arm curl. Familiarization with the individual exercises and the proper techniques must proceed testing. The weight required for testing must be calculated. The leg extension exercise is tested first, using 50% of body weight. This is followed by bench press and latissimus dorsi pull-downs at 45% of body weight, and the leg curl at 25%. The last exercise is the arm curl using 18% of body weight. For example, a woman weighing 120 pounds would multiply her weight by the percentage necessary for testing procedures. Thus, the leg extension calculation would be $120 \times 0.5 = 60$ pounds; bench press and pull-downs would be $120 \times .45 = 54$ pounds; leg curl would be $120 \times .25 = 30$ pounds; and the arm curl would be $120 \times .18 = 21.6$ pounds. During the assessment, a woman performs as many repetitions as possible of each exercise. The number of repetitions performed is then compared with set standards. Standards are as follows: (1) leg extension — 10 repetitions; (2) bench press and pull-downs — 11 repetitions; (3) leg curl — 7 repetitions; and (4) arm curl — 12 repetitions.[2] This is the minimal suggested number of repetitions. Higher repetitions reflect greater muscular strength and endurance capabilities.

21.2.2.3   Body Composition

Body composition can be divided into fat and fat-free weight (FFW). FFW includes all of the tissues of the body — muscle, bone, skin, blood, and organs minus the extractable fat. Chemically, FFW is composed of water, proteins, and bone mineral. The fat component of the body includes both storage and essential fat. Storage fat includes subcutaneous adipose tissues and the fat surrounding the internal organs. Essential fat includes the fat in the bone marrow, central nervous system, cell membranes, heart, lungs, liver, spleen, kidneys, intestines, and muscles. In the female, essential fat includes sex-specific or sex-characteristic fat. This component of essential fat is important for childbearing and other hormone-related functions. Many times the terms LBM and FFW are used interchangeably, but technically, they are not identical. LBM includes essential fat and FFW does not.

TABLE 21.5

Standard Values for Percent Body Fat for Women[a]

Rating	Age				
	18–29	30–39	40–49	50–59	60+
Excellent	<16	<17	<18	<19	<20
Good	16–19	17–20	18–21	19–22	20–23
Average	20–28	21–29	22–30	23–31	24–32
Fair	29–31	30–32	31–33	32–34	33–35
Poor	>31	>32	>33	>34	>35

[a] Adapted from Jackson, A.S. et al., *Br. J. Nutr.* 40, 497, 1978; and Jackson, A.S. et al., *Med. Sci. Sports Exercise* 12, 175, 1980.

21.2.2.3.1 *Normative Values for Girls and Women*

Methods of assessing body composition are beyond the scope of this book. However, for children, skin fold data estimating body composition seem to be most accurately analyzed. Research has shown a systematic increase in skin fold thickness among 6- to 9-year-old girls from the 1960s to the 1980s. Body composition values in the 6 to 11 age group increased from 17.6% between 1963 and 1965 to 27.1% between 1976 and 1980.[3] Standards from the Prudential FITNESSGRAM showing healthy scores for percent of body fat for girls ranges from 17% to 32% from ages 5 through 17.[4]

For women ages, 18 to 60 and over, standards for desirable body composition depend on health goals, athletic performance goals, and aesthetic goals. Standard values for health and fitness for percent body fat are presented in Table 21.5. However, these values must be interpreted in light of goals. For example, if the goal is athletic prowess in a specific sport, a lower percentage of acceptable body fat may be the standard. If the objective is health rather than fitness or, for example, the resumption of normal menstrual cycles, values in the average category are acceptable and should be promoted. Educators must make recommendations of acceptable levels of body fat depending on the needs and goals of their clients.

A simple, yet crude method for assessing body fatness is the BMI or body mass index. However, the BMI score should not be confused with an actual body fat percentage score. The BMI score simply enables one to assess level of risk for disease based on body fatness. A higher score is associated with a high prevalence of mortality from heart disease, diabetics, and cancer. This measurement tool utilizes the height and weight of a person to estimate body fat values. To calculate your BMI multiply your weight in pounds by 705 and divide this number by the square of your height in inches. For example, if a person weighed 120 pounds and was 63 inches tall her BMI would be calculated as follows: (a) $120 \times 705 = 84,600$; (b) $63 \times 63 = 3,969$; and (c) $84,600/3,969 = 21.32$. Table 21.6 classifies the acceptable ranges of BMI for females according to age.

TABLE 21.6

Body Mass Index Standards for Females

Age	BMI Value	Classification
5–11	14–21	Acceptable`
12–13	15–23	Acceptable
14–17	17–24	Acceptable
> 18	<20	Underweight
	20–25	Acceptable
	25–30	Overweight
	>30	Obese

21.2.2.4 *Flexibility*

Flexibility is the ability of a joint to move through its full range of motion (ROM). Static flexibility is the total ROM at the joint. Dynamic flexibility is a measure of the torque or resistance to movement. Flexibility is related to age, sex, and physical activity. However, the major limitation to both static and dynamic flexibility is the tightness of soft tissue structures. The relative contribution of soft tissues to the total resistance encountered by a joint during movement is estimated to be: (1) joint capsule — 47%; (2) muscle and its fascia — 41%; (3) tendons and ligaments — 10%; and (4) skin — 2%.[5] Inactivity is a major cause of inflexibility but it can also be associated with the aging process as well. Flexibility increases with age until puberty and thereafter begins to decline through the teenage and adult years.[6]

21.2.2.4.1 *Normative Values for Girls and Women*

Flexibility is a joint-specific attribute of fitness. In order to achieve a total flexibility score, one should perform a battery of flexibility tests. However, time and resources often are limited. Thus, the sit-and-reach test has become widely accepted as a general test for flexibility. This test primarily measures flexibility of two main groups of muscles, the hamstrings and lower back muscles, and one joint, the hip. To perform the sit-and-reach test, one should sit on the floor with the back against a wall, legs straight, and arms and feet extended directly in front. A box is placed in front of the extended legs with the bottom of the feet resting on the end of the box. A ruler is placed on top of the box parallel to the length of the box and to the extended arms and legs. The end of the ruler nearest the extended fingertips should read 0 cm. A partner holds the ruler in place and reads the measurement as the participant leans forward and reaches as far as possible down the length of the ruler without bouncing. The final position reached and held for 2 s is the score. Between the ages of 5 and 17, girls should be able to reach a minimum of 25 cm with a progression of 1 cm for every year after age 5. After age 18, girls should be able to reach 40.6 cm. Women of ages between 19 and 35 should be able to reach 40.1 cm; 36 to 49, 36.8 cm; and over 50, 31.2cm. Reaching further indicates greater flexibility.[2]

21.3   Exercise Prescription for Girls

A fitness testing program sponsored by the Chrysler Fund Amateur Athletic Union found that children between the ages of 6 and 17 are becoming slower in endurance running and weaker as a population. Other studies have shown the children of today are becoming more overweight, and spend more hours watching TV than exercising. The union's Web site is http://www.amhrt.org/Health/Lifestyle/Physical_Activity/ChildFac.html.

21.3.1   Why Exercise So Young?

A general consensus among researchers is that the predisposition for osteoporosis begins in childhood, and it is readily altered through childhood activity.[7-9] These alterations were shown by Bass et. al[9] to be maintained into adulthood, and may even reduce the risk of fractures occurring in women after menopause. Cooper et. al[6] demonstrated that pre-pubescent activity largely modulates skeletal mineral density and may add to the consolidation of bone following the end of linear growth. Carrie and Bonjour[7] add that the events occurring in the first two decades of life are large determinants for osteoporosis risk. Bailey, Faulkner, Kimber, Dzus, and Yong-Hing[10] found that mechanical loading of the skeleton during the growing years is an important factor in bone mineral density (BMD).

21.3.2   Are There Risks of Exercising for Children?

A cautionary note must accompany the promotion of exercise training for children. Certain physiological and psychological factors in children increase the inherent risks in terms of the rate of injury and the severity of the injury. Ligamentous structures in children are two to five times stronger than the cartilage and bone at the epiphyseal plate. Since ligaments are attached to the area of and around the epiphyseal plate, a child has a predisposition for a fracture of the epiphyseal-metaphysical junction, whereas in an adult, similar strains would more commonly injure the ligament.[11] Once injured, recovery periods may last from several days for mild overuse, to 10 months for a displaced medial epicondyle fracture,[12] or 4.2 years for juvenile osteochondritis dissecans.[13] Harvey and Tanner[14] say some factors predispose young athletes to back injuries. These factors include the growth spurt, abrupt increases in training intensity or frequency, improper technique, unsuitable sports equipment, and leg-length inequality. Though these were listed primarily as factors for low back pain, it is fairly obvious that they do in fact have implications over a far greater range of injuries. Another aspect that often leads to injury of preadolescent children is due to coaching attitudes and the vulnerability of children. Coaches often forget that children are not mini adults and are far more fragile and developing individuals.

Can childhood injuries be prevented or at least minimized? Webb[15] states that the incidence and severity of childhood injuries can be minimized by proper supervision and attention to proper technique. He also suggests pre-rehabilitative exercises that would include training of often-forgotten and untrained muscles, like the rotator cuff. Attention to complaints of joint pain is also strongly recommended by Webb. Studies have demonstrated that at least 60% of all osteochondrosis injuries were in direct relation to training and could have been prevented with changes in the training programs.[11] Orava[16] stated that 50% of the typical overuse injuries in this category also bothered adult athletes.

21.3.3   Cardiorespiratory Endurance

What are the recommended guidelines for cardiorespiratory fitness for children? Children should be encouraged to participate in physical activity which is rhythmic in nature, such as walking or running, of a moderate intensity, most, if not all, days of the week for a total duration of 30 min a day for health gains. At the preadolescent ages, cardiovascular exercise should be fun. Children will develop a sense of purpose in exercise and are more likely to continue with exercise programs well into their adult years if exercise is fun. Continual engagement in physical activity throughout life will help to prevent injuries and diseases in advanced age. Exercise does not have to be strenuous to be beneficial. In fact, Lindhold, Hagenfeldt, and Ringertz[8] remind us that intense physical exercise and diet restriction could result in delayed puberty and have a negative influence on the acquisition of peak bone mass during puberty. However, a decrease in activity level and the resumption of normal menstrual cycles may provide a possible catch-up phase for these female athletes in terms of bone mineral density.

TABLE 21.7

Resistance Training Guidelines for Children

- Before initiating a resistance training program, preadolescents should be examined by a physician and declared fit.
- Resistance training should be encouraged as only one of a variety of normal recreational and sport activities.
- Children involved in the program must be mature enough to accept coaching and instruction.
- Thorough warm-up and cool-down periods should be included in any resistance training session.
- Resistance training using body weight should be encouraged.
- If weight training machines are used, only those specifically designed for children, or those for which the loads and levers can be easily adjusted to accommodate the reduced strength capacity and size of children, should be used.
- Extremely high intensity efforts, such as maximal or near-maximal lifts with free weights or machines, should be avoided.
- Children must be capable of performing at least eight repetitions of a weight in an exercise set.
- Training session should consist of 1 to 2 sets of 8 to 10 different exercises (with 8–12 repetitions) which include all major muscle groups.
- Strength training sessions should be limited to twice per week.
- Eccentric training involving isolated muscles should be avoided, and the emphasis should be on dynamic concentric and eccentric contractions performed in a controlled manner through the full range of motion.
- Balance should be achieved between upper- and lower-body development and between agonistic and antagonistic muscles.
- Children should only begin training if they believe it to be beneficial and should continue training only as long as they find it fun, challenging, and satisfying.

In summary, it is of utmost importance for parents and educators to provide safe environments where children can play. The American Heart Association states:

> Healthy children, when in an environment conducive to physical activity, will be active. Emphasis should be placed on play (rather than exercise) and on activities that the child enjoys, that are consistent with the child's skill level, and that can be accomplished given the family's personal resources and interests. Children are remarkably able to adjust their levels of activity to their individual capability. Maximum heart rate in healthy children is about 200 beats per minute, and there is no need to arbitrarily restrict them to lower heart rates. Therefore, taking target heart rates in healthy children is neither recommended nor necessary.

The association's Web site is http://www.amhrt.org/Heart_and_Stroke_A_Z_Guide/exercisek.html.

21.3.4 Muscular Strength and Endurance

Resistance training for children has been controversial. However, given proper supervision and appropriate guidelines, benefits can be reaped through moderate exercise whether weight-bearing cardiovascular activities or sensible resistance training programs designed for adolescents. It must be noted that optimal loading parameters in terms of number of repetitions, sets, and training sessions per week have not been firmly established for children. It has been established that strength gains during preadolescence can be attributed primarily to improvements in neuromuscular activation and motor coordination, not hypertrophy. Furthermore, the risk of musculoskeletal injury resulting from resistance training during preadolescence cannot be excluded, but the risk is low in competently supervised training conditions where competition among subjects is prohibited. Table 21.7 offers general guidelines for coaches and parents concerning resistance training during preadolescence. For more information, please view, http://www.coach.ca/articles/sport_e.html or visit your local library for sports-specific references.

21.3.5 Achieving Healthy Body Composition Values

The premises or bases for healthy body composition are similar for children and women. Healthy body composition for girls can be maintained by balancing energy intake with caloric expenditure; exercise is a vital part of this balance.

Children should be encouraged to be active and play in games or sports that are rhythmic in nature, i.e., walking, running, bicycling, etc. These activities should be done on most if not all days of the week for a total of 30 min daily. Activities which develop lean body mass should also be a vital part of a children's exercise program. For the more structured child who is involved in sports, a safe resistance training program may be appropriate. Many activities promote lean body mass through resistance including swimming, gymnastics, and judo.

21.3.6 Flexibility

The general principles for flexibility apply to individuals of all ages. Flexibility exercises should be performed in a slow, controlled manner with gradual progression to a full range of motion. Static stretches should be performed at least 3 days a week. A stretch to a position of mild discomfort should be held for 10 to 30 s. The exercise should be repeated 3 to 5 times for each stretch. A series of easy-to-understand stretches are published in Hoeger and Hoeger.[2]

Children have much shorter attention spans and may not be able to hold stretches for as long or do as many stretches in one session as an adult. For this reason, stretching routines should be made fun and lively. Activities that more closely resemble games are preferred by children and will be better accepted and have higher participation rates. Another point to remember is that when children learn new skills, the concepts need to be taught in a way that they understand. For instance, instead of telling a child to stretch to a position of mild discomfort, it is better to have the child stretch to a point where she can feel the muscle pull in a certain area.

21.4 Exercise Prescription for Women

21.4.1 Cardiorespiratory Endurance

Four components must be considered when designing a cardiorespiratory conditioning exercise program: frequency, intensity, duration, and mode. The variability in these components depends on an individual's level of conditioning. Ideally, an individual should exercise 3 to 5 days a week, at 50% to 85% of heart rate reserve using Karvonen's Formula (VO_{2max}) or 60 to 90% of max heart rate, for 20 to 60 min. Activities that use large muscle groups and can be sustained continuously are suggested.

Heart rate should be monitored during the exercise program. This can be done by palpating the carotid artery with the index and middle fingers for 6 sec and then adding zero to determine beats per min. Heart rate may be counted for 10 s and then

TABLE 21.8

Karvonen's Formula to Determine Exercise Intensity Using Heart Rate Reserve

Steps	Procedure
1	220 – age = estimated maximum heart rate (MHR)
2	MHR – resting heart rate = heart rate reserve (HRR)
3	HRR × desired % (i.e. 50%)
4	Add resting heart rate to answer in step 3; this is lower limit
5	HRR × desired % (i.e. 85%)
6	Add resting heart rate to answer in step 5; this is upper limit
7	Target heart rate would then range from lower limit to upper limit

multiplied by 6 to get a more accurate beat per minute count. Initially heart rate should be monitored frequently until the individual is familiar with the appropriate exercise intensity. If the heart rate is above 100 beats per min before the individual begins exercising and stays elevated after 15 min of rest, he or she should not exercise. This elevation is probably caused by medication, but the individual should check with his or her doctor.

Exercise prescription should be conservative and gradual. Exercise should begin with a mild warm-up, continue with the aerobic conditioning phase, and end with a cool-down. If an individual is unaccustomed to exercising and has a low exercise tolerance, initially exercise can begin with 3 to 5 min of exercise followed by rest bouts. Depending on the level of exercise tolerance, this 3 to 5 min exercise bout can be repeated until mild fatigue sets in. The goal should be 30 min of exercise, i.e., walk for 5 min, rest for 1 min, and repeat this sequence 5 times. It is preferable for the individual to continue walking at a decreased intensity during the rest period since a complete stop may cause a dangerous drop in blood pressure.

Four methods to determine intensity will be described. The first method is called the heart rate reserve method. In order to use this method, the individual must ascertain her resting heart rate. Resting heart rate can be determined by palpating the radial (on the thumb side of the wrist) or carotid artery (in the neck, below the jaw, next to the Adam's apple) with the index and middle fingers slightly pressed on the artery in order to feel the pulse for 1 min in the morning before rising. It is best if this is done three mornings in a row and the average recording is used. Karvonen's formula is then used to determine the appropriate training zone (see Table 21.8). The individual may choose a training zone anywhere from 50% (for the lower limit) to 85% (for the upper limit) depending on level of conditioning. When beginning a cardiorespiratory program, it is suggested that if the individual cannot talk during this level of exercise intensity, the upper limit should be lowered in order to achieve a more comfortable training zone.

An easier method that can be used to determine exercise intensity is the max heart rate formula. The advantage of this method is that one does not need to know his or her resting heart rate. This method slightly underestimates the intensity at which one should exercise in order to achieve a comparable level of fitness using the heart rate reserve method; therefore, a higher intensity level must be chosen. The level of intensity for this method ranges from 60% to 90% of max heart rate. The formula for this method can be found in Table 21.9.

Two other useful methods to prescribe exercise intensity are the ratings of perceived exertion (RPE) and the ratings of perceived breathlessness (RPB) scales. The RPE scale has been found to be a valuable and reliable means to monitor exercise intensity. A rating of moderate (3) to very strong (6 to 9) has been shown to correlate with an intensity level of 50% to 85% using the heart rate reserve method or 60% to 90% using the max heart rate method (see Tables 21.8 and 21.9).[17] If individuals have moderate to severe

TABLE 21.9

Maximum Heart Rate Formula to Determine Exercise Intensity[a]

Steps	Procedure
1	220 – age = estimated maximum heart rate (MHR)
2	MHR × desired % (i.e., 60% lower limit)[a]
3	HRR × desired % (i.e., 75% upper limit)
4	Target heart rate would then range from lower limit to upper limit

[a] Training zone ranges from 60% to 90%.

TABLE 21.10

Borg Scales[a]

Rating of Perceived Exertion (RPE)		Rating of Perceived Breathlessness (RPB)	
0	None	0	None
0.5	Very, very weak	0.5	Very, very slight
1	Very weak	1	Very slight
2	Weak	2	Slight
3	Moderate	3	Moderate
4	Somewhat strong	4	Somewhat severe
5	Strong	5	Severe
6		6	
7	Very severe	7	Very severe
8		8	
9	Very, very strong	9	Very, very severe
10	Maximal	10	Maximal

[a] Use only one of these scales as a monitoring device during exercise. If fatigue tends to limit you during aerobic workouts, use the exertion scale on the left.

Source: From Borg, G.A., *Med. Sci. Sports Exercise* 14, 387, 1982; and Wilson, R.C. et al., *Clin. Sci.* 76, 277, 1989.

respiratory diseases, such as asthma, they may want to use the dyspnea scale to choose an appropriate conditioning level (see Table 21.10). The target range for breathlessness is 3 for exercise intensity at 50% and 6 for training at an intensity of 85%.

21.4.2 Muscular Strength and Endurance

Muscular strength and endurance can be developed through isotonic, isometric, and isokinetic exercise programs. Isotonic strength training involves concentric and eccentric contractions of the muscle groups throughout the full range of motion against a variable or constant resistance. Examples of these types of exercise programs are basic body-weight exercises, free weights, and use of variable resistance machines such as Nautilus equipment. When variable resistance is used and a constant speed is maintained, the term used to describe the training is isokinetic. Isometric training is normally used in rehabilitation settings. Isokinetic training involves concentric and eccentric contractions against an accommodating resistance that matches the force produced by the muscle group throughout the full range of motion. Isometric training is also referred to as static contractions and strength gains are specific to the joint angle used during training. Exercise prescription guidelines for these methods of training can be found in Table 21.11. However, certain basic terms, considerations, and exercise guidelines must be understood and adhered to for safe, effective, and efficient strength training.

TABLE 21.11

Example Guidelines for Designing Strength and Endurance Programs

Type	Sets	Intensity	Repetitions	Frequency/Duration/Speed
Isotonic Strength Program	3	85% 1, RM[a]	6	3 days a week
Isotonic Endurance Program	3	60% 1, RM	15	3 days a week
Isokinetic Strength Program	3	Maximum contraction	2–15	3 days a week — 24°–80°/s
Isokinetic Endurance Program	1	Maximum contraction	Until fatigued; at least 180°/s	3 days a week
Isometric Strength Program		100% MVC[b]	5–10	5 days a week
Isometric Endurance Program		60% MVC or less	Until fatigued	5 days a week

[a] RM Repetition maximum
[b] MVC Maximum voluntary contraction

The basic terms and considerations used in designing resistance training programs are *Range of Motion (ROM), Repetition Maximum (RM), Repetition, Sets, Frequency, Maximal Voluntary Contraction (MVC), Duration,* and *Exercise Speed. ROM* includes both the lifting (concentric) and lowering (eccentric) phases of an exercise and should be performed in a controlled manner. *Repetition* is the number of times a movement is performed. *RM* is the greatest weight that can be lifted for a given number of repetitions of an exercise. A *Set* consists of a given number of consecutive repetitions of an exercise. *Frequency* is the number of days per week the exercises should be performed. Because high-resistance exercises may produce tissue microtrauma, it is advisable to allow at least 48 hours between work-outs. *MVC* is the maximal resistance that can be held in a in one 6-s static contraction. *Duration* is the time needed to sustain the static contraction for strength or endurance gains. *Exercise Speed* is the time it takes to complete a concentric or eccentric contraction. A reasonable training recommendation for isotonic strength training is 1 to 2 s for each lifting movement and 3 to 4 s for each lowering movement. Isokinetic speeds vary between 24° to 300° per second depending on the individual's needs, i.e., endurance versus explosive power.

Basic resistance training guidelines are specificity, overload, progressive resistance, and order of exercises.[18] Specificity means that the development of muscular strength and endurance is specific to the muscle group exercised, the type of contraction, and the training intensity. Overload means that in order to achieve strength gains, the muscle must be worked by at least 60% RM.[19] For endurance gains, the overload can be as minimal as 30% RM. Progressive resistance means that as the muscle adapts to a specific exercise resistance, the resistance must be gradually increased to stimulate further strength gains. Order of exercise means that one should arrange the exercises so that successive exercises do not involve the same muscle groups. It is also advised to proceed from the larger muscle groups such as the legs to the smaller muscle groups of the torso, arms, and neck. The major muscle groups that should be exercised include the quadriceps, hamstrings, hip adductors, hip abductors, low-back, abdominals, pectoralis major, latissimus dorsi, deltoid, biceps, triceps, neck flexors, and neck extensors.[20]

When choosing a resistance training program, it is important to choose a program that will be adhered to based on the time demands imposed on most individuals. The American College of Sports Medicine[21] promotes a muscular fitness program that encompasses both resistance training guidelines and personal/societal time limitations. Two basic premises to keep in mind while designing strength and endurance program are (1) programs lasting longer than an hour are associated with higher drop-out rates, and (2) while more frequent training and additional sets or combinations of sets will elicit larger strength gains, the additional improvement is relatively small. Guidelines for muscular fitness can be found in Table 21.12.

TABLE 21.12

Guidelines for Muscular Fitness

Perform a minimum of 8 to 10 separate exercises that train the major muscle groups in a rotating order in order to prevent muscle fatigue (thighs and hips, chest and upper arms, back and posterior thighs, legs and ankles, shoulders and upper arms, abdomen, forearms, wrists).

Perform 1 to 3 sets of 8 to 12 percentages of repetition maximums (RM) of each of these exercises. For example, if you only perform 1 set of the exercise, for maximum benefits you should perform the set at 90–100% of RM after your warm-up. If you are performing 2–3 sets, use the first set as a warm-up by only doing 40–50% RM. The second set could be done at 60–75% RM and the third set 90–100% of RM. RM is the greatest weight that can be safely lifted for a given number of repetitions.

Perform these exercises at least 2 days a week. You should not work the same muscle groups 2 days in a row. Because high- resistance exercises may produce tissue microtrauma, it is advisable to allow at least 48 hours between work-outs. Therefore, the maximum lifting frequency if you are working the same muscle group is every other day.

Perform these exercises through the full range of motion.

Maintain a normal breathing pattern since breath-holding can induce excessive increases in blood pressure.

21.4.3   Achieving Healthy Body Composition Values

Table 21.5 lists categories of body fat percentages such as excellent, good, average, fair, and poor. These categories must be interpreted in light of goals. If the goal is athletic prowess in sports that emphasize thinness, the "excellent" category may be the target percentage body fat. However, these tables must be interpreted with caution. For the average adult female, the healthy level of body fat is 18% to 22%.[22] For women with anorexia nervosa, especially, it is important to emphasize the importance of healthy values of body composition. Low body fat is associated with alteration in estrogen metabolism.[23,24] It has been suggested that anorexics use internal fat as a means of providing calories,[25] possibly decreasing the role it plays in converting androgen to estrogen since fat tissue is an estrogen formation and storage site. In the human female, adipose tissue of the breasts, abdomen, omentum, and fatty marrow of the long bones convert androgen to estrogen, therefore, adipose tissue is a significant extragonadal source of estrogen.[26] Additionally, a critical level of body fat has also been emphasized as a potential contributor to menstrual irregularity by many.[27-29] The proponents of the theory that low body fat is related to menstrual irregularity base that on Frisch's findings.[30] Frisch contends that the onset and maintenance of regular menstrual function is dependent on a critical weight for height representing a critical lean to fat ratio or percent body fat. Frisch also states that the minimal amount of body fat needed to begin menarche is approximately 17%, and after age 16, at least 22% of body fat is needed to maintain normal menstruating cycles. Since a characteristic of anorexia nervosa is the absence of menstruation for at least 6 months, normal levels of body fat must be emphasized in the recovery process.

While body composition is determined by a complex set of genetic and behavioral factors, healthy values of body composition for women can be maintained by balancing energy intake with energy expenditure. If energy intake exceeds expenditure, body weight will increase. Conversely, weight is lost when the opposite situation occurs. An exercise-induced negative caloric balance results in weight loss consisting primarily of fat. One pound of fat equals 3500 kcal of energy.

When the goal is the attainment of healthy body composition, it is important to augment the activities or behaviors that will increase the basal metabolic rate (BMR) of an individual. BMR is the level of energy required to sustain the body's vital functions. Approximately 60% to 70% of our energy cost is determined by BMR.[20] If an individual consumes 2000 kcal a day, approximately 1200 to 1400 kcal will be used to support

TABLE 21.13

Recommendations for Safe Weight Loss

In order to increase loss of body fat, it is advisable to combine decreased caloric intake with increased caloric expenditure through an exercise program.

Caloric intake should not be lower than 1200 kcal per day. These calories should come from the food groups recommended by the NDA. Furthermore, negative caloric balances should not exceed 500–1000 kcal per day. Since 1 pound of fat equals 3500 calories, one can expect to lose 1 pound of weight by decreasing caloric intake by 500 calories a day. The caloric balance theory has strengths and limitations. Many factors contribute to weight loss. Be patient and persevere, even if you do not lose 1 pound a week every week, and you consistently decrease your caloric intake by 500 calories a day. Patience pays off with weight loss programs.

Weight loss must be gradual. Loss of 1–2 pounds a week is recommended.

Exercise is a vital part of a prudent weight loss program. It is advisable to engage in activities that promote a daily caloric expenditure of 300 kcal a day. Walking is a prudent exercise choice. However, exercises at lower intensities must be continued for a longer duration. A 150-pound person would have to walk at a normal pace for approximately 55 minutes to burn 300 calories.

A resistance training program should also be an important part of a program that has as its goal the loss of fat-weight. A resistance training program, while increasing lean body mass and possibly total weight, also increases resting metabolic rate. For every pound of muscle gained, approximately 30–50 additional calories a day will be burned during rest.

Since approximately 70% of your caloric costs per day result from your resting metabolic rate, your daily energy expenditure will increase because of additional lean body mass.

Most importantly, the program chosen should be a program that can be maintained for life.

Yo-yo diets with severe calorie restriction only make it harder in the long run for you lose weight and keep it off because your resting metabolic rate decreases because of severe food restriction. When you begin eating normally again, you may gain weight. Be sensible and choose a balanced approach to weight loss.

---

the BMR. A person's BMR is influenced by a number of factors, including exercise, diet, age, height, gender, and environmental temperature. Only the roles diet and exercise play in influencing an individual's BMR for optimal body composition will be discussed in this section.

The American Council on Exercise (ACE)[20] and the American College of Sports Medicine (ACSM)[21,31] recommend the following guidelines for caloric restriction for weight loss purposes. The intention of these guidelines is to enhance the loss of body fat rather than lean body tissue. Normal adults should consume at least 1200 kcal per day. This requirement may not be appropriate for athletes or older individuals. If the caloric intake is less than 1200 kcal per day, metabolic rate can drop as low as 20%. This drop is caused by the loss of lean tissue and the body's efforts to conserve energy by slowing the BMR. Negative caloric balance should not exceed 500 to 1000 kcal per day. To get an estimation of energy needs, use the worksheet in Appendix 21-B. Intake should not be less than 1000 kcal of energy expenditure. The maximum weight that should be lost per week is 1 kg or 2.2 pounds. The diet should consist of foods that are acceptable to the dieter in terms of sociocultural background and usual eating habits, providing that the nutrient intake is adequate. These habits should be sustainable for life. Safe weight loss guidelines have been summarized in Table 21.13.

Exercise is extremely valuable in maintaining healthy levels of body fat. Various web sites allow you to determine the energy cost of your activities. Appendix 21-C shows the caloric costs of selected recreational activities, but the list is not exhaustive. For a more extensive caloric expenditure activity list, please log on to the Web addresses listed in Appendix 21-C. For weight loss purposes, it is suggested that daily exercise expenditure should be approximately 300 or more kcal per day. The goal should be to expend 2000 kcal per week through exercise. This can be accomplished through a balanced exercise program consisting of cardiorespiratory, muscular strength, and endurance exercises tailored to meet an individual's needs and interests. For example, in

TABLE 21.14

Guidelines for Flexibility

Parameter	Guideline
Frequency	3–5 days a week
Intensity	To a position of mild discomfort
Duration	10–30 s for each stretch
Repetitions	3–5 for each stretch
Type	Static, with a major emphasis on the lower back and thigh area

order to use 2000 kcal per week through exercise, a 130-pound person could walk at a normal pace for 60 min 5 times a week and perform resistance exercises twice a week for 45 min. The effectiveness of a combined aerobic/strength training program in aiding weight loss was demonstrated by Wescott.[32] Wescott compared two groups of exercisers. One group performed aerobic exercises for 30 min three times a week. The other performed 15 min of aerobic exercises and 15 min of strength training exercises 3 days a week. Both groups spent the same amount of time exercising. The group that combined aerobic exercise with resistance exercises lost more fat than the group who only performed aerobic exercise, and also gained more lean muscle mass. Therefore, a resistance program using body weight or additional weights should be a vital part of achieving optimal body composition. Each additional pound of muscle tissue can raise the BMR 30 to 50 kcal a day.[33]

When using skin fold methods to estimate body fat, it is imperative to use equations that have been developed for a particular population or a similar population. Equations that have been developed for eumenorrheic females (normal menstruating females) may overestimate percentage of body fat because the bone mineral content levels of eumenorrheic females may be higher than those of amenorrheic females.[34,35]

21.4.4 Flexibility

Three types of stretching exercises are generally used to increase flexibility: (1) ballistic stretching, (2) static stretching, and (3) proprioceptive neuromuscular facilitation (PNF). Ballistic stretching uses a bouncing movement to produce stretch and produces the greatest risk of injury. In slow, static stretching, the joint is positioned at the desired range of motion and the muscle is stretched while maintaining the lengthened position. This type of stretching has the lowest risk of injury. The third type, PNF, involves isometric contraction of the muscle group being stretched, followed by static stretching of the same group. This type involves a low to medium risk of injury. Static stretching is the most commonly recommended program because (1) the risk of injury is low, (2) it requires little time and assistance, and (3) it is effective. The exercise prescription for static stretching can be found in Table 21.14.

21.5 Application of Research Question

21.5.1 What Is an Appropriately Balanced Exercise Prescription (A Program Attentive to All Five Components of Physical Fitness) That Maximizes Fitness and Health Gains?

An appropriately balanced exercise prescription is attentive to all five components of fitness but more importantly, it is practical and fits into the lifestyle of an individual. In

TABLE 21.15

A Comparison of the Guidelines for Cardiorespiratory Fitness Recommended by the
American College of Sports Medicine and the Surgeon General's Report

Agency	ACSM
Guidelines	Cardiorespiratory Fitness
Frequency	3–5 days a week
Intensity	60–90% of maximum heart rate or
	50–85% of heart rate reserve or max VO$_2$
Duration	20–60 min of continuous aerobic activity. Duration is dependent on intensity, thus, lower intensity exercises should be maintained for a longer period of time.
Agencies	U.S. Department of Health and Human Services
	Centers for Disease Control and Prevention
	National Center for Chronic Disease Prevention and Health Promotion
	The President's Council on Physical Fitness and Sports
Guidelines	Cardiorespiratory Health
Key messages	Physical activity need not be strenuous to achieve health benefits.
	Women of all ages benefit from a moderate amount of physical activity, preferably daily. The same moderate amount of activity can be obtained in longer sessions of moderately intense activities (such as 30 minutes of brisk walking) as in shorter sessions of more strenuous activities (such as 15–20 minutes of jogging). Additional health benefits can be gained through greater amounts of physical activity. Women who can maintain a regular routine of physical activity that is of longer duration or of greater intensity are likely to derive greater benefit. However, excessive amounts of activity should be avoided, because risk of injury increases with greater amounts of activity, as do the risks of menstrual abnormalities and bone weakening. Previously sedentary women who begin physical activity programs should start with short intervals (5–10 minutes) and gradually build up to the desired level of activity. Women with chronic health problems, such as heart disease, diabetes, or obesity, or women at high risk for these conditions should first consult a physician before beginning a new program of physical activity. Women over age 50 who plan to begin a new program of vigorous physical activity should first consult a physician to be sure they do not have heart disease or other health problems. The emphasis on moderate amounts of physical activity make it possible to vary activities to meet individual needs, preferences, and life circumstances. See Web site http://www.cdc.gov/nccdphp/sgr/women.htm

this chapter, we have focused on exercise prescription for fitness. Exercise prescription for health purposes is less demanding the exercise prescription for fitness. A comparison of guidelines for cardiorespiratory fitness and a summary of key messages for cardiorespiratory health for women from *Physical Activity and Health: A Report of the Surgeon General* can be found in Table 21.15 or downloaded at http://www.cdc.gov/nccdphp/sgr/women.htm. The important message is to be physically active. If an exercise program is too demanding in time, intensity, or equipment, the program must be simplified so it is practical and easily incorporated into one's lifestyle. In the 1970s, the American College of Sports Medicine (ACSM), the American Heart Association (AHA), and other national organizations began issuing physical activity recommendations to the public. These recommendations generally focused on cardiorespiratory endurance and specified sustained periods of vigorous physical activity involving large muscle groups lasting at least 20 min on 3 or more days per week. As understanding of the benefits of less vigorous activity grew, further recommendations followed suit.

During the past few years, ACSM, the Centers for Disease Control, AHA, and the National Institutes of Health have all recommended regular, moderate-intensity physical activity as an option for those who get little or no exercise. Interest has been developing in ways to differentiate between physical activity that improves health and activity that has been shown to improve cardiorespiratory endurance. It remains to be determined how the interrelations of amount, intensity, duration, frequency, type, and pattern of physical activity are related to specific health or disease outcomes. Attention has been drawn recently to findings from three studies showing that cardiorespiratory fitness gains are similar from physical activity in several short sessions (e.g., 10 min) and from the same amount and intensity of activity in one longer session (e.g., 30 min). Moreover, for people who are unable to set aside 30 min for physical activity, shorter episodes are clearly better than none. An ideal exercise program that is attentive to flexibility, body composition, cardiovascular endurance, and muscular strength and/or endurance is outlined below. An exercise program should allow time for relaxation techniques as discussed in Chapter 7. This is only a sample program. The ideal program is one that matches the goals and time restraints necessary to maximize adherence to the program.

21.5.1.1 Sample Exercise Program for Maximizing Physical Fitness and Health for Women

Monday (1 hour total)	Tuesday (1 hour total)	Wednesday (1 hour total)	Thursday (1 hour total)	Friday (1 hour total)	Saturday (1 hour total)
Warm-Up Exercises 5–10 min Legs & ankles Thighs & hips Back & torso Chest & upper arm Forearms & wrists Shoulder & neck	*Warm-Up Exercises* 5–10 min Legs & ankles Thighs & hips Back & torso Chest & upper arm Forearms & wrists Shoulder & neck	*Warm-Up Exercises* 5–10 min Legs & ankles Thighs & hips Back & torso Chest & upper arm Forearms & wrists Shoulder & neck	*Warm-Up Exercises* 5–10 min Legs & ankles Thighs & hips Back & torso Chest & upper arm Forearms & wrists Shoulder & neck	*Warm-Up Exercises* 5–10 min Legs & ankles Thighs & hips Back & torso Chest & upper arm Forearms & wrists Shoulder & neck	*Warm-Up Exercises* 5–10 min Legs & ankles Thighs & hips Back & torso Chest & upper arm Forearms & wrists Shoulder & neck
Aerobic Exercise 30–45 min Continuous Rhythmic Exercise using large muscle groups 60–75% Max HR 3–5 RPE	*Strength Resistance Training Program* 30–40 min Work major muscle groups in alternating sequence 3 sets/10 reps 85% RM	*Aerobic Exercise* 30–45 min Continuous rhythmic exercise using large muscle groups 60–75% Max HR 3–5 RPE	*Strength Resistance Training Program* 30–40 min Work major muscle groups in alternating sequence 3 sets/10 reps 85% RM	*Aerobic Exercise* 30–45 min Continuous Rhythmic Exercise using large muscle groups 60–75% Max HR 3–5 RPE	*Group Yoga Exercises* Look in your community for instructed program
Cool-Down 5–10 min Same muscle groups as warm-up	*Flexibility Exercises* 10–15 min Concentrate on worked muscles	*Cool-Down* Same muscle group as warm-up	*Flexibility Exercises* 10–15 min Concentrate on worked muscles	*Cool-Down* Same muscle group as warm-up	*Cool-Down* Same muscle group as warm-up
Flexibility Exercises 10–15 min Concentrate on lower back and posterior thigh area To a position of mild discomfort 10–30 s for each stretch	*Relaxation Exercises* 10–20 min Body scan meditation	*Flexibility Exercises* Concentrate on lower back and posterior thigh area To a position of mild discomfort 10–30 s for each stretch	*Relaxation Exercises* 10–20 min Body scan meditation	*Flexibility Exercises* 10–15 min Concentrate on lower back and posterior thigh area To a position of mild discomfort 10–30 s for each stretch	*Relaxation Exercises* Breathing meditation

21.5.1.2 Sample Cardiorespiratory Training Program for Women

21.5.1.2.1 Sample Stationary Cycling Program

This program is designed for the development of cardiorespiratory fitness for extremely unconditioned individuals. It is based on the rate of perceived exertion (RPE) scale (1 to 10).

Week	Session Duration	Daily Frequency	Weekly Frequency	RPE
1	3–5 min exercise/1 min rest	2–3 times	3–5 times	3–4
2	3–5 min exercise/1 min rest	3–5 times	3–5 times	3–4
3	5 min exercise/1 min rest	2–3 times	3–5 times	3–4
4	5 min exercise/1 min rest	3–5 times	3–5 times	3–4
5	5 min exercise/1 min rest	4–6 times	3–5 times	3–4
6	5 min exercise/1 min rest	5–6 times	3–5 times	3–5
7	5 min exercise/1 min rest	6 times	3–5 times	3–5
8	15 min exercise	1 time	3–5 times	3–4
9	20 min exercise	1 time	3–5 times	3–4
10	25 min exercise	1 time	3–5 times	3–4
11	30 min exercise	1 time	3–5 times	3–4
12	30 min exercise	1 time	3–5 times	3–5

21.5.1.2.2 Sample Walking Program

This program is designed to develop cardiorespiratory fitness for moderately unconditioned individuals. It is based on the heart rate reserve method.

Week	Session Duration	Daily Frequency	Weekly Frequency	Intensity
1	15 min exercise/5 min rest	1–2 times	3–5 times	50–55%
2	15 min exercise/5 min rest	1–2 times	3–5 times	55–60%
3	30 min exercise	1 time	3–5 times	50–55%
4	30 min exercise	1 time	3–5 times	55–60%
5	30–45 min exercise	1 time	3–5 times	50–60%
6	30–45 min exercise	1 time	3–5 times	50–60%
7	30–45 min exercise	1 time	3–5 times	55–65%
8	30–45 min exercise	1 time	3–5 times	55–65%
9	45–60 min exercise	1 time	3–5 times	50–60%
10	45–60 min exercise	1 time	3–5 times	50–60%
11	45–60 min exercise	1 time	3–5 times	55–60%
12	45–60 min exercise	1 time	3–5 times	55–65%

21.5.1.2.3 Sample Jogging Program

This program is designed to develop cardiorespiratory fitness for highly conditioned individuals. It uses the maximum heart rate formula.

Week	Session Duration	Daily Frequency	Weekly Frequency	Intensity
1	30–45 min exercise	1 time	3–5 times	60–75%
2	30–45 min exercise	1 time	3–5 times	60–75%
3	30–45 min exercise	1 time	3–5 times	60–75%
4	30–45 min exercise	1 time	3–5 times	60–75%
5	40–50 min exercise	1 time	3–5 times	70–80%
6	40–50 min exercise	1 time	3–5 times	70–80%
7	40–50 min exercise	1 time	3–5 times	70–80%
8	40–50 min exercise	1 time	3–5 times	70–80%
9	45–60 min exercise	1 time	3–5 times	75–85%
10	45–60 min exercise	1 time	3–5 times	75–85%
11	45–60 min exercise	1 time	3–5 times	75–85%
12	45–60 min exercise	1 time	3–5 times	75–85%

21.5.1.3 Sample Resistance Training Program for Women

An easy method of achieving a total body workout with resistance training is the circuit room. A circuit room is a specially designed weight room in which a person moves from machine to machine in an orderly fashion. The machines are placed so that each part of the body is worked but has time to recover before the next exercise.

Individuals can work on hypertrophy, strength, or endurance just by changing the number of repetitions performed. One to eight repetitions before muscle fatigue (when you can no longer push the weight up again) will primarily increase the size of a muscle, both minimally for women. About 8 to 12 repetitions before fatigue will increase strength (6 are generally recommended), and over 12 repetitions before fatigue will increase endurance (15 are generally recommended).

Below is a sample resistance circuit training program. In order to maximize the benefits of the circuit room, each exercise should be performed to the set number of repetitions throughout the circuit. Rest periods between sets should range from 1 to 3 min. Depending on goals and time constraints, a second and possibly a third circuit should be made. Thus each exercise should be performed ideally two to three times a visit. In addition, the circuit room workout should be performed two to three times per week.

Machine Number	Machine Name	Muscles Used
1	Leg press	Hamstrings, gluteal group, quadriceps
2	Chest press	Triceps, pectoralis group, deltoids
3	Leg extension	Quadriceps
4	Lat pull-downs	Rhomboids, latissimus dorsi, biceps
5	Seated leg curl	Hamstrings
6	Chest fly	Pectoralis group
7	Standing calf raise	Soleus, plantaris, gastrocnemius
8	Rowing	Rhomboids, latissimus dorsi, trapezius
9	Abdominal crunches	Rectus abdominis
10	Shoulder press	Triceps, deltoids
11	Back extension	Erector spinae
12	Arm curls	Biceps
13	Lateral raise	Deltoids
14	Tricep extension	Triceps

The number of repetitions and sets will depend on goals. See Table 21.11.

References

1. McSwegin, P., Pemberton, C., Petray, C., and Going, S., *Physical Best*, AAPHERD, Reston, VA, 1989.
2. Hoeger, W.K. and Hoeger, S.A., *Principles and Labs for Physical Fitness*, Morton, Englewood, CO, 1999.
3. Gortmaker S.L., Dietz, W.H., Sobol, A.M., and Wehler, C.A., Increasing pediatric obesity in the United States, *Am. J. Dis. Child*, 141, 553, 1987.
4. Meredith M.D., *FITNESSGRAM User's Manual*, Institute for Aerobics Research, Dallas, TX, 1987.
5. Johns, R.J. and Wright, V., Relative importance of various tissues in joint stiffness, *J. Appl. Physiol.*, 17, 824, 1962.
6. Cooper, C., Cawley, M., Bhalla, A., Egger, P., Ring, F., Morton, L., and Barker, D., Childhood growth, physical activity, and peak bone mass in women, *J. Bone Miner. Res.*, 10, 940, 1995.
7. Carrie-Fassler, A.L. and Bonjour, J.P., Osteoporosis as a pediatric problem, *Pediatr. Clin. N. Am.*, 42, 811, 1995.
8. Lindholm, C., Hagenfeldt, K., and Ringertz, H., Bone mineral content of young female former gymnasts, *Acta Paediatr.*, 84, 1109, 1995.
9. Bass, S., Pearce, G., Bradney, M., Hendrich, E., Delmas, P.D., Harding, A., and Seeman, E., Exercise before puberty may confer residual benefits in bone density in adulthood: studies in active prepubertal and retired female gymnasts, *J. Bone Miner. Res.*, 13, 500, 1998.

10. Bailey, D.A., Faulkner, R.A., Kimber, K., Dzus, A., and Yong-Hing, K., Altered loading patterns and femoral bone mineral density in children with unilateral Legg-Calve-Perthes disease, *Med. Sci. Sports Medicine*, 29, 1395, 1997.

11. Maffulli, N. and Helms, P., Controversies about intensive training in young athletes, *Arch. Dis. Child.*, 63, 1405, 1988.

12. Case, S.L. and Hennrikus, W.L., Surgical treatment of displaced medial epicondyle fractures in adolescent athletes, *Am. J. Sports Med.*, 25, 682, 1997.

13. Cahill, B.R., Phillips, M.R., and Navarro, R., The results of conservative management of juvenile osteochondritis dissecans using joint scintigraphy: a prospective study, *Am. J. Sports Med.*, 17, 601, 1989.

14. Harvey, J. and Tanner, S., Low back pain in young athletes. A practical approach, *Sports Med.*, 12, 394, 1991.

15. Webb, D.R., Strength training in children and adolescents, *Pediatr. Clin. N. Am.*, 37, 1187, 1990.

16. Orava, S. and Puranen, J., Exertion injuries in adolescent athletes, *Br. J. Sports Med.*, 12, 4, 1978).

17. Pollock, M.L. and Wilmore, J.H., *Exercise in Health and Disease: Evaluation and Prescription for Prevention and Rehabilitation*, W.B. Saunders, Philadelphia,1990.

18. Heyward, V., *Advanced Fitness Assessment and Exercise Prescription*, Human Kinetics, Champaign, IL, 1991.

19. McArdle, W.D., Katch, F.I., and Katch, V., *Exercise Physiology*, Lea & Febiger, Philadelphia, 1981.

20. American Council on Exercise, *Personal Trainer Manual*, Reebok University Press, Boston, 1991.

21. American College of Sports Medicine, *Guidelines for Exercise Testing and Prescription*, Williams & Wilkins, Baltimore, 1995.

22. Williams, M., *Nutrition for Fitness and Sport*, William C. Brown, Dubuque, IA, 1988.

23. Fishman, J., Boyar, R.M., and Hellman, L., Influence of body weight on estradiol metabolism in young women, *J. Clin. Endocrinol. Metabol.*, 41, 989, 1975.

24. Petterson, F., Fries, H., and Nillius, S., Epidemiology of secondary amenorrhea: incidence and prevalence rates, *Am. J. Obstetr. Gynecol.*, 117, 80, 1973.

25. Bale, P., Doust, D., and Dawson, D., Gymnasts, distance runners, anorexics, body composition and menstrual status, *J. Sports Med. Phys. Fitness*, 36, 49, 1996.

26. Frisch, E.R., Gotz-Welbergen, A.V., McArthur, J.W., Albright, T., Witschi, J., Bullen, B., Binholz, J., Reed, R.B., and Herman, H., Delayed menarche and amenorrhea of college athletes in relation to age of onset of training, *JAMA*, 246, 1559, 1981.

27. Brooks-Gunn, J., Warren, M.P., and Hamilton, L.H., The relation of eating problems and amenorrhea in ballet dancers, *Med. Sci. Sports Exercise*, 19, 41, 1987.

28. Myerson, M., Gutin, B., Warren, M., May, M., Contento, I., Lee, M., Pi-Sunyer, F., Pierson, R., and Brooks-Gunn, J., Resting metabolic rate and energy balance in amenorrheic and eumenorrheic runners, *Med. Sci. Sports Exercise*, 23, 15, 1991.

29. Walberg, J. and Johnston, C., Menstrual function and eating behavior in female international weight lifters and competitive body builders, *Med. Sci. Sports Exercise*, 23, 30, 1991.

30. Frisch, R. and MacArthur, J., Menstrual cycles: fatness as a determinant of minimum weight for height necessary for their maintenance or onset, *Science*, 185, 949, 1974.

31. American College of Sports Medicine, *Resource Manual for Guidelines for Exercise Testing and Prescription*, Lea & Febiger, Baltimore,1993.

32. Wescott, W.L., You can sell exercise for weight loss, *Fitness Management*, 7, 33, 1991.

33. Hafen, B. and Hoeger, W., *Wellness Guidelines for a Healthy Lifestyle*, Morton, Englewood, CO, 1994.

34. Barrow, G. and Saha, S. Menstrual irregularity and stress fractures in collegiate female distance runners, *Am. J. Sports Med.*, 16, 209, 1988.

35. Drinkwater, B. L., Nilson, K., Chestnut, C., Bremner, W., Shainholtz, S., and Southworth, M., Bone mineral content of amenorrheic and eumenorrheic athletes, *New England J. Med.*, 311, 277, 1984.

Appendix 21-A: Health History Questionnaire

Last name _____   First name _____   Middle initial_____

Date of birth _____   Sex _____   Home phone _____   Work phone _____

Address_____

City _____   State _____   Zip_____

Dietary habits_____

1. What is your current weight? _____ lb.   height? _____ in.
2. What would you like to weigh? _____ lb.
3. What is the most you ever weighed as an adult? _____ lb.
4. What is the least you ever weighed as an adult? _____ lb.
5. What weight loss methods have you tried?
6. Which do you eat regularly?
   - ☐ Breakfast
   - ☐ Midmorning snack
   - ☐ Lunch
   - ☐ Midafternoon snack
   - ☐ Dinner
   - ☐ After-dinner snack
7. Do you occasionally go all day without eating, followed by a large dinner later in the evening?   ☐ Yes ☐ No
8. What size portions do you normally have?
   - ☐ Small   ☐ Moderate   ☐ Large   ☐ Extra large   ☐ Uncertain
9. How often do you eat more than one serving?
   - ☐ Always   ☐ Usually   ☐ Sometimes   ☐ Never
10. Do you usually eat at least 1200 calories a day?   ☐ Yes ☐ No
11. When you snack, how many times a week do you eat the following?
    Cookies, cake, pie _____   Candy _____   Diet soda _____
    Soft drinks _____   Doughnuts _____   Fruit _____
    Milk or milk beverage _____   Potato chips, pretzels, etc. _____

Medical History

12. When was the last time you had a physical examination?

13. If you are allergic to any medications, food, or other substances, please name them.

14. If you have been told that you have any chronic or serious illnesses, please list them.

15. Give the following information pertaining to your last three hospitalizations. Do not list normal pregnancies.

	Hospitalization 1	Hospitalization 2	Hospitalization 3
Type of operation			
Month and year hospitalized			
Name of hospital			
City and state			
During the past 12 months			

16. Has a physician prescribed any form of medication for you? Yes ☐ No ☐
17. Has your weight fluctuated more than a few pounds? Yes ☐ No ☐
18. Did you attempt to bring about this weight change through diet or exercise? Yes ☐ No ☐
19. Have you experienced any faintness, light-headedness, or blackouts? Yes ☐ No ☐
20. Have you occasionally had trouble sleeping? Yes ☐ No ☐
21. Have you experienced any blurred vision? Yes ☐ No ☐
22. Have you had any severe headaches? Yes ☐ No ☐
23. Have you experienced chronic morning cough? Yes ☐ No ☐
24. Have you experienced any temporary change in your speech pattern, such as slurring or loss of speech? Yes ☐ No ☐
25. Have you felt unusually nervous or anxious for no apparent reason? Yes ☐ No ☐
26. Have you experienced unusual heartbeats such as skipped beats or palpitations? Yes ☐ No ☐
27. Have you experienced periods in which your heart felt as though it were racing for no apparent reason? Yes ☐ No ☐

At present:

28. Do you experience shortness of breath or loss of breath while walking with others your own age? Yes ☐ No ☐
29. Do you experience sudden tingling, numbness, or loss of feeling in your arms, hands, legs, feet, or face? Yes ☐ No ☐
30. Have you ever noticed that your hands or feet sometimes feel cooler than other parts of your body? Yes ☐ No ☐
31. Do you experience swelling of your feet or ankles? Yes ☐ No ☐
32. Do you get pains or cramps in your legs? Yes ☐ No ☐
33. Do you experience any pain or discomfort in your chest? Yes ☐ No ☐
34. Do you experience any pressure or heaviness in your chest? Yes ☐ No ☐
35. Have you ever been told that your blood pressure was abnormal? Yes ☐ No ☐

36. Have you ever been told that your serum cholesterol or
    triglyceride level was high?   Yes ☐ No ☐

37. Do you have diabetes?
    If yes, how is it controlled?
    ☐ Dietary means   ☐ Insulin injection   ☐ Oral medication   ☐ Uncontrolled

38. How often would you characterize your stress level as being high?
    ☐ Occasionally   ☐ Frequently   ☐ Constantly

39. Have you ever been told that you have any of the following illnesses?
    ☐ Myocardial infarction ☐ Arteriosclerosis ☐ Heart disease ☐ Heart block
    ☐ Coronary thrombosis ☐ Rheumatic heart ☐ Heart attack ☐ Aneurysm
    ☐ Coronary occlusion ☐ Heart failure ☐ Heart murmur ☐ Angina

40. Has any member of your immediate family been treated for or suspected to
    have had any of these conditions? Please identify their relationship to you
    (father, mother, sister, brother, etc.).
    ☐ Diabetes   ☐ Heart disease   ☐ Stroke   ☐ High blood pressure
    Relationship   Relationship   Relationship   Relationship

    _____   _____   _____   _____

Appendix 21-B: Estimating Your Daily Energy Needs

Your weight in pounds = _____

Your weight in kilograms = _____ = $\dfrac{\text{wt (lbs)}}{2.2}$

1. Calculate your BMR:

   Males: multiply your wt. (kg) × 1 kcal/kg/hr × 24 hr/day = _____ kcal/day

   Females: multiply your wt (kg) × .9 kcal/kg/hr × 24 hr/day = _____ kcal/day

2. Account for slower metabolism during sleep:

   Subtract from your BMR: .1 kcal/kg/hr sleep × your wt (kg) × hours of sleep.
   Adjusted BMR = _____ kcal/day

3. Add the appropriate activity increment:

	Males	Females
Sedentary/light	225 kcal	225 kcal
Moderate	750	500
Heavy	1500	1000
Very heavy	2500	1750

   Energy Expenditure – Adjusted BMR + Activity Increment = _____ kcal/day

4. Add 10% to the value in 3 for the increased metabolism due to digestion.
   Total expenditure = kcal/day (from 3) _____ + 10% of kcal/day (from 3)
   _____ = kcal/day.

5. How does this energy expenditure compare with your daily kcal consumption?

6. Please finish the sentence:

   To increase weight I must...

   To decrease weight I must...

   To maintain weight I must...

Appendix 21-C: Estimation of the Energy Expenditure in Selected Recreational and Sport Activities

Instructions: To estimate the total caloric cost of your activity, please multiply the listed value next to the activity by the time in minutes you engaged in the activity and your body weight in pounds. Please access these Web addresses for a more comprehensive list of activities.

Activity Calorie Calculator — http://www.primusweb.com/fitnesspartner/jumpsite/calculat.htm. Calculate the number of calories you burn for 158 activities.

Burning off the Fat — wysiwyg://5/http://www.msnbc.com/modules/quizzes/caloriecalc.asp. Activities range from aerobics to yoga, also included are daily living activities.

Calorie — http://www.home.connectnet.com/eoinf/cal.html. Estimate the number of calories you burn at a given running pace.

Activity	kcal min⁻¹ lb⁻¹	Multiply by weight in lbs	Multiply by time in min	Cost of Activity
Aerobic dance	(.054)	× weights in lbs ( )	X time in min ( ) =	_____ kal
Circuit training				
Free weights	(.0391)	× weights in lbs ( )	× time in min ( ) =	_____ kal
Nautilus	(.0418)	× weights in lbs ( )	× time in min ( ) =	_____ kal
Universal	(.0527)	× weights in lbs ( )	× time in min ( ) =	_____ kal
Cycling				
Leisure, 5.5 mph	(.0291)	× weights in lbs ( )	× time in min ( ) =	_____ kal
Leisure, 9.5 mph	(.0455)	× weights in lbs ( )	× time in min ( ) =	_____ kal
Racing	(.0768)	× weights in lbs ( )	× time in min ( ) =	_____ kal
Gymnastics	(.03)	× weights in lbs ( )	× time in min ( ) =	_____ kal
Jumping rope				
70 per min	(.0736)	× weights in lbs ( )	× time in min ( ) =	_____ kal
80 per min	(.0745)	× weights in lbs ( )	× time in min ( ) =	_____ kal
145 per min	(.0895)	× weights in lbs ( )	× time in min ( ) =	_____ kal
Running				
11 min per mile	(.0614)	× weights in lbs ( )	× time in min ( ) =	_____ kal
9 min per mile	(.0877)	× weights in lbs ( )	× time in min ( ) =	_____ kal
7 min per mile	(.1036)	× weights in lbs ( )	× time in min ( ) =	_____ kal
Scuba diving	(.1095)	× weights in lbs ( )	× time in min ( ) =	_____ kal
Snow skiing-leisure				
Hard snow (level)	(.0595)	× weights in lbs ( )	× time in min ( ) =	_____ kal
Soft snow	(.0475)	× weights in lbs ( )	× time in min ( ) =	_____ kal
Swimming				
Back stroke	(.0768)	× weights in lbs ( )	× time in min ( ) =	_____ kal
Breast stroke	(.0736)	× weights in lbs ( )	× time in min ( ) =	_____ kal
Crawl	(.0646)	× weights in lbs ( )	× time in min ( ) =	_____ kal
Side stroke	(.0555)	× weights in lbs ( )	× time in min ( ) =	_____ kal
Treading water	(.0526)	× weights in lbs ( )	× time in min ( ) =	_____ kal
Tennis	(.0495)	× weights in lbs ( )	× time in min ( ) =	_____ kal
Volleyball	(.0227)	× weights in lbs ( )	× time in min ( ) =	_____ kal
Walking	(.0368)	× weights in lbs ( )	× time in min ( ) =	_____ kal

Part VI

Therapeutic Approaches to the Treatment of Eating Disorders

22

Contact Movement Therapy for Clients with Eating Disorders

Adwoa Lemieux

CONTENTS

22.1 Learning Objectives

After reading this chapter you should be able to:

- Understand the concept of contact movement therapy;
- Understand the concept and vocabulary of contact improvisation;
- Understand the use of the paradigm as used in two case studies;
- Have tools that might help a therapist begin contact based work with a client.

22.2 Introduction

In working with women with eating disorders for nearly 20 years in an inpatient advanced eating disorder clinic and with outpatients in private contact work, I have found a paradigm that has worked well for my clients. It addresses areas that are critical in the process to recovery. These areas include intimacy, contacting one's own center, maintaining a relationship with another and still honoring one's self, touch and boundaries, sensing an accurate body image, letting go of control, being able to receive and give support, and learning to take risks and be spontaneous.

Contact movement therapy is the unity of two forms that overlap. I am a dance/movement therapist and a contact improvisation dancer. Contact movement therapy has its roots in movement therapy and in contact improvisation. Marion Chace, Mary Whitehouse, Steve Paxton, and Nancy Stark Smith built the foundation for this work. My teachers, contact partners, students, and clients inspired and influenced the creation of this work. Using the groundwork of contact improvisation and the fundamentals of dance/movement therapy, I have brought these two forms together in a program called contact movement therapy.

In this chapter, I will define contact movement therapy, outline the paradigm, describe how I use the paradigm with an eating disorder client, offer one case study of a woman in a phase of anorexia/bulimia, and present tools for the therapist's use. It is my intention in this chapter to describe a method that is useful for the eating disorder therapist. I use this model with groups and in individual sessions. Since the majority of the people that I have worked with who have had eating disorders were women, for purposes of simplicity, the feminine pronouns will be used in this chapter.

Contact movement therapy may be difficult initially for many people with eating disorders. By proceeding with sensitivity and openness and continuing to listen through each moment, contact movement therapy can break through patterns of isolation and fears of being touched or of touching. It can increase comfort in one's body, increase the accuracy of one's body image, and bring clarity to one's boundaries. It can teach a woman to receive support by letting go of her own weight and give support by taking others' weight. Women can also learn to let go of control, trust their bodies, and improvise in the moment. While this work may be very new, Steve Paxton said, "If you want to get to a new place, you can't know where you are going."[1]

22.3 Research Background

22.3.1 What Is Contact Improvisation?

Some ambiguity has always accompanied the concept of contact improvisation. In 1972, a group of dancers began work on contact improvisation by studying the way communication was possible through touch. The movement which resulted from contact improvisation was intuitive, based upon intimate communication. It is a movement form that works with the physical forces of gravity, momentum, and inertia. Contact improvisation is an approach in which the student moves from the motivations of reflex and intuition. It includes learning skills such as rolling, falling, taking and giving weight, playing with gravity and momentum, discovering ledges and levels, and exploring textures and depths of touch. The technique is learned in a duet form; it is not done alone. The dancers maintain physical touch, mutually supporting and initiating the dance, while playing with the physical laws relating to gravity, momentum, inertia, and friction. The dance is about the discoveries in the moment, remaining curious about what is happening in the dance rather than upon achieving a result. Although the movement is primarily a physical contact, there is the sense that one participant is contacting the other in other ways as well. The two people create a spontaneous, unplanned dance. Both people in the dance are equals.

Although the technique has no set technique, guidelines developed over the years have aided beginners to learn to give their weight, experience gravity, experience disorientation, and create a place of safety for their partners and themselves by learning to fall, roll, and relax. The form itself is the real teacher. Each person learns from her own body, gathering information from each dance and from each partner. The leader guides this process. It is important for the leader to create an environment that is physically and emotionally safe for the group or the individual. It is best in beginning sessions to match partners with people similar in size. Warm-up activities that feel safe and familiar to the group should be included. Progression of skills should be within the realm of the group's or individual's ability. Each person's emotional state should be respected and hopefully her accepted range of emotions will expand.

The contact improvisation partner responds to the movement of her partner. The feedback is immediate, direct, and physical. This communication is often in relation to a partner's weight or touch. The participants form a sensitive relationship in which they are aware of themselves and their partners and create a dialogue. Something happens through this awareness. Both people in the dance often move in new ways. The movement frequently affects a person physically and emotionally.

The dance follows a cycle. To begin, the partners make some sort of contact (not necessarily physical). They build trust through respecting each other during the dance. A connection or partnership evolves, possibly following a point of contact and weight exchange. Both people in the dance improvise until the dance feels complete. This can happen in a short time but can take longer. The dance can continue for minute to an hour or more. Contact improvisation derives its moves from spontaneous responses. The movement is felt physically through the point of contact with a partner. The partner remains open and sensitive to the other person and follows the path of least resistance.

22.3.2 Contact Vocabulary

Contact improvisation has a vocabulary familiar to contact dancers. The terms and concepts are presented for your greater understanding. These terms and concepts will be discussed further in the section on contact movement therapy.

The *personal warm-up* in a contact improvisation class is the time when a person enters the studio and begins moving in a way that enables her body to *arrive* or bring her whole self to the class. This might mean lying on the floor for a time, running, or slowly stretching. Although everyone works individually, the group often begins to establish a "group mind," or shared energy.

As people begin making contact with others in the room they develop an intention to exchange or communicate. Sometimes this is done through duets or through a group movement in which different kinds of contact might be explored (e.g., using glances or eye contact, using movement in a small space, using a light physical touch, falling together). This may develop naturally or may be guided by a teacher or leader.

One exercise, called the *stand* or the *small dance* that was originated by Steve Paxton[2] is an exercise in sensitizing the self to the inner movement of one's own body and experiencing the pull of gravity while remaining grounded. Body weight falls through the feet into the ground. A person starts by simply standing and feeling the body as it stands. She feels her skeleton as it supports the body, and allows the muscles to release while she still remains standing. She is in a condition of vertical rest. Some small adjustments and rebalancings may occur, some of which are not distinguishable to an onlooker.

Another term that is familiar to contactors is *states*. A state is an energetic, sometimes emotional quality that is reflective in the movement. Most often a state arises from a physical movement that creates an atmosphere or environment. Examples might be a heavy state, an oceanic state, a light playful state, or more abstract images such as the five elements (earth, air, water, fire, ether).

Counter-balancing is another frequently used term. This is usually done by two people and they share control. The movement may be done with arms or other body parts. The two people balance their weights by creating a tension through pulling away from or pushing toward each other. A balance is found. That means either person falls without the support of the other's weight. The two play by slowly shifting the point of balance.

Another important concept is *depth of touch*. This is the level at which one person contacts another. Contact may be at skin level or more deeply by contacting the musculature. Although depth of touch refers to the physical contact of one person with another, energetic contact may be experienced as well. A sample of an exercise is to have one person stand while the other places a hand somewhere on the first person's body. Both allow energy to pour into the point of touch, then let the point open to the touch. Other points are selected. This may lead to a duet which involving light touch. A light touch dance is one in which a point of contact is maintained between two people. It involves little or no weight bearing.

Giving weight is another term common in the contact language. One might lie on the floor, feeling her weight slowly pouring into the floor. This also can be done by partners. In that situation, one person pours her weight into a point of contact in her partner. The image is that sand is pouring through the body. A participant can sense the sand spilling through her body and pouring into the floor or into another's body.

Another technique is receiving weight or being a support. There are different ways of practicing this movement. One way is *surfing*. One person does a log roll (literally rolling like a log); the other rolls or glides as if catching a wave, and gets a ride. Another move is called *sluffing*. One person stands; the other leans into the person and slides off, maintaining a point of contact as her weight falls by gravity toward the floor. One other practice is the *table* or posting. This is done on various levels. One person is on all fours. The other drapes all of her weight on the table and then rolls off. This move can also be done in a standing position, or by taking the weight on a hip or shoulder.

A *jam* is a practice environment in which these concepts or techniques are improvised. No one leads. Everyone practices and improvises. A jam can be unstructured dance time, for practicing what has been learned in a class or exploring one's own dance with peers. Sometimes a *round robin* is included in a jam. A round robin is a form used to change or rotate partners. The group forms a circle. A dancer begins moving in the center, another enters, and they begin a duet. At some point a third dancer enters. The first dancer leaves and the second and the third continue to dance. This structure continues as a fourth person joins and the second person leaves, and so on. The dance is always changing. Each dance transitions into the next. This allows dancers to practice beginnings and endings. Because of the round robin structure, the dancers are obliged to let these endings occur. The dances are not prearranged and all dancing is improvised.

The preceding explanations cover exercises and vocabulary that are familiar to most contactors. Contact improvisation is moving without knowing or planning the next step. Being in contact with another person, feeling both weights physically, and allowing the physical forces to be present allows mutual freedom of movement by body and mind. When one frees the body, the mind and the emotions are also freed.

22.3.3 Application: The Contact Movement Therapy Paradigm

Contact movement therapy has eight steps or stages. These can be utilized in individual sessions or throughout a therapy program. Each stage may not be reached in every session and it is possible that the steps will not follow this specific order. Additionally, some step or stage may not be appropriate for a particular client. The stages are making contact, building trust, developing trust, creating a duet, working with touch, receiving support, taking risks, spontaneity/round robin, and closure. Appendix 22-A lists tools for the therapist working with the technique.

22.3.3.1 *Making Contact*

Making contact is the touching or meeting of two people in association or relationship. It is the prerequisite for receiving information and communicating. The environment should be safe and at the same time invoke the curiosity of a client. Making contact with a client may take a minute, may be instantaneous, or may take more than half the session. However, contact is a vital step in the recovery process. In the initial stages of therapy, the contact may not have depth until trust is established.

It is also essential that the therapist maintain contact with herself or himself during this process. Self-contact is required before one can make contact with another. Contact with oneself can be accomplished through the process of centering. Centering may be achieved through attention to breathing, gentle stretching or movement, or simply a state of inner awareness. In making contact, the boundaries between client and therapist are softened. One feels the other's presence while still maintaining an awareness of her own body and feelings.

22.3.3.2 *Developing Trust*

The next stage is developing trust with the client. Trust is the unquestioning belief in the integrity, strength, or ability of a person. The purpose of this step is to establish a sense of safety in which to work and develop a ground or a base on which to work. It is important to firmly establish trust before continuing. Without trust, a client cannot be in contact with the depth of feelings and emotions or the depth of process needed to continue working. It is important that the therapist feels trust in herself, that the client feels trust in herself, and that they trust each other. Nancy Stark Smith talks of the need to develop trust and yet remain open to new possibilities, "It seems the edge is movable — that by sensing the limit, respecting it, you encourage it to open ... but if you go only as far as you are welcome, you are invited back."[3]

Trust or lack of trust is a key issue for many clients with eating disorders. They do not trust their bodies. They do not trust themselves to stop eating, to control sexual responses, or manage their responses related to intimacy and boundaries. It may be important to work on body trust first. This may take many sessions. For some clients, it is easier to trust someone else (i.e., the therapist). Although this could develop into dependency, it may be useful as a developmental step. Clients can and will break away. Some learn to trust themselves through trusting another. In developing trust, a client gains a deeper awareness of herself. She gains confidence in herself and in others. The client and therapist will notice small changes during this process. The client will experience a softening of the body, more steady and continuous breathing, relaxed body posturing, and softer muscle tone.

Randy Warshaw, a teacher of contact improvisation, remarks on the importance of trust in a class:

> "It's important that students notice the trust and confidence they gain in themselves and their partners to stay with a moment, and meet the needs of each changing moment. Trust, patiently nurtured through confidence and familiarity, prepares the way for diversity. Through trust, awkward, uncomfortable moments of vulnerability, and powerful moments of virtuosity become equally rich."[4]

For trust to be developed, it also needs to be given. At some point the client takes a leap of faith (I trust you). This can be seen in a client's body; her body is relaxed and open to being seen (this is me). As with any dance; the ground is tested. The client's space must be respected and must not be pushed any further than she needs or wants to allow. She must feel safe while remaining ready for a further invitation.

A tool to use to develop trust is enabling the client to move on the floor. The experience of releasing her weight into the floor and trusting the support of the floor builds her trust in herself. Through rolling and sinking into the floor, she develops the foundation to push upward and to stand on her own feet. This step also establishes the ground for later work. Soft pillows or mats may be used to assure a client has safe soft ground to explore.

Another way to develop trust is through sensitizing a client to her own body needs and having her satisfy those needs, for example, making herself more comfortable and taking time to lie on a soft mat and breathe. Trust in oneself develops through experiencing one's own ability to take care of oneself. Some clients may feel safer working for a while with closed eyes; for others that is too risky.

Trust develops through time and experience. A client may learn to trust by taking a risk and being supported. Taking a risk means having safe boundaries stretched. However, a client must not be pushed before she is ready. Respecting the safe boundaries of the client develops trust. A therapist must also trust his or her impulses, intuition, and the process of the work. Trust must be established for a client to work in a duet, to be touched, to be supported, to take risks, and to be spontaneous. It also must be firmly established before a client can leave the session or therapy. In summary, Mary Whitehouse reflected upon trust in a dance movement session:

> It seems to me the most important element in private movement sessions has to do with trust; the client's trust of you and your trust in yourself and also your trust of your client and the client's trust of herself. Mutual trust allows both of you to say 'yes' or 'no' according to the way she really feels. This relationship is not transference, which is compelled by the unconscious. The more human — the more your actual self — you manage to be in your movement sessions, the less chance there is of confusion never resolved. One cannot provide reassurance, caring, approving, listening, directing until safety has been established. Trust arises as soon as the individual feels there will be no betrayal; then it truly doesn't matter how quickly or how much she responds.[5]

22.3.3.3 Creating a Duet

A duet is a relationship two people share. It is a partnership. In contact movement therapy, the duet is between the therapist and the client. The duet occurs merely because the client and therapist are in the same space. One responds to the other; a dialogue or conversation occurs in the interaction. This may be entirely nonverbal. The duet breaks the pattern of isolation for a client. By simply entering into a therapeutic relationship, her isolation is broken; someone knows. This is an opportunity for her to develop and work on a healthy relationship. For some clients this may be a new experience. Also, in working in this form, other kinds of patterns from past relationships often surface. Through moving, responding, and dialoguing, there is a possibility the client can work through old patterns and develop new pathways. This occurs on a movement level. It can then be integrated into other parts of a client's life.

Eye contact can be used to develop the client/therapist duet. Being seen and maintaining contact are difficult for many clients. Sometimes a client may hide, run, or cover parts of her body. The client realizes that she has been seen and waits for a response. It is important to respond to that particular client in the moment. This may be done by waiting for her to move, without interfering, by adding music, or even by joining her under pillows. This may establish a playful relationship and let her know that she is not alone. For some clients this is a new experience.

Another tool to establish a duet with a client is drawing — having a conversation on paper. After a relationship is established, the drawing may be taken into the movement. Mirroring or reflecting similar movement or shadowing the other person can also be used. In mirroring, a client's movement is reflected back to her as if she were looking into a mirror. For some clients, mirroring the therapist is safer. Shadowing is moving similarly but generally to the side of or behind the client. It is important not to interfere with the client's movement. This establishes a duet. Sculpted relationships can also be created. The client sets up the physical distance in the relationship through posture, gesture, or a phrase. Using movement, the client may mold the therapist into the person she is in a relationship with; the client assumes her own role in the relationship. This gives her a new perception of her role in that relationship and other relationships.

Communicating fears, joys, conflicts, and other feelings through these tools with another person present is often a new experience for clients. They gain a sense of intimacy. Especially for people with eating disorders, these steps are difficult and play a part in healing.

22.3.3.4 Touching

The next step is touching. Touching is a basic human need. When we speak of being touched, we are describing the feeling of being emotionally moved. "To touch" has come to mean to be sensitive to human feeling. To be "touchy" means to be oversensitive. "To keep in touch" means that however far we may be removed, we remain in communication."[6]

Most children will begin to explore a new environment by touching. It is the action of reaching into the environment and feeling what the environment actually is. Touching is extending oneself out into the world, to make contact. Ashley Montagu, in his book, *Touching*, defines touching as:

> The action, or act, of feeling something with the hand, etc. Although touch is not an emotion, its sensory elements induce those neural, glandular, muscular, and mental changes that in combination we call an emotion.

We need touch for survival. In our culture people feel a deprivation of touch. Being held, being stroked, and feeling a body nearby are healing factors. Physical touch can facilitate deep emotional feelings and allow someone to feel touched. The above statement by Ashley Montagu clearly states the reason the use of touch in therapy is important, and "The communications we transmit through touch constitute the most powerful means of establishing human relationships, the foundation of experience."[6]

Stephen Thayer also confirms the healing power of touch in an article in *Psychology Today*:

> People who were comfortable with touching were more talkative, cheerful, socially dominant and nonconforming; those discomforted by touch tended to be more emotionally unstable and socially withdrawn. People who were less comfortable about touching were also more apprehensive about communicating and had lower self-esteem. Not surprisingly, another study showed that those comfortable with touch were likely to be more satisfied with their bodies and physical appearance.[7]

Most clients long to be touched, to be held. A gentle touch often brings feelings to the surface. If a client acknowledges, "I want to be held," her sadness, pain, or loneliness may surface.

For a client with an eating disorder, this step is critical in her healing process. However, she must be ready to be touched. It is important to explore the need for touching as a therapeutic tool. A therapist may ask a client, "Is this okay?" If the client needs more time, her wish should be respected. The client should clearly have the power to say "no" and to talk about feelings that surface around touching and being touched.

There are many kinds of touch. A therapist needs to be clear about her intention with touching. Touch can be nurturing and supportive, it can be healing, or it can be directive, like an instruction to "breathe into this part of your body." Touch can give a clear message of a boundary. A therapist may push against a client's arms or legs to provide resistance or to enable her to feel a boundary. Touch is an invitation for a client to feel support and caring — a client may be held in the therapist's arms while she sobs. The intention of healing, of dancing, or of simply being with a person can elicit a natural touch or contact that is separate from sexual touching or being violated. Stephen Thayer comments on the importance of touch in creating intimacy, "Other means of communication can take place at a distance, but touch is the language of physical intimacy. And because it is, touch is the most powerful of all the communication channels."[7]

Touch may not always serve as the language of physical intimacy or sexual excitement. Touch may also elicit sexual fears or fears related to earlier physical abuse. For certain individuals, touch has a strong meaning that can be frightening. However, withholding touch often reinforces the feeling that she does not deserve to be touched and held, or that touch is not safe. The therapist must listen carefully and move as slowly as is needed.

22.3.3.5 *Giving and Receiving Support*

Touch is one way of supporting a client. Giving and receiving support is the next step. "To support" means to hold up, to sustain or withstand [weight], or to help or comfort. In the support stage, a client practices both giving weight and receiving weight; most people have a preference. This refers not only to physical weight, but also to emotional weight. The transfer of weight is translated into the fluidity of giving and taking in a relationship. Being comfortable in both roles, giving and receiving, is important.

Playing with the physicality and the reality of weight is a frightening and revealing experience for most people who have eating disorders. The practice of feeling one's weight and allowing another to support that weight is a vulnerable time transition. In giving weight, a client needs to surrender and not seek control. She receives support physically by literally placing her body on another's. In learning and practicing to give weight, she clearly receives the message that she can be supported. It is important to work slowly and safely into different levels of giving weight. For a person with a distorted body image or a person who has always felt too big, this is a powerful experience. It can also be very frightening — "I've never given all my weight to anyone. I didn't think anyone could support all of me." An emotional release like sobbing often follows a physical release.

It is also important for the client to be in the role of supporter. By receiving weight, she has the opportunity to feel her personal strength. She can feel her own support and experience an ease in taking another's weight and supporting that person. A client may need to realize that she can support another person and that she is strong. In learning to support, one also develops a stronger trust in oneself. However, it is important to practice receiving the weight that can be handled and not invite too much.

A give-and-take technique is the passive/active exercise in which one person surrenders totally to another's control. One person lies down and allows the other person to move her around. It can be frightening to surrender control, and it can be nurturing to feel cared for. It is important that the active person is trustworthy. As the active person, one gets to experience nurturing and controlling another. For some people, being the active person is valuable. For others who have difficulty receiving, the passive role is more important to experience. This exercise can extend to exchanging roles and creating a balance between letting go and taking charge.

22.3.3.6 Taking Risks

Each stage of this work may be a risk for a client. However, the purpose of the risk taking stage is to experience full range of movement and full emotional expression. By taking a risk, a client is exposing herself to vulnerability, loss, or the unknown. Attention should be drawn to the chance of vulnerability by the therapist. This stage is specific to each individual — a risk for one is not a risk for another. For some clients, being strong and direct is a risk that might produce anger or a feeling of potential power. For others being spontaneous, indirect, or giving all of their weight produces fear of loss of control.

It is important that the client clearly make the choice to take a risk. This is the stage of change that often leads to transformation. Change may not occur in each session or may occur on a smaller scale. The ability to take risks may have to be developed over time in small increments. After a risk is taken, a client may reach a tentative stage and need more support and nurturance. After time, this new possibility becomes integrated. This is not a time for the therapist to push; it is a time to give encouragement. A client needs the space to move into taking risks by her choice when she is ready. The momentum of the previous work provides the impetus for the risk.

Falling may be used as a tool to explore risk taking — falling through space. Another way to work on risk taking is through total weight exchanges — giving all of oneself to the moment. Range of movement can also be used to explore risks; for example, being as wide as one can be or as small, as fast or as slow.

22.3.3.7 Round Robin/Spontaneity

The next stage, the round robin, works with the fluidity of change, or rather, changing states. A state is an expression of a particular emotional condition or a response to an environment. In changing states, one plays with inspiration, impulse, and spontaneous expression. As an emotion or feeling surfaces, a client is encouraged to move with that feeling, let it go, then move on to the next feeling or state, and so on. The technique involves letting the experience move freely, letting each moment be fully experienced for what it is and can be, and allowing simple transitions. Kinetic rather than static energy is used. Kinetic energy is changing or moving on; static means staying the same. Round robin is a practice in beginning and ending. It represents the integration of the session's work; what has already surfaced in the session is practiced. Round robin is a time of practicing endings and letting go. It means preparing for the unknown by being spontaneous, responding without inhibition, and then letting go to move on.

22.3.3.8 *Closure or Warm-Down*

The last stage is closure or warm-down. This is the time just before the session is to end, but reaching this stage may take a few weeks. A client needs time to warm-down physically and emotionally. It is important to allow enough time, so that this stage is not hurried or cut short. The closure or warm-down needs to feel clear, grounded, and spacious. The pace should be slowed down gradually. There should be time for a verbal exchange. For example, a therapist may say, "We need to end soon," before the end of the session, and then let the client ask for and get what she needs before ending. Talk is sometimes lighter and more animated at the end of a session. It is important that the client is ready to move out into the world.

22.4   Application of Research Question

An individual who is in a phase of an eating disorder is starved for love. The reasons for this insatiable hunger vary. Ages of victims vary from 13 to 50; weights range from 70 pounds to 250 pounds; most people with eating disorders are female. Individuals who have anorexia have certain issues in common. These issues may manifest in different degrees or ways. Some of these issues include personal power and strength, a need for space, or fear of space. Fears center around control — feeling out of control or feeling a need to control. Issues of inaccurate body image, low self-esteem, and lack of personal power are common among all women in our culture and they often appear in the form of eating disorders. Rather than love their bodies as they are, women are often critical of their bodies and try to change them. Women sometimes abuse their bodies in response to a culture that disempowers them.

Geneen Roth, in her book, *Breaking Free from Compulsive Eating,* speaks of how women use their bodies, "They use their bodies as their battlegrounds; they know that in our culture women's voices may not always be heard, but their bodies will still be noticed."[8] A woman may fear her impulses. Boundaries are often unclear. A woman often feels a need for protection. Kim Chernin says, "Thinness becomes a statement of power."[9] The need for protection sometimes can be met by extra weight or through the protective shell of anorexia. The shell may be isolating, yet it feels safe. A woman feels a need for nurturance and fears that there will not be enough. She may feel that her needs are too much and that she will overwhelm people with her needs. People frequently feel a need for control and often fear spontaneity. People at times feel a need for protection and have unclear boundaries or very rigid boundaries. People sometimes isolate themselves, feel lonely, and need nurturance. They may have been subjected to unhealthy relationships, physical abuse, sexual abuse, or alcohol or drug abuse. Rage and sadness are often present. A person in a phase of an eating disorder frequently does not want to be seen. Intimacy is difficult. She may have had no experience with intimacy. Geneen Roth states, "When a person is focusing and obsessing on food, it is difficult to find time for intimate relationships."[9] A woman's obsession with food can take over her life.

A self-consciousness has developed through our cultural consciousness. A woman's body often expresses how she feels about herself. Kim Chernin in her book, *The Obsession,* states, "Her body will have to express whatever uneasiness she feels about her life."[10] Women's images of what they should look like are created by multimillion dollar industries that have a lot at stake. Fashion businesses, the diet industry, diet salons, diet foods, and exercise and aerobic clubs all profit when women try to fit an ideal image. Little girls are clearly given the same message. Growing into a woman's body is not necessarily an attractive prospect. Girls receive a mixed message — be strong, yet be petite and feminine. The idea of femininity seems confusing because of conflicting ideas about what a woman's body should look like. Should she have little breasts or large breasts, no hips or round hips? Should she be tall or short? Anne Cameron, in her book, *Daughters of Copper Woman,* observes the damage imposed by our culture:

> "Instead of being raised and educated by women who told them the truth about their bodies, the girls were taken from their villages and put in schools where they were taught to keep their breasts bound, to hide their arms and legs, to never look a brother in the eye, but to look down at the ground as if ashamed of something. Instead of learning that once a month their bodies would become sacred, they were taught they would become filthy. Instead of going to the waiting house to meditate, pray, and celebrate the fullness of the moon and their own bodies, they were taught they were sick. They were taught the waves and surgings of their bodies were sinful and must never be indulged or enjoyed. By the time the girls were allowed home to their villages, their minds were poisoned, their spirits damaged, their souls contaminated."[11]

An anorexic may have learned that she has some control over her life through restricting her food. She may be doing what is needed to survive. She is often responding to a dysfunctional family system. That was the situation in the case study presented in this chapter. Whatever her age, an anorexic is surviving the only way she can. She clearly is asking for help; she wants to be fed. She does not know how to nurture and feed herself. She is starving physically and emotionally. Her self-perceptions are usually inaccurate. She is often out of touch with her feelings and with others. She does not know how to receive support. She is afraid. Her life has become a series of rituals so that she can survive. She is, however, slowly killing herself. A diagnostic pamphlet presented by the American Dance Therapy Association states:

> Characteristic of those with eating disorders is a distortion of body-image, and a misperception regarding body size and body boundaries, accompanied by impoverished self-esteem and resultant problems with interpersonal relationships. These disorders often are compounded by difficulties in identifying feeling states, or by the individual's efforts to disassociate from bodily sensations and the attendant loss of body functions.[12]

Contact movement therapy addresses the body directly by breaking through the pattern of isolation and establishing a relationship that involves trust, intimacy, and support. The therapy helps to establish boundaries, more realistic body perceptions, and a stronger sense of self. It provides an opportunity to experience the spontaneous expression of the body by responding to and adjusting to the movement of feelings. Making contact with oneself, developing trust in oneself and in another, sharing with another, giving and receiving support, taking risks, improvising, and having clear endings are ways the body learns to practice and trust in a relationship.

The next section presents a case study of Anna, who was diagnosed with bulimarexia. What has become clear in my healing and in my work with Anna, is the need to trust the basic wisdom of the body and the need for protection of the self. The body responds with intelligence in surviving emotionally and physically. At some point, the body screams for help. It is then ready. Many clinical settings do a violent injustice to their clients by labeling or categorizing them, pushing them, restraining them, or numbing them with medication. Some clients may need interventions medically and physically. My client was denied her voice, her wisdom, and her experiences of her body by being generalized, labeled, and medicated. The injustice was that she believed her therapists. She struggled with the disparity between her bodily experiences and what they told her to believe.

Contact movement therapy clearly acknowledges and affirms a client's body experiences. It recognizes differences in each person and allows space for a client to explore her needs and pace and feel her body and emotions. For Anna, allowing movement in her body was transforming. By simply being with her and accepting her, I gave her an experience she needed desperately. Working with contact movement therapy gave her the opportunity to physically feel the support of another and to move a relationship with another without losing herself. I respected Anna's process by taking into account her needs, fears, and energy level as I directed and improvised during a particular session. Anna clearly affirmed this work. She remarked, "This is the most powerful and healing work that I'm doing or have ever done."

22.5 Case Study

I worked with Anna for 8 1/2 months. We began working while she was involved in an inpatient treatment setting for advanced eating disorders and continued with outpatient treatment in individual sessions. I was drawn to work with Anna from the first time I saw her. She was withdrawn, weighed 90 pounds, wore loose clothing, and had darting eyes. Her body posture was distinctly down and drawn inward as if she were hiding and protecting herself. She appeared very scared. She joined my movement therapy group about 3 weeks later. She has been anorexic/bulimic for 17 years. She has had conflicts with her mother as long as she can remember. Being touched was threatening to her. She remarked in our first session that she would die if her skin was touched. She did not trust me or any other person in the group. The group setting was extremely difficult for Anna. She withdrew into a corner, looked terrorized, and would not move. She refused to talk to anyone, except to say, "I'm scared, leave me alone."

After 2 weeks I began individual sessions with Anna. She was angry, and asked "Why are you doing this to me?" At the end of the second session, she was crying in my arms. She felt very young. I was aware that her developmental needs were not met. She was scared, yet she had made contact and was working with me.

The third individual session was in a different setting due to weather. Anna was anxious when I arrived. Although she did not admit it, she had questioned the nurses because she was afraid I would not come. Abandonment was a key issue for her. In this session, the work centered around trust. She became frightened and hid under a blanket. Again she seemed very young. She refused to move during the next group session. She approached me after the session in tears. She was afraid that I was angry and would not continue to work with her. The pattern was familiar: anger followed by abandonment. She was testing this issue with me.

In our next session she began to move more. This frightened her. It broke her pattern of believing "I cannot move." Her body withdrew. She told me that she was confused about whether she should or could trust me. She recently suffered a number of losses in her life. Predominant issues for Anna were fear of abandonment, fear of loss, emptiness, emotional splits (good/bad), harsh self-judgments, undirected anger, deep wounds related to her mother, fear of intimacy, lack of support, fear of trusting, lack of spontaneity, and unclear boundaries.

Anna was 40 years old. She had been in only one intimate relationship in which she felt betrayed and angry. She was unable to bear the thought that she might be alone. She had many short-term relationships with friends, employers, and others. None had been intimate. She also does volunteer work with people who have been abused and works 40 hours a week teaching school. Her time is filled. She is afraid of her own neediness. If she is in control, she can get by. She is afraid of what might happen if she is not in charge. Her anorexia/bulimia began 17 years ago when she weighed 210 pounds. She feels she was born "wrong." Anna's mother wanted a cute, graceful little girl and got a "fat, clumsy, stupid" one. She describes her mother as having two distinct sides: one side is wildly intelligent and humorous, the other is angry. Anna distrusts one side and hates the other. Her mother was abusive both physically and emotionally.

In a series of art therapy drawings, Anna drew herself before and after she ate. The first drawing is a faceless character that is reaching into emptiness. A tiny dot of bright color is in the corner of the page, out of reach. The other drawing is a faceless person curled up with a red hole in the middle of her body, with black arrows pointing to the body. This person is in a box or a cave with no room to move. It is black all around. Anna said that reaching out makes her too vulnerable. If she reaches for what she wants, it will go away. As she said this, she covered her stomach and chest with a red pillow. She would not reach out or even begin to move. When she eats, she is filling a hole — an emptiness. Afterward she is afraid; she hides so she does not feel the pain. If she eats, she purges; she needs to be in control.

Anna's relationship to her eating disorder is similar to her relationships with people. She is feeding her hungry heart but cannot take the nourishment and throws it up. She does not make nurturing, healthy food choices. She snacks and nibbles and does not explore possibilities that might be satisfying. Similarly she is afraid to explore the possibility of trusting herself to explore the depth of a relationship. She is afraid to try new ideas with food. As with her other relationships, she is obsessed with food. She is not eating because of hunger for food. She eats when she is alone. She eats to fill an emptiness and is not satisfied. She eats to numb herself from her feelings. She eats to insulate herself from her rage, her anger, her uncontrollable feelings, and her deep sadness.

Anna will not let herself keep the food in. She purges, then feels emptier and lonelier. She controls her relationship with food. She will not eat for days or weeks, restricting all contacts with food. She is in control; she chooses but still feels out of control. She is terrified of letting go. She names food as her problem. She cannot leave it. It engulfs her life but it does not give her what she needs. Anna's life is a cycle of emptiness and unexpressed rage. She continues to rage against her own body, passively hurting and killing herself. A good girl doesn't eat. A bad girl eats and purges. This conflict sets up a split in her self-perception. Anna isolates herself from food and relationships. She is afraid to keep food in or to bring people close to her. She is afraid of being rejected or abandoned so she pushes away first.

My therapeutic relationship with Anna was an unfamiliar one for her. She was afraid to like or trust me, yet she continued to work with me. The unfamiliar part of the relationship was that I did not leave her or push her away. I remained consistently available to her during sessions. I remained in contact (not necessarily physical contact) with her. Our sessions were often about playing together. I followed her movement, responding to the child in her that seemed to want to come out and be loved. Part of our work was reclaiming that child and actually moving through the developmental stages of a child to allow Anna to experience the separation and individuation stages of child development. Since we are client and therapist, not mother and child, we create ways to work that are appropriate to our present relationship and Anna's age.

22.5.1   Questions

1. What tools from contact movement therapy could have been used to help Anna with her eating disorder?
2. How can contact movement therapy tools help a person recover from an eating disorder?
3. Please describe tools you would use and for what specific issues you would use them with Anna. How would you expect Anna to respond?

22.5.2   Answers

Question 1

There are many tools that can be used from Contact Movement Therapy to address the issues relevant to the individual person with an eating disorder. Some of the tools are making contact, movement, duet, touch, support, risk taking, round robin, and the closure or warm-down.

Question 2

Contact/Movement Therapy clearly acknowledges and affirms a client's body experience. It recognizes differences in each person and allows space for a client to explore her needs, pace and to feel her body and emotions. This particular dance form also works specifically well with central issues, relationship issues through the duet, normally a central issue for this population.

Question 3

Tools that can be used to help Anna address specific issues are: (1) making contact; (2) building trust; (3) the duet; (4) touch; (5) support; (6) risk taking; the round robin; and finally (7) closure/warm-down.

References

1. Paxton, S., Chute transcript, *Contact Quarterly*, vol. 7, Spring/Summer 1982.
2. Paxton, S., The small dance, *Contact Quarterly*, vol. 3, Fall 1978.
3. Smith, N. S., Editor's report, *Contact Quarterly*, vol. 2, Spring 1978.
4. Warshaw, R., What are we teaching?, *Contact Quarterly*, vol. 7, Spring/Summer 1982.
5. Whitehouse, M., *Transference and Dance Therapy*, unpublished.
6. Montagu, A., *Touching*, Harper & Row, New York, 1978, 128, xv.
7. Thayer, S., Close encounters, *Psychology Today*, March, 31, 1988, 33.
8. Roth, G., *Breaking Free from Compulsive Eating*, Signet Books, New York, 1984, 213.
9. Roth, G., *Feeding the Hungry Heart*, Signet Books, New York, 1982, 36.
10. Chernin, K., *The Obsession*, Harper & Row, New York, 1981, 67, 48.
11. Cameron, A., *Daughters of Copper Woman*, Press Gang Publishers, 1981, 61.
12. American Dance Therapy Association, diagnostic pamphlet (out of print), Columbia, MD.

Appendix 22-A: Tools for the Therapist Working with Contact Movement Therapy

I have found the skills of Contact Improvisation invaluable in my training as a dance/movement therapist. They have helped me both personally and in my therapeutic relationship with clients. It has affected my body awareness and sense of confidence in myself. I have learned to trust myself and my spontaneous impulses through experience and practice on a physical level. I have learned to feel a deep level of intimacy with others that is not sexual. I have become aware of what I need to be present and ready with myself and with another. I have learned to be comfortable with disorientation. This allows me to see the world from many angles and sides while continuing to be aware of myself and another while still moving. My peripheral vision has expanded. This enables me to see and include what is occurring in the entire room while still being in touch with myself. Most important in practicing Contact Improvisation, I have learned to play and to create and to move spontaneously while being in relationship with another.

— Adwoa Lemieux

Please use Chapter 22 as a reference for the context of these exercises and use only those exercises with which you as a therapist are comfortable.

Weight Release

This is an exercise for letting go of one's weight. I would use it in the beginning of a session to relax, to release tensions of the day, to allow the client time for herself to arrive at the session. I might also use it at an end of a session to allow the client time to process or debrief the session.

To begin, guide the client or group to lie on the floor. Have the client or group take their time to let their body or bodies release into the floor. Rather than lie, allow the body to fall into the floor. Let it fall, let it go, and simply breathe. Let several minutes go by, giving the body time to release. You might use image of sand pouring through the body to give the sensation of weight.

The Stand or the Small Dance

This exercise could be used anytime in a session. It is useful to guide a client into focusing inward, to feel herself more fully. This is an exercise in sensitizing the self to the inner movement of the body and experiencing the pull of gravity while remaining grounded. One's weight falls through the feet into the ground.

A person starts simply by standing and feeling the body as it adjusts to the stillness of standing. She feels the skeleton as it supports her body, allowing the muscles to release while she remains standing. This is a condition of vertical rest. Small adjustments and rebalancings occur, some of which are not distinguishable to an onlooker. I guide the client through my voice to feel the small adjustments, to notice the breath, to be aware of the fluids moving in the body, to feel the small dance inside her body even as she is standing. You might feel like doing something more and encourage her to simply notice what is happening. I would initially have the person do the small dance for about a minute or two. Eventually I would stretch her comfort level into four or five minutes.

The Hand Dance
This is a good exercise in breaking through isolation and making contact. One needs to release control for this to work and to follow the point of contact. Each partner needs to listen and not lead; both follow.

Each partner uses one hand. The partners find a point of contact, a place where their hands touch. They begin by listening to each other. A conversation begins. Both partners follow a point of contact on the hand. A point on each person's hand remains in contact with the other. The partners might pause or there might be a lot of activity for a while. The rest of the body can move to accommodate the dance as long as the hands remain in contact. I usually let this continue for ten minutes or more. This exercise can be done using other body parts as well, e.g. heads or elbows.

Counter-balancing
Two people share control. This exercise builds trust in oneself and in one's partner and allows one to feel weight shifts in the body.

The partners hold hands. They stand in a relaxed stance with the knees slightly bent. Each allows her weight to fall off balance so that each partner is supported by the other. The partners balance their weights by creating a tension through pulling away from or pushing toward each other. A balance is found in which either person alone would fall without the support of the other's weight. The two play with slow shifts, changing the points of balance. Each person will adjust her weight to accommodate the other. This will not work if one person gives too much or too little.

Following a Point of Contact or the Orange Dance
This could be used later in a session to encourage full body integration and to open more pathways in the body.

Begin back to back with a partner. Imagine an orange between a point of contact on your backs. Feel it. Let it slowly begin to move. Breathe. Take your time and follow the orange as it moves, letting your body move so that the orange doesn't fall. A certain amount of pressure keeps the orange from moving, falling, or being squashed. Play with this. If the orange falls, simply pick it up and start again. The point can begin to move around your body and not just stay on your back. Let the orange roll. Feel the dance between you and your partner.

Passive/Active
This exercise works through give and take of weight. One person surrenders totally to the other's control. A level of trust must be developed before this exercise is undertaken.

The first person lies down and allows her weight to fall into the floor. The second person will slowly begin testing the first person's release of weight in each body part by lifting an arm and letting it drop into her hand. Eventually the second person will move the first around by totally supporting her partner's weight with her body. It can be frightening for one letting go of control or it can be nurturing. It is important that the active person is trustworthy. As the active person, one gets to experience nurturing and/or controlling another. For some people, being the active person is valuable and for others who have difficulty receiving, the passive role is more important to experience. This exercise can extend to exchanging roles and to creating a balance of letting go and taking charge.

Depth of Touch

This is an exercise to experience the depth or layers of the body and the levels at which one person contacts another. This takes the contact from the superficial layer into the depths or layers of the body. More options become available. One may contact another through the touch of skin, or deeper contact by opening to feeling the layer of muscles of a partner. Although this exercise involves the physical contact of one person to another, one can experience energetic contact as well. This exercise could be used after several sessions in building trust and confidence.

To begin, one partner starts the small dance. Both people breathe. One will warm her hands and feel the energy between them. She will begin by placing her hand on the other person who simply stands, breathes, and allows the area beneath the hand to open. Both partners focus on opening — feeling the layers of the body, skin, tissue, and bone without pushing into the point of contact. Another point is chosen and the standing partner shifts, emptying the energy from one point and filling the next point with energy. This continues. At some point the partners exchange roles. An extension of this would be to have the toucher also use other body parts such as elbow, knee, head, or hip. Eventually the partners could connect the dots between the spots and devise a dance of following the point of contact, taking time to pause in the dance and to deepen.

23

Dance/Movement Treatment Perspectives

Lucy Ramsey DuBose

CONTENTS

23.1 Learning Objectives

After completing this chapter you should be able to:

- Define the concept of body image and understand how dance/movement activities affect body image;
- Learn how dance/movement and other creative arts activities enhance self-awareness, including ability to sense and feel emotions as well as other body sensations such as hunger, satiety, tension, and relaxation;
- Learn how thinking and imaging patterns contribute to positive or negative thoughts and feelings about oneself and influence body states such as tension and relaxation;
- Understand how dance/movement and other creative arts activities can promote the creative process and enhance healing capacity.

23.2 Introduction

As a dance/movement therapist and licensed counselor, I worked in in-patient psychiatric hospitals for 7 years. I met many people who were diagnosed with eating disorders. That was my first clinical experience with people with eating problems and I was surprised at the extent of their suffering. Sadly, one person in the hospital died as a result of her eating disorder. Never again would I take the issue lightly. As I began to realize the seriousness of this problem, I became intrigued with the psychological profiles of people with eating disorders and began to learn about the complex family, societal and cultural aspects of this disorder.

I then joined the staff of an out-patient eating disorders clinic, which was directed by a psychiatrist. In this setting I worked almost exclusively with individuals diagnosed with eating disorders. I began to relate much of the written research about people with eating disorders to in the attitudes and behaviors of the people with whom I regularly worked.

23.3 Research Background

As noted by C. Philip Wilson in *Fear of Being Fat*, nearly all people with eating disorders display certain family characteristics. They often face parental overconcern and fears of being fat; perfectionism tends to be pervasive in the family; and emotions are often repressed (for example, many parents do not quarrel in front of their children and aggressive behavior is not tolerated). Children in these families usually find it difficult to grow up and become independent because they are so over-controlled.[1]

These characteristics seem to manifest themselves physically and through behavior in general. Very often in groups and in individual sessions, patients exhibit tense, constricted body postures and shallow breathing. Low self-esteem and an inability to be assertive and act in their own best interests, are common complaints. They also are quite naive and ignorant about their own emotions, and have surprisingly limited knowledge concerning their own physical needs related to hunger, satiety, tension, and relaxation.

In addition to the family and individual dynamics of girls with eating disorders, the enormous complexity of cultural and historical influences surfaces. In spite of the resurgence of the Women's Movement in the 1960s and 1970s, women are still bombarded with messages that beckon them to conform to some impossibly thin ideal. Hutchinson says, "We live in a culture that places a very high premium on physical appearance. If this is true for the culture as a whole, it is doubly true for women who have been brought up believing that their chief, perhaps their only role in life, is as ornament, wife, and mother."[2] Movies, television commercials, magazine advertisements, and billboards tout the ideal of the tall, thin, young woman.

A major cultural factor in middle-class American families that contributes to our attitudes about beauty and the body is the idea that equates mind and spirit with masculinity, and body and evil with femininity. These ideas about the body and femininity, stemming from ancient Judeo-Christian religious ideas, are subtle yet powerful cultural persuasions, that contribute to our attitudes and feelings about ourselves. M. D. Hutchinson wrote:

> Man has soared the spiritual heights while Woman has remained mistress of the dark, mysterious, and powerful realm of the flesh, her body associated with instinct, irrationality, unpredictability, sensuality, uncleanness, evil, the power to give and take life itself. Because woman has been seen as essential but feared, she has been controlled.... In breaking free of the narrow and unnatural standards of our culture we are going against a very powerful historical current.[3]

Clarissa Pinkola Estes said in *Women Who Run With the Wolves*, "When women are relegated to moods, mannerisms, and contours that conform to a single ideal of beauty and behavior, they are captured in both body and soul, and are no longer free."[4]

The general public has a lack of understanding and information about eating disorders. Numbers of eating disorder cases are increasing, yet treatment remains complicated and controversial. Although research on eating disorders was abundant in the early to mid 1980s, the general public still understands little about the problem in the new millennium. Many eating disorder patients are high-school and college-age active competitive athletes. It is not uncommon to encounter athletes, even Olympic athletes, such as swimmers, who have been diagnosed with bulimarexia. The athletes continue to listen to their swimming coaches who strongly encourage them to keep their weight down and eat less. Little does the coach realize that he or she is inadvertently contributing to an athlete's attitudes toward eating and competitive play.

Educational curricula and teacher training programs in the U.S. from the 1950s through the late 1970s did not include body awareness, stress management, or the importance of developing keen kinesthetic sensory awareness. Of course, many teachers and coaches kept up with the latest research and incorporated these ideas into their teaching programs; however, it was not until the late 1970s that universities began to include wellness education, fitness training, and stress management in their teacher training programs.

The changes in the late 1970s encompassed dance therapy programs. Dance therapy students spent countless hours studying and learning anatomy, physiology, and concepts of body awareness. These concepts had not been introduced in high school or even undergraduate college for students in the 1960s. Training in dance therapy helps one to notice her body in new and helpful ways.

Clinicians began to realize that educating people — especially girls — about body image, body awareness and body sensations, deep relaxation, and stress management was one way to begin to approach the serious issue of eating disorders. Armed with the knowledge of family and individual characteristics of people with eating disorders, the growing body of literature discussing the historical and cultural influences that promote eating problems, and the lack of public awareness about eating disorders (including inadequate teacher training), clinicians began to devise practical techniques for educating girls and women about eating disorders and treating them.

These techniques centered around the concepts of (1) body image; (2) self-awareness (including feeling the sensations of hunger, satiety, tension and relaxation); (3) thinking patterns and how they relate to negative or positive feelings about oneself and to increased or decreased levels of tension; and (4) the influence of individual creativity on positive self-esteem and control over the healing process.

Vital modes of intervention that utilize these concepts are dance/movement therapy and other creative arts techniques such as drawing, working with clay, and creative writing. Perhaps it is paradoxical that the popular art form of dance has been a major culprit in touting the tall, thin, young body as ideal and the therapeutic techniques of dance therapy seek to help girls and women appreciate their bodies regardless of size, form, or age.

Activities should be developed to lead women from highly structured activities along a continuum into more free, creative dance and art experiences. These activities can be varied and utilized by teachers, clinicians, and educational leaders in a variety of settings.

The first of the four learning objectives to be presented in this chapter is to define the present concept of body image and understand how dance/movement and other creative art activities might affect one's perceptions of her own body. Paul Schilder in his now classic work, *The Image and Appearance of the Human Body*, defines the image of the body as "the picture of our own body which we form in our mind, that is to say the way in which our body appears to ourselves.... The body schema is the tri-dimensional image everybody has about himself."[5] The body image is a part of the larger self-image that develops through life.

A brilliant young psychoanalyst who came to the United States in 1930 to escape the Nazis, Shilder was one of the first people to seriously study and write about body image. Shilder understood body image as a constantly changing, shifting process affected by all aspects of life. He said, "The body-image is based not merely on associations, memory and experience, but also on intentions, will, aims, and tendencies."[5]

Shilder's work helped pave the way for the therapeutic use of dance/movement. According to Shilder, "There is another way of dissolving or weakening the rigid form of the postural model of the body, and that is movement and dance."[6] Although a complicated concept, movement obviously affects the body and the body image. Perhaps you remember playing spinning games when you were a child and the exhilarated, heightened sense of awareness and often distorted sense of reality that resulted from fast, furious spinning. This is a small example of how movement affects body image. Whenever we move, the postural model of the body changes. Dance, in particular, seems to have a loosening and changing effect on the body.

In addition, dance activities represent practical and wonderful ways to learn about non-verbal communication and observe how others communicate without words. Research indicates that a great deal of all our communication is non-verbal.[7] The more we learn about our own communication styles, the better we are able to communicate with others. Extensive modern dance studies enables one to understand what Barbara Mettler calls "the language of movement."[8] Anne Green Gilbert, author of *Creative Dance for All Ages*, makes a case for teaching the basic concepts of dance, rather than dance steps. Many dance educators and dance therapists agree that dance has the capacity to build healthy self-esteem and promote interpersonal communication.[9]

Furthermore, simple facts about anatomy and physiology can give students practical information, which they can utilize on their own — without the need for a doctor or a therapist. For example, information about interaction of breath, the spine and the rib cage often surprises and delights students. Everything they learn gives them more tools for their "coping bags."

Tension and relaxation of muscles, moving the body with and against gravity and centrifugal forces, may have an enormous influence on the body image.[10] This is confirmation for not only the active dance/movement activities, but activities involving deep relaxation and gentle breathing as well.

There is a tendency to over-simplify the concept of the body image. One can only hope that more research will be done in this area. The development of body image is a complex process influenced by all the inner and outer experiences a human being has. For purposes of reducing and managing stress through dance/movement activities, it is best to think of the body image as the reported experience — including thoughts, pictures, feelings, and sensations — a student has at any given time.

The second objective of enhancing self-awareness through dance/movement and other creative arts activities is often a major goal in psychotherapy and is often indicated for people with eating disorders. This includes helping students sense and feel emotions and other sensations such as hunger, satiety, excessive tension, and relaxation.

Many dance/movement activities engage the kinesthetic and proprioceptive sensory mechanisms of the body. These are physical processes that constantly operate in the body, but little attention is paid to what these physical processes tell us. The kinesthetic sense helps one to know where she is in space and sense movement. The proprioceptive receptors are located in muscles, tendons, joints and the inner ear. These receptors provide feedback about position, vibration, deep pressure, and pain.[11]

Dance therapy training also incorporates other creative arts techniques, such as drawing, clay modeling, and creative writing. Dance therapy students immerse themselves in many creative activities. Understanding the tools that heal helps one to nurture others. A keener awareness of feedback (feeling tense, tired, hungry, and full) the body so willingly provides is developed through the use of creative art activities.

The third objective concerns thinking patterns and how they influence negative and positive feelings about self as well as how thoughts and images can influence postural and muscular patterns of tension and relaxation. This objective leads one to the literature in the field of cognitive and behavioral psychology as well as biological research on the phenomenon of stress.[12] A noted author and researcher, Jean Houston, conducts workshops on how thinking patterns can affect feelings. She shares the ancient Buddhist meditation technique of repeating a word or phrase (a mantra) over and over. Repetition of these simple words and phrases is positive, uplifting, and designed to bring one closer to a state of inner peace. At one of her many workshops Jean recounted an example of a very contemporary mantra. She told of a woman who went around for days thinking, "Oh, I'm not good enough, I'm not good enough, I'm not good enough," until she believed it even more emphatically.[13] One can easily see that by the end of the day, this type of negative thinking would profoundly effect a person. By thinking negative mantras in our day-to-day existence, we program ourselves for failure. Negative thought patterns are prevalent for girls and women with eating disorders. In addition to the impact individual thought patterns have, research indicates that the images one carries and perpetuates can also be beneficial or detrimental.

In the field of dance, several people have pioneered important work utilizing imagery to promote body alignment and enhance movement capacities.[14] Joan Skinner uses a highly developed program which she calls Skinner Releasing Technique.[15] Her work has paramount significance in stress management, tension release, and the development of physical flexibility. Stephanie Skura, a choreographer who teaches the Skinner Release Technique, says:

> Letting go is a crucial preparation for allowing an image to truly move you. Releasing does not have to do with moving softly; it has to do with a constant flux without grabbing onto anything. You get your orientation not by holding onto some center, but by letting the energy flow within you, through you, and around you.[16]

These are tremendously important ideas for young girls and women to explore, especially those who are afraid of losing control. Many women and children with eating disorders do not feel they can control their environments, so they rely on controlling their bodies through appetite suppression. Whether you are a therapist or educator, you can teach girls and women activities and techniques for changing their negative thoughts and images into more positive, uplifting thinking. Self-awareness is the key, because most people pay little attention to their thinking patterns.

The fourth objective relates to understanding how dance/movement activities promote the creative process, reach the artist within each person, and enhance healing capacities. In addition to the practical and clinical aspects of dance therapy, another, more elusive, aspect is related to the creative process. The creative process has long been considered an avenue to healing and good health. The famous psychologist Carl Jung thought that creative play was a healing factor that operated in adults and children. Louis H. Stewart, a Jungian analyst, said, "By playing again like a child, with all the seriousness of a child at play, the adult revives lost memories, releases unconscious fantasies, and in the course of time, constellates the image of reconciliation and wholeness of the individuation process."[17]

Often, after an individual or group activity, my clients reported joy and wonder at their own creativity. As they symbolized their hurt, pain, and despair through, dance, drawing, or writing, something deep within shifted, and they experienced their own abilities to guide their healing processes. I think this symbolic process is at the heart of the transcendent function of the arts. We have thousands of years of countless examples of how the creative process has afforded humans a way to face the often frightening and painful realities of life through transforming this reality symbolically into dance, literature, music and painting. Even though it can seem magical, I believe there is a healthy, growing part in many people, which can be activated by the creative process. When our own efforts and strivings for health reach a deep part of the psyche through a creative art experience, feelings of hope and strength often permeate a person's entire emotional state. This can be quite powerful.

23.4 Application of Research Question

This part of the chapter is divided into four sections: (1) the warm-up; (2) activities designed to meet the four objectives outlined in the learning objectives; (3) suggestions for group leaders, teachers, and therapists; and (4) conclusions.

23.4.1 Warm-Up

23.4.1.1 Beginning and Ending

It is preferable to begin and end most groups with clients standing or seated in a circle. The circle is an ancient formation for humans and it is an arrangement which insures that everyone can see everyone else. The leader may do a "go round" and have each person share her name and something she hopes to get from the group. Depending on the group and the type of room, it is best for people to take off their shoes and socks. The feet have many sensory receptors and the stimulation often promotes a general good feeling. Every group leader must develop group rules, such as determining who can leave the group and for what reasons.

23.4.1.2 Warm-Up Activities

- Using music, one can talk the group through a movement warm-up beginning with the fingers and hands, then wrists, elbows, shoulders, torso, hips knees, ankles, feet and toes, ending with the face. Group participants should be encouraged to move each body part in any way they prefer in order to wake up the movement-feeling or kinesthetic sense in each part.
- Move one body part any way you want, then move two parts, then three.
- Find a new place in the circle while you move your hands, arms, shoulders, head, etc.
- While still in the circle, work with someone standing next to you; without touching, move your hands as though you were doing a duet. Then move your head, elbows, shoulders, and feet.
- After the group begins to solidify, the leader may have the participants pair up and give each other shoulder pats.
- The warm-up is also a good time to teach or reinforce knowledge about the body's anatomy — locating the ribs and scapulae, sensing and feeling the abdominal diaphragm, counting the number of spinal vertebrae, and learning about bones in the feet. Passing around pictures of the anatomy or posting pictures of the anatomy can be very helpful.

23.4.2 Activities Designed to Meet the Four Learning Objectives

23.4.2.1 Body Scan

In the early 1980s, Moshe Feldenkrais[18] introduced the body scan exercise to many dance therapists. Each time one does a body scan, the experience is different. There is no right or wrong information gleaned from a body scan. One simply notices as much as possible about all aspects of the body. It is best done lying down; however, the scan can be done seated or even standing. Group participants are asked to remain stationary in their designated postures.

The typical sequence of a body scan is as follows:

Close your eyes.

Notice your feet.

Notice whether your toes turn in or out.

Notice whether one foot feels different from the other.

Notice what parts of your legs rest fully on the floor and what parts seem to be raised off the floor.

Scan your entire spine from bottom to top. Parts of the spine may not be clear in your imaging. This is quite natural.

Move on to your shoulders, arms, and hands.

Notice your neck and throat.

Scan your tongue and the inside of your mouth.

Notice your jaw and face including your eyes.

Go back and scan your whole body. Don't strain or strive.

The scanning should be easy, even restful. The group should sit up slowly and easily and discuss what was noticed. A body scan has no generalized meanings. It is important to allow each person to interpret the meaning of his or her own scan.

23.4.2.2   Body Picture

Draw a picture of your body. It does not have to be representational. This is not about drawing an art product. The intent is to gain information about yourself. Review what you drew. Notice what parts you included and excluded and what colors you used.

23.4.2.3   Modeling with Clay

With eyes closed (or using a blindfold), mold a representation of your body with clay. Again, it can be lifelike or not. A person might mold a bowl and then explain how her body is like a bowl. Look at your finished clay piece and notice what parts of your body you emphasized and what parts you paid little attention to. What meanings, if any, do you make of your clay piece? How does it relate to your thoughts and images of your body?

23.4.2.4   Spine Visualization

Sit or lie down. Close your eyes and breathe easily. Do not take big, fast deep breaths when attempting to relax. That will cause more tension. Let your breathing be easy and gentle. Concentrate on relaxing the muscles of the lower abdomen. Think about your spine. Starting at the bottom of the spine, begin to imagine space between each vertebra. Allow yourself to think of beautiful, drifting clouds and imagine these clouds flowing easily in and out among your vertebrae. Imagine the vertebrae releasing, relaxing and letting go of tension. Continue this relaxed feeling for a while. When you are ready to sit up, draw a picture of your relaxed spine and/or discuss the experience with the group.

23.4.2.5   Body Part Visualization

Relax by sitting or lying down. Allow your body to relax from top to bottom and then from bottom to back. A good way to relax is to think of your body as relaxing, releasing all tension, and becoming calm and relaxed. Picture yourself walking on a beach. The day is just the way you like it — not too hot or too cold. Imagine yourself feeling alert, strong, carefree, and happy. As you stroll down the beach feeling your feet on the warm, damp sand, you reach a beautiful pile of rocks. You sit down and then you stretch out on one of the large rocks and relax even more deeply. You become aware of a part of your body that troubles you, a part which you don't like or perhaps you find unattractive. Begin a dialog with this body part. Ask the part to talk with you, to tell you how it feels and what it needs from you. Let this dialog continue for 2 min. (At the end of 2 min the leader should begin speaking again.) Say good-bye to this body part and be aware that you can talk again whenever you like. Feel yourself beginning to stretch and sit up on a large rock. Now begin your walk back down the beach. Know that you have had a profound and deep encounter with a part of yourself. Take your time and gently come to a sitting position and bring your awareness back to the group. The leader may want to lead a discussion and ask people to share what they learned or each person could write about her experience of dialoging with a body part.

23.4.2.6 Body Part Drawing

Draw a picture of some part of your body which often seems tense. Perhaps you would like to use shapes, symbols, or specific colors. When you have finished, decide whether you want to add words to your drawing. After this exercise, thoughts may be shared with the group.

23.4.2.7 Breathing

Sit or lie down. Perhaps you want a pillow under your head or your knees. Make sure you are as comfortable as possible. Notice your breathing. Do not change it. What do you notice? What moves when you breathe? Can you think of any metaphors that seem to fit your breathing? Is it like a gentle breeze, a noisy, slow train, an ocean wave? There are no right or wrong answers. Continue breathing for 5 to 10 min, then sit up and discuss what you discovered.

23.4.2.8 Breathing for Tension Release

Think of a particular part of your body that carries tension. Perhaps your shoulders or neck feel tense. Sit or lie in a comfortable position. Allow yourself to relax as much as possible. Without straining, begin to bring your breath deeply into your abdomen. See whether you can easily breathe in through your nose and out through parted lips. Allow your breath to be smooth, slow, and easy. Stop and rest any time. When you feel ready, begin to imagine that you are directing your breath, into a part of your body that is tense or painful. Imagine the breath permeating this body part. Imagine the breath bringing a special feeling of calmness and peace to the area. Think of the area as loose, wide, spacious, and very relaxed. Continue this exercise for a few minutes. After about 10 to 15 min, stop, rest, and return to a sitting position. Notice how you feel and share your thoughts and feelings with the group.

23.4.2.9 Exploring Basic Locomotor Movements

Play music with a good, steady beat. Invite each participant to explore the basic movements of walking, running, skipping, leaping, jumping, hopping, sliding, and galloping. Give people plenty of time to rest. Sometimes instead of recorded music, it is interesting to use a small drum to produce rhythm as the people move. After exploring these movements, sit down and discuss what thoughts and feelings these movements evoked.

23.4.2.10 Exploring Movements in Place

After a warm-up, invite each person to fully explore making these movements: wiggle, writhe, squirm, stretch, bend, twist, turn, flop, collapse, fall, shake, swing, sway, rock, spring, bounce, bob, jump, undulate, whirl, spin, lurch, sag, slump, pounce, and jostle.[19] Rest and then discuss what effects (if any) these movements had on each person.

23.4.2.11   Exploring Movements from Place to Place

After a warm-up, call out these movements for people to explore: creep, crawl, roll, walk, skip, run, gallop, leap, hop, stride, prance, strut, stroll, stagger, march, scurry, trudge, stalk, race, scramble, and hustle.[19] Rest and discuss the experience.

23.4.2.12   Creative Writing for Discovery

Ask the participants to sit or lie in a comfortable position. Ask each person to keep pen and paper nearby. Engage the participants in a short relaxation activity. For example, suggest that the group members relax from head to toe, and again, from toe to head. Participants may picture a calming, soft light of any color they choose. Suggest that the light travels down through their heads and fills every cell in their bodies, bringing deep relaxation to all parts of their bodies. Following this short relaxation activity, ask each person to write a list of negative phrases they often think about concerning their own bodies. After 5 min, ask them to pick three phrases from their lists. Show the group how to create an affirmation from a negative phrase. For example, if someone wrote, "I can't stop eating too much," a positive version might read, "Every time I eat, I eat a healthy amount." Affirmations should be stated in a positive way in the present tense. "I will stop eating too much" applies to the future and is not a present-tense affirmation. Affirmations work better if the person writes or says the affirmation many times and floods her consciousness with the positive statement. I generally write an affirmation a minimum of 15 times. Another effective strategy is to imagine the affirmation is true as stated. For example, a participant could imagine herself eating a healthy amount of food she writes, "Every time I eat, I eat a healthy amount."

23.4.2.13   Practicing Imagery

Imagery is an activity that improves with practice. You can help group members to increase their skills by asking them to participate in imagery exercises. Have the members sit or lie in a comfortable position, close their eyes, and imagine that they are looking at a movie screen. Suggest that they picture a soft, black kitten on the screen, let that go, then see a beautiful, snow-capped mountain on the screen, followed by a marching band in a parade. As that image dissolves, they can picture a large tree with beautiful green leaves, followed by a red rose, and a field of wheat waving in the wind. They can imagine smelling newly mown grass and think about hearing church bells ringing in the distance or a small kitten walking on piano keys. Other suggested images are running hands down the rough bark of a tree, petting soft kitten's fur, the smell of a fresh wood fire, the smell of freshly baked bread, the taste of a fresh orange, too much salt on a bite of potato, and a taste of fresh spring water. This imaging activity can be repeated.

23.4.2.14   Exploring Tension and Relaxation through Movement

After a warm-up, have the group explore the polarity between tension and relaxation through movement. They should lie on the floor and make tense movements with their bodies. They should try to make every part of their bodies tense. The next step is to make more tense movements while sitting or squatting followed by making these movements while standing and moving through space. After a rest, they can explore making relaxed movements while lying, sitting, standing, and moving through space. After another rest, the group should sit in a circle and discuss what they discovered with the therapist.

23.4.2.15   *Exploring other Polarities through Movement*

The intent is to explore through movement the polarity of large and small, up and down, fast and slow and any other parameters you choose. Give the participants an opportunity to discuss what they discover.

23.4.2.16   *Making Shapes*

After a warm-up, another technique is to explore making shapes: Make a shape with the whole body, then let it dissolve and make another shape. Keep this up for a while. Try to use the whole body, not only the arms and hands, but also the torso, shoulders, and knees. Make the shapes first at low level (lying down), then at mid-level (sitting, squatting, or kneeling), and then at high or standing level. Shapes can be made in one place or while moving throughout the room. After a rest, reactions can be discussed.

23.4.2.17   *Movement and Stillness*

After a warm-up, introduce the idea of moving freely through space, then freezing into a still shape, then continuing to repeat the cycle — movement followed by stillness. Emphasize the freedom of this activity so that participants can move and be still whenever they choose. Encourage people to experience the stillness as an important part of the activity. After exploring this activity, the group can rest and discuss the responses.

23.4.2.18   *Movements and Emotions*

After a warm-up, ask participants to move freely, exploring movements with their bodies that express sadness, then joy, then anger, then fear, or any other emotions you or they choose. Rest and discuss the results.

23.4.2.19   *Shapes Pertaining to Certain Times of Life*

After a warm-up, ask the participants to make shapes related to certain times in their lives, for example, the past, the present, the future, first grade, or high school. This can be a very creative activity that allows imaginations to soar. The group participants will probably want to choose shape topics.

23.4.2.20   *Putting Movements Together*

Ask the participants to make up three movements that have some meaning for them, for example, a movement pertaining to the past, present, and future. Ask them to move for 5 to 10 min, molding the movements into one long phrase. The movement becomes a very short dance. The idea, again, is not about a finished product, but about how they think and feel about what they do. This might be a good time for group members to witness each other's movements. Only the mover speaks after moving, because the experience is intended to discover how she thinks and feels about what she creates, without facing criticism.

23.4.2.21   *Witnessing*

After a warm-up, divide the group into two parts. Half of the group moves, and half of the group witnesses. After the first group moves for an agreed amount of time (5 to 10 min is recommended for beginners), they then sit in a circle. Allow only the movers to speak. Repeat this process after the second group moves.[20] Time for drawing, writing, and clay work after each movement round can make this an even more deeply meaningful activity. Witnessing is part of a dance form called authentic movement by some and contemplative dance by others.*

23.4.3 Suggestions for Group Leaders, Teachers, and Therapists

- Start and end the groups in a familiar way.
- Give members as much freedom as possible to participate or sit out and observe (except during the witnessing activity). Encourage group members to share only what they feel comfortable sharing when they discuss the activities.
- Do not become too dependent on music for the warm-up. Allow group participants to find their own rhythms.
- Constantly emphasize the neutrality of activities, thoughts, and images. There are no right or wrong thoughts or images. Group members may need encouragement to think positive, healing thoughts and images, but their thoughts are not wrong.
- Encourage the group members to be as detailed as possible in their discussions about body sensations, increased body awareness, moments of hunger, and times of feeling full. Areas of the body that carry excess tension should be explored in times of sensations and at times when the body feels calm and relaxed. Helping the group members to make connections between what they do and learn in the group and what they think and feel outside the group is important.

23.4.4 Conclusions

Because of a vast amount of writing in the area of stress management, imagery, creative arts therapies, body-mind interaction and psycho-educational groups, a resourceful leader will never run out of material. Leaders may feel that their techniques have failed as often as they feel that their methods have been successful. This is not unusual. A group leader should keep striving to offer creative activities because the experience can make a difference in the lives of the participants even if the leader does not see immediate, remarkable results. Human nature is difficult to change, but people continue to learn. Continue your efforts and become creative with your leadership. The activities that have been presented are only suggestions and springboards for your own creative exercises. A modern dance pioneer, Ruth St. Denis, profoundly stated, "I see the dance being used as a means of communication between soul and soul — to express what is too deep, too fine for words."[21]

References

1. Wilson, C.P., The family psychological profile and its therapeutic implications, in *Fear of Being Fat*, Wilson C.P., Hogan C.C., and Mintz I.L., Eds., Jason Aronson, Inc., New York, 1985, chap. 2.

* I am especially grateful for my studies with Mary Ramsay and Alton Wasson for this technique.

2. Hutchinson, M.G., *Transforming Body Image*, The Crossing Press, Trumansburg, NY, 1985, 63.
3. Hutchinson, M.D., *Transforming Body Image*, The Crossing Press, Trumansburg, NY, 1985, 147.
4. Estes, C.P., *Women Who Run with the Wolves*, Ballantine Books, New York, 1992, 200.
5. Shilder, P., *The Image and Appearance of the Human Body*, John Wiley & Sons, New York, 1964, 206.
6. Feldenkrais, M., personal communication, February, 1980.
7. Knapp, M.L., *Nonverbal Communication in Human Interaction*, Holt, Rinehart & Winston, New York, 1972, 12.
8. Mettler, B., Personal communication, 1987.
9. Gilbert, A.G., *Creative Dance for All Ages*, American Alliance for Health, Physical Education, Recreation and Dance, 1992, 3–4.
10. Shilder, P., *The Image and Appearance of the Human Body*, John Wiley & Sons, New York, 1964, 208.
11. Anthony, C.P. and Thibodeau, G.A., *Textbook of Anatomy and Physiology*, 10th ed., C.V. Mosby, St. Louis, 1979, 290.
12. Pelletier, K. R., *Mind as Healer, Mind as Slayer*, Dell Publishing, New York, 1977, 124–291.
13. Houston, J., lecture, Houston, 1987.
14. Todd, M.E., *The Thinking Body*, Dance Horizons, New York, 1937 (reprinted 1975).
15. Skinner, J., personal communication, 1998.
16. Skura, S., in *Dynamic Alignment through Imagery*, Franklin, E., Ed., Human Kinetics, 1996, 9.
17. Stewart, L.H. et al., *Sandplay Studies*, C.G. Jung Institute, San Francisco, CA, 1981, 36.
18. Feldenkrais, M., personal communication, 1981.
19. Mettler, B., personal communication, 1988.
20. Ramsay, M. and Wasson, A., personal communications, 1996–1997.
21. St. Denis, R., in *Dance Lovers' Quotations*, Exley, H., ed., Exley Giftbooks, New York, 1994.

24

The Role of Nutrition in the Treatment of an Eating Disorder Patient

Jan Hamilton

CONTENTS

24.1 Learning Objectives

After completing this chapter you should be able to:

- Understand new biochemical markers;
- Comprehend the effects of hormonal imbalances;
- Assess and evaluate physiological parameters relating to eating disorders;
- Apply new knowledge in diagnosing and treating eating disorders.

24.2   Research Background

24.2.1   Introduction

Is it possible to treat eating disorders (EDs) from a platform of total acceptance through nurturing and nutritional balance and to lead patients to become inwardly motivated to live a lifestyle that includes meeting their own nutritional needs? If this is possible, how can it be done? An individual network of biochemical, hormonal, physiological, and psychological factors comprises the nutritional equilibrium or imbalance of every person and thus the appetite and food choices of an eating disorder patient. When these systems develop irregular patterns, anorexia nervosa (AN), bulimia nervosa (BN), binge eating disorders (BD) and obesity are potential outcomes.

Nutrition influences etiologies and outcomes of most disease processes. This is certainly true for EDs. ED cannot be addressed without incorporating the nutritional needs of the individual. Although ED is widely accepted as a psychological disease the disease was not listed in the *Diagnostic and Statistical Manual of Mental Disorders* until 1987. ED was included under several other categories for 300 years before that.[1,2] One example of an early dilemma recognized by healthcare professionals was exercise-induced anorexia. It was challenging to differentiate between the purely psychological and the physiologically induced components of the anorectic condition. Effective nutritional programs for individuals with AN, BN, and ED can be implemented, but until an endogenous balance of psychological and physiological components occurs, success is often not achieved.

For many individuals with ED and other imbalances, a more ephemeral balance, one of spirit, mind, and body, must be achieved for the necessary healing to occur. The body is designed to heal itself when all necessary components are in synergy. This is also the case with healing ED, despite the substantial psychological aspects. The unique personality, background, and biochemistry of each eating behavior patient must be analyzed, so no stereotyped design for nutritional programs can be written.

Basic nutritional programs should address the typical needs of all components of the Recommended Daily Dietary Allowances including vitamins, minerals, and energy needs as listed in Appendices 24 A-D. However, an individual cannot be forced to meet these needs. If overt coercion is a factor in the behavioral change process, negative outcomes are likely. Within the decision making process of each individual lies the perception that he or she is fat and that consuming excessive amounts of food is detrimental. In order to overcome those perceptions, new biochemical nutritional tests can show physiological markers of each individual, revealing new insights. The power of such assessments lies in their objective nature; such information is inherently much more persuasive than a subjective evaluation of body dimensions, particularly if subjective information is at odds with a patient's view of her own needs.

New laboratory tests are designed to measure hormonal levels, antioxidant status, and the adequacy of nutritional intake, and thus determine deficiencies in nutritional status. See Appendix 24-E for Clinical Signs Associated with Nutritional Deficiencies. Test results can then be used to measure profiles and determine the extent to which a patient deviates from healthy ranges of nutrient assimilation. With this information, healthcare professionals can advise ED patients with greater accuracy and with a greater element of trust, which is perhaps the greatest advantage to such an objective approach. Patients can also see signs of progress, and thereby turn to proactive approaches to their health.

24.3 Physiological Markers in Eating Disorders

The obvious physiological disturbances of patients with ED have led to speculation that their profoundly abnormal behavior is caused by primary biological abnormalities. Disruptions of the gastrointestinal tract, the pituitary, the adrenals, and neurotransmitters have been proposed as causal factors in the development of nutritionally based diseases. Recent studies in AN patients reveal new physiological systems relevant to eating behavior. An increase in serotonin leads to reductions in food intake. Decreased amino acids such as tryptophan, a serotonin precursor, in the brain are associated with depression. Increased levels of serotonin reflect decreased relative intake of carbohydrates and a decrease in blood glucose levels.[3] These indicators show a direct correlation to increased levels of depression and food intake abnormalities.

Leptin is a hormone secreted by fat cells that appears to play an important role in regulation by the hypothalamus of body fat stores. Consistent with reduced fat tissue, underweight individuals with AN have low serum levels of leptin, which increase as body weight increases. Along with hormonal effects on food intake and body weight are changes in levels of female sex hormones measured throughout the menstrual cycle — particularly in the luteal phase. Additionally, disturbances in the insulin-like growth factor hormone balance have been shown in ED patients.[4,5] Recently, female sex hormones have been shown to affect eating behavior and food choices. Higher levels of progesterone can correlate to increased intake of chocolate, fat, and sugar. A nurturing balance of endogenous chemistry with the awareness of potential outcomes is essential to the design of nutritional programs for eating-disordered individuals. Abnormalities triggered by endogenous and exogenous sources should be examined and addressed in the care and treatment of these patients.

24.3.1 Eating Patterns

Eating is a necessary part of the survival of all species and is a well-established pattern of behavior from birth to death. Therefore, the individual pattern of what, when, where, and how much to eat is the product of a complex pattern of habit and socialization and body chemistry. The conflicting feelings and debilitating nature of AN and BN have been reported in the *Harvard Mental Health Letter*.[6] When normal patterns go amiss from ages 15 to 30, the years of optimal hormonal function, we must measure and address the entire chemistry of the body, not only food intake. The influences on these choices are many. The choices surrounding eating patterns and quantities remain within the power of the individual. This makes ED a very complicated disease process.

Eating choices often become a battlefield on which the patient expresses a personal need for control of her own body and the world outside. Personal habits are formed by each individual — ranging from the refusal to ingest even a simple food to restriction at minimal intake, or relieving the body of food already ingested through purging. Since a patient typically begins therapy in a state of profound imbalance consequent to a prolonged period of sub-optimal nutrition, the analysis and treatment of her basic nutritional needs through the early and critical stages are imperative for her survival. With attentive nurturing through all avenues of healing, an individual can be led to self-healing through personal motivation to become more aware of her value and become more motivated to return to optimal health.

24.3.2   Therapeutic Modalities with Emphasis on the Team Approach

We do not yet have a cure for ED. There are more questions than answers surrounding the diagnosis and treatment of ED in the fields of psychiatry, medicine, and nutrition.[2] However, current reports reveal that the first image a healthcare professional portrays becomes established in the mind of the patient. This provides the basis for the unique and individual treatment of each patient in a positive relationship. Caregivers must remain cognizant of the fact that a patient's own eating patterns reflect her unique decision and express a very deep need. A team of healthcare professionals from various disciplines is necessary to formulate a network of care through which an individual can realize her value and begin to have a happy life. Healthcare professionals must foster and preserve this gallant effort and demonstrate that the individuality of each patient has merit and significance. As vital members of this team of healthcare professionals, we must educate ourselves and stay open to all treatment options.

Early attention to nutritional needs of the ED patient is necessary to prevent the onset of atrophy of the whole body. A study reported in the March 16, 1996 edition of *Dagens Nyheter*, the largest newspaper in Sweden, suggests that psychiatric treatment of anorexia is typically a first line of treatment that has not proven successful according to the parents of formerly anorexic girls who were treated successfully at the Center for Eating Disorders, Karolinska Institute, Huddinge University Hospital, Stockholm. The successful treatments included spirituality, nurturing, and close physical contact. Parents faced much opposition because they believed empirically that it was a mistake to classify anorexia as a purely psychological or mental illness. These parents clearly believe that the disease goes beyond the purely psychological dimension, and that current medical approaches in the U.S. are very different and often ineffective.

Regardless of the official classification of the disease state created for ED, we know that the ravaging effects of starvation (whatever the causes) are life threatening.[1] The diagnosis is often suspected by the family first, and is typically confirmed by a physician as the evidence of atrophy appears. Atrophy in general is related to changes in nutrition and metabolic activities of cells and tissues. The unavailability of certain essential protein components and vitamins disturbs the metabolic processes, and that leads to atrophy of cells and tissues. In certain conditions of protein starvation, the body protein is broken down into constituent amino acids, which serve to provide energy and help maintain the integrity of the most essential organs. See Appendix 24-C for data on estimated safe and adequate daily dietary intakes of selected vitamins and minerals. Atrophy accounts for the loss in muscle tissue after fat stores are depleted in the ED patient. When the diagnosis is made late in this disease, the metabolic impact of starvation and malnutrition must be treated very carefully and skillfully because the body is very fragile.[7]

Nutritional needs are often discussed and implemented as a first line of defense but due to the absence of an integration of treatment approaches, continued success is not often achieved. The delay often occurs from sporadic compliance with nutritional interventions that are forced or mandated during the course of treatment, causing the patient to feel out of control. The patient's avoidance of medical care creates the extreme manifestation seen when the patient is admitted to the emergency room and requires parenteral therapy.[7] This can occur at the onset of the disease, during treatment, or as a relapse if success is inaccurately perceived. By then, the nutritional needs of the patient are acute and must be addressed abruptly through intravenous feeding to keep her alive. This typically occurs when enteral therapy has already failed. Clearly at this point, it is appropriate to address the basic needs for nurture through nourishment as a first line of treatment.

The life-threatening nature of eating disorders makes the measurement of basic hormonal and nutritional biomarkers in urine and serum by laboratory analysis an essential and imperative component of comprehensive patient care. Detailed nutritional analysis allows the team of the nutritionist and the physician to function optimally, as soon as the disease is suspected or diagnosed.[8] New tests developed at the Johnson Space Center by Dr. Richard Cutler to assess the normal levels of nutritional biomarkers of astronauts now provide heretofore unavailable details of analytical biochemistry. These biomarkers were designed to assess oxidative stress, hormonal levels, anti-oxidant levels, vitamin and mineral levels, and toxicity denoting imbalances, which could lower autoimmune response. Levels were compared to those of a well population entered in the database of the Centers for Disease Control in Atlanta, Georgia. Based on the latest NHANES studies, this information provides healthcare professionals with new data on the nutritional biochemistry of the ED patient.

24.3.3 Biochemistry Assessment

According to the Harvard Mental Health Letter,[6] the level of female hormones in the blood and urine of an anorexic woman falls drastically, and her menses and sexual function may be delayed. Exogenous hormone administration for purposes of contraception, disease management in osteoporosis, cardiovascular disease, and anti-aging therapy has become a major therapeutic approach. The largest potential benefit of estrogen replacement therapy is the prevention of heart disease, the major cause of death in females. In countries where relatively high risk of heart disease exists, current studies suggest that estrogen reduces that risk by 50%.[9] The decline in estrogen in the ED patient may also play a role in her survival. After recent clinical trials showed the protective cardiovascular effects of hormone replacement therapy, a large number of women in the U.S. and other developed countries may be prescribed extended estrogen replacement therapy to reduce cardiovascular disease.[10]

However, very little is known about the effects of exogenous hormones on energy balance in women. Such research is needed related to females with ED. If measurements are not taken, healthcare professionals cannot be sure whether the hormonal imbalance induces the illness or the illness initiates the hormonal imbalance. Between puberty and menopause, serum estrogen and progesterone levels vary throughout the menstrual cycle. According to Becker in *Principles and Practice of Endocrinology and Metabolism*,[11] the follicular phase is estrogen dominant with high concentrations of estrogen and low progesterone levels. During the luteal phase, the progesterone levels rise to a level where neither hormone is dominant. With ED, the level of estradiol, produced primarily by the ovaries, falls and is replaced by a less active estrogen, estrone, produced primarily by conversion of androstendione in adipose tissue. The decline in adipose tissue in the ED patient may inhibit an otherwise normal event. After the onset of ED, endogenous estrogen production by the ovaries can further decrease. Progesterone appears to decline at the same ratio as estrogens. Women with ED have a widespread perception that increased food intake and body weight are marks of weakness and that deprivation is indicative of strength and stamina. Those who are already underweight and those who continue to lose weight by increasing caloric expenditure through excessive exercise both subscribe to this fallacy. Insofar as education can be implemented to dissuade patients from their fallacious beliefs, the assessment and discussion of critical biomarkers — hormonal and nutritional — are imperative in the treatment of the ED patient.

24.3.4   Impacts of Societal Concern with Thinness

Among women who are already at medical risk for ED, steps need to be taken to minimize the impacts of media advertisements on weight loss, especially in the vulnerable age groups between 15 and 30. A report by Manson et al.[12] in the Nurses' Health Study cited norms for weight at age 18 and said weight beyond that baseline can be considered excessive. Body weight management to reduce health risks is prudent. However, this kind of reporting can create often negative health behaviors, particularly in the younger female population. Normal weight gain as one matures and enters childbearing years may protect against the increased caloric expenditure of nursing babies. In women of puberty and early childbearing ages, the rates of anorexia nervosa and bulimia are increasing. Body weight increase has become a national paranoia.

This attitude is manifested by the fact that $33 billion is spent yearly on weight control in this country.[13] Low fat diets and body weight reduction in the female segment of the population have become national obsessions. Therefore, the issue of whether health perceptions correlate to thinness must be examined critically. It is important to know the impacts hormone levels have on food choices and weight gain due to use of contraceptives and hormone replacement. Due to the current emphasis on thinness and low fat diets,[14] women often resist use of exogenous agents that could lead to weight gain regardless of the potential positive effects. Therapeutic use of certain pharmaceutical agents during an illness may be ignored because of perceived body weight implications. Some reports in the early 1990s on the effects of contraceptives on health risks in women show that after adjustments for age and smoking, the risk of ED is 3.3 times higher in a woman with a body mass index (BMI) of <19.0 compared to a woman with a BMI of >24.0. Therefore, if a female feels that prescriptions can cause body weight increases, she may decline their use or fail to comply with a physician's orders for care.

24.4   Application of Research Question

24.4.1   Compliance Issues

What can be done to increase the compliance rates in therapeutic treatment modalities? Recent publications have cited reasons for the wide range of compliance problems, with body weight as one of the most prevalent. However, with increased general awareness of new information regarding the effects of decreased body weight on increased risk of osteoporosis, the overall rate of dietary therapeutic intervention has become surprisingly high. In the case of bone density, clearly more than calcium intake is implicated; the intake of certain synthetic hormones also affects the loss of bone. Body weight increase is the primary reason for noncompliance with therapeutic orders for contraceptives and hormone replacement therapy.

Among the list of negative side effects are persistent food intake complications and cravings, severe mood changes, and lack of adaptation and response to manipulation of therapy programs. Projected new clinical research trials will provide guidance on clinical evaluation of combinations containing drug interventions and dietary supplements. The earliest reports by leaders in the field state that, in clinical trials, the new drugs and dietary supplements should: (1) initially compare the rate of weight increase or decrease in the treated group to that of a placebo group; (2) report the lowest dose that ensures that daily dietary intake needs are met; and (3) establish the minimum effective dose of a specific dietary supplement for any given physiological marker.[15–17] Perhaps these new dietary supplement guidelines will address earlier misconceptions, decrease negative physiological side effects of some pharmaceutical agents, and ultimately increase compliance rates among those who are at risk and in need of medical nutritional therapy. However, if the perception of increased body weight is one of those side effects, the problem is often greater to overcome. More than vanity is at stake. A study to investigate the impact of dietary deficiencies in 15- to 39-year-old females and the correlation to ED is needed to assess the impact of dietary deficiencies as an increased risk factor for ED. According to the National Institutes of Health, up to 3% of all American females are underweight due to ED, and the numbers appear to be increasing yearly.[18]

24.4.2 Relevant Research Issues

Health implications surrounding ED and body weight are also relevant because it is known that the chemistry associated with ED contributes to additional appetite decline and decreased nutritional intake. The problem of taking dietary supplements is compounded if the perception also exists that the protective effect will be offset by the increased weight gain. The issue of whether medical nutritional therapy through dietary supplementation contributes to additional body weight gain should be scientifically measured and reported.

Currently, the use of IV nutrition with more than glucose in the critically ill ED patient is yielding positive outcomes in clinical trials. A multiplicity of nutritional needs can be met through IV therapy that can restore the ED patient to a state of nutritional balance when oral intake is impossible. Formulations can be compounded by a pharmacy or purchased in prepared vitamin-rich dosages ready for IV administration. The current emphasis on dietary fat intake has created a concern regarding anything that might trigger an appetite for fat. The perception exists that the higher levels of fat intake may contribute to additional weight increases. Fat intake has also been correlated to satiety and absorption of essential fatty acids necessary for nutritional balance and metabolic harmony. Dietary fat from the proper sources, consumed at appropriate levels of intake, can actually decrease cravings for uncontrolled caloric intake through carbohydrate consumption.

Another research question that has recently surfaced is of whether synthetic dietary supplements and plant sources (often called natural forms) of vitamins and minerals have different metabolic effects. Dietary supplement intake may be driven by biological factors as well as biochemical indices of deficiencies. Dietary supplementation intake may be needed in ED patients with a number of nutrition-related disorders. Additionally, the consumption of calorie-rich foods may relate to palatability, high energy density, and the ultimate positive physiological effects. Body weight increase may be induced by a decrease in exercise and/or increased caloric intake. Additional research is needed to understand metabolic implications of dietary supplementation and how the sensory qualities of foods and individual differences in preferences for dietary supplement intake influence subsequent human food intake, body composition and general health.[19] Changes in food intake during ED disease may also change the nutrient intake patterns related to the process.[20] Metabolic demands and hormonal levels can affect the ratio of the intake of fats, carbohydrates and proteins. Clearly, exercise, resting metabolic rate, and the ratio at which calories are converted into body weight under the influence of additional demands of ED must be examined as part of the body weight profile.[21]

Malnutrition in elderly patients with ED is an equally challenging eating behavior concern. The choice of high calorie sweet foods is often a preference both for their palatability and practicality, since they typically need little or no preparation time. Research must be designed to address the state of malnutrition surrounding these perplexing questions. More information is needed to provide preliminary data on the biochemistry, endocrinology, and metabolic implications for the elderly ED patient. The focus of future research should involve the body weight implications of the relationship between macronutrient food choices, body weight, and dietary supplements. The body weight consequences of changes in physiological status through excessive exercise with and without dietary supplementation should be examined. Changes in macronutrient preference, caloric conversion ratios, and the measurement of body composition should be examined. Contemporary models of the regulation of energy balance should investigate and emphasize the physiological signals such as appetite, increase or decrease in energy expenditure, and lethargy. See Appendix 24-D for data on median heights and weights and recommended energy intake.

Female research subjects should be studied to obtain data on body weight, caloric regulation, and macronutrient choices at measured hormonal levels in a controlled environment. Future studies of biochemical markers in the ED patient will provide an arena in which to examine questions that could otherwise not be investigated and answered in human subjects. The tests developed for astronauts at the National Institutes of Health by Dr. Richard Cutler[8] provide the most comprehensive nutritional profile currently available through the analysis of the serum and urine. Newly released laboratory tests are in use at the Johnson Space Center. What will the results of these tests portend in terms of current body weight increase concepts reported by television and the popular press, and taught in weight control clinics across the country? We may learn that metabolic regulators affecting body weight go beyond merely counting calories. It may be that at certain times of the month in the normally cycling female or the aging postmenopausal female on cyclical hormone replacement therapy, food intake is converted into body weight at different ratios. It may be the case that energy expenditure changes or hormonally induced lethargy occur cyclically or even that a totally different dynamic exists and has not yet been fully discovered.

For the female human population, it is the desire of this scientist to propose new individualized assessments of dosage levels of hormone replacement therapy to protect against ED, osteoporosis, cardiovascular disease, and cancer. Risk assessments calculated for each female individually, based on her stress levels, genetic predisposition to these diseases prior to prescribing exogenous supplementation would seem to be an appropriate system of analysis. With this information, she can then make decisions based on medical and scientific evidence. Negative symptoms of ED that impact compliance rates of medical nutrition therapy are typically not measured in humans.[22] Further investigations are needed to measure hormonal effects on macronutrient food choice, caloric regulation, food intake, and subsequent impacts on body weight and composition in humans.

The following questions need to be researched. Do calories convert into body weight at different ratios under the influences of various hormone levels? Is change in body weight evidence of a malfunction in the set point hypothesis? Is the human system that has worked well for centuries being altered by exogenous xenobiotics from the environment, progestins, estrogens, or endogenous hormones, which could cause the set point to be altered in unexpected, unpredicted, and undesirable ways? Is all of this the result of a biological survival mechanism that provides additional energy during the luteal phase when the body is potentially preparing to support new life? New information collected in an aging model that is designed to investigate female body weight increase will provide insights in this area, and hopefully provide a basis for more extensive investigation in ED in the future. Additionally further information will assist in answering the perplexing question of the impact of female sex hormones on body weight and food intake. The hormonal phase (endogenous levels) in the normally cycling female may affect food intake and body weight data, and should therefore be measured and documented in all future ED research studies.

ED may cause metabolic differences in the way calories are converted into body weight; the conversion may be affected by both endogenous and exogenous female sex hormones. Eating behavior, food choices, and caloric regulation may also be affected by endogenous and exogenous female sex hormones. Higher protein intake through the consumption of red meat by the postmenopausal female during breakthrough bleeding can be of value if she is deficient in heme iron. New research is needed to reset the set point at which stress and genetic or environmental factors violate or disturb this hypothesized metabolic mechanism.[23]

The larger question encompassing all previously discussed parameters is "What determines body weight fluctuations?" Body weight gain and loss by ED patients can relate to hormonal profiles; individual levels should be measured. Research findings in the aging rat model do not agree with earlier findings in the young rat model. In older rats, additional food intake resulting in additional body weight gain correlated to higher progesterone levels. Increased levels of progesterone have been shown to increase caloric intake and alter macronutrient sources[24] with an accompanying increase in percent body fat stores.

Clearly, more than eating behavior is involved in the study of the ED patient. New biochemical markers are capable of providing additional laboratory values that heretofore have not been utilized. New information may appear as individual levels of hormones and nutritional biomarkers are measured and evaluated by a team of healthcare professionals. The unlocked mysteries may be solved through new biochemical investigations.

References

1. Walsh, B.T. and Devlin, M.J., Eating disorders: progress and problems, *Science*, 280, 13870, 1998.
2. Hamilton J.B., Satiety of protein sources, *FASEB*, 11, 1276, 1993.
3. Wurtman R.J. and Wurtman J.J., Brain serotonin, carbohydrate-craving, obesity and depression, *Obesity Research*, Suppl. 4, 477S, 1994.
4. Eckert, E.D., Pomeroy, C., Raymond, N., Kohler, P.F., Thuras, P., and Bowers, C.Y., Leptin in anorexia nervosa, *Journal of Clinical Endocrinology and Metabolism*, 83, 791, 1998.
5. Argente, J., Caballo, N., Barrios, V., Munoz, M. T., Pozo, J., Chowen, J. A., and Hernandez, M., Disturbance in the growth hormone insulin-like growth factor axis in children and adolescents with different eating disorders, *Hormone Research*, 48, Suppl. 4, 16, 1997.
6. *Harvard Mental Health Letter*, parts II and III, October/November, 1997.
7. Mehler, P.S. and Weiner, K.L., Anorexia nervosa and total parenteral nutrition, *International Journal of Eating Disorders*, 14, 297, 1993.
8. Cutler R., *The Genox Oxidative Stress Profile: An Overview on its Assessment and Application*, Birkhauser Verlag, Basel, 1998.
9. World Health Organization, *World Health Statistics Annual*, World Health Organization, Geneva, 1989.

10. Writing Group for the PEPI Trial, Effects of estrogen/progestin regimens on heart disease risk factors in postmenopausal women, *Journal of the American Association*, 273, 199, 1995.
11. Becker, K.L., Principles and practice of endocrinology and metabolism, Lippincott, Philadelphia, 1990.
12. Manson, J.E., Willett, W.C., Stampfer, M.J., Colditz, G.A., Hunter, D.J., Hankinson, S.E., Hennekens, C.H., and Speizer, F.E., Body weight and mortality among women, *New England Journal of Medicine*, 333, 677, 1995.
13. Atkinson, R.L., Cost effectiveness of the treatment of obesity: treatment of the patient with medically significant obesity, North American Workshop on Study of Obesity, Atlanta, December, 1990.
14. Ley, C.J., Lees, B., and Stevenson, J.C., Sex and menopause-associated changes in body fat distribution, *American Journal for Clinical Nutrition*, 55, 950, 1992.
15. Grady, D. and Cummings, S.R., Postmenopausal hormone therapy; ethical and efficient drug studies, *Journal of the North American Menopause Society*, 2, 123, 1995.
16. Andrews, W.C., FDA guidance for development of combination estrogen-progestin products. *Journal of the North American Menopause Society*, 2, 121, 1995.
17. Gambrell, R.D., FDA guidance for development of combination estrogen-progestogen products, *Journal of the North American Menopause Society*, 2, 127, 1995.
18. Barinaga, M., "Obese" protein slims mice, *Science*, 269, 475, 1995.
19. Rolls, B.J., Aging and appetite, *Nutrition Reviews*, 50, 422, 1992.
20. Kimura, S., Taste and nutrition, *Nutrition Reviews*, 50, 888, 1992.
21. Hamilton J.B., Effects of exogenous female sex hormones on food intake, macronutrients and body weight in the ovariectomized postbreeder female rat, Ph.D. dissertation, Louisiana State University and Agricultural and Mechanical College, Baton Rouge, 1996.
22. Lerner, J., Counseling the patient at menopause concerning hormone replacement therapy, *Journal of the North American Menopause Society*, 2, 175, 1995.
23. Roush, W., Can "resetting" hormonal rhythms treat illness? *Science*, 269, 1220, 1995.
24. Hamilton J.B., Hegsted, M., and Keenan, M., Do exogenous female sex hormones affect body weight and intake of sweet, fat and chocolate? Louisiana State University, Pennington Biomedical Research Center, Baton Rouge, 1997.

Appendix 24-A: Recommended Dietary Allowances[a]

Category	Age (years or Condition)	(kg)	(lb)	(cm)	(in)	(g)	(µg RE)[c]	(µg)[d]	(mg a·TE)[e]	(µg)
Infants	0.0–0.5	6	13	60	24	13	375	7.5	3	5
	0.5–1.0	9	20	71	28	14	375	10	4	10
Children	1–3	13	29	90	35	16	400	10	6	15
	4–6	20	44	112	44	24	500	10	7	20
	7–10	28	62	132	52	28	700	10	7	30
Males	11–14	45	99	157	62	45	1,000	10	10	45
	15–18	66	145	176	69	59	1,000	10	10	65
	19–24	72	160	177	70	58	1,000	10	10	70
	25–50	79	174	176	70	63	1,000	5	10	80
	51+	77	170	173	68	63	1,000	5	10	80
Females	11–14	46	101	157	62	46	800	10	8	45
	15–18	55	120	163	64	44	800	10	8	55
	19–24	58	128	164	65	46	800	0	8	60
	25–50	63	138	163	64	50	800	5	8	65
	51+	65	143	160	63	50	800	5	8	65
Pregnant						60	800	10	10	65
Lactating	1st 6 Months					65	1,300	10	12	5
	2nd 6 Months					62	1,200	10	11	65

Water-Soluble Vitamins							Minerals						
Vitamin C (mg)	Thiamin (mg)	Riboflavin (mg)	Niacin/ND (mg)[f]	Vitamin B6 (mg)	Folate (µg)	Vitamin B12 (µg)	Calcium (mg)	Phosphorus (mg)	Magnesium (mg)	Iron (mg)	Zinc (mg)	Iodine (µg)	Selenium (µg)
30	0.3	0.4	5	0.3	25	0.3	400	300	40	6	5	40	10
35	0.4	0.5	6	0.6	35	0.5	600	500	60	10	5	50	15
40	0.7	0.8	9	10.0	50	0.7	800	800	80	10	10	70	20
45	0.9	1.1	12	1.1	75	1.0	800	800	120	10	10	90	20
45	1.0	1.2	13	1.4	100	1.4	800	800	170	10	10	120	30
50	1.3	1.5	17	1.7	150	2.0	1,200	1,200	270	12	15	150	40
60	1.5	1.8	20	2.0	200	2.0	1,200	1,200	400	12	15	150	50
60	1.5	1.7	19	2.0	200	2.0	1,200	1,200	350	10	15	150	70
60	1.5	1.7	19	2.0	200	2.0	800	800	350	10	15	150	70
60	1.2	1.4	15	2.0	200	2.0	800	800	350	10	15	150	45
50	1.1	1.3	15	1.4	150	2.0	1,200	1,200	280	15	12	150	45
60	1.1	1.3	15	1.5	180	2.0	1,200	1,200	300	15	12	150	50
60	1.1	1.3	15	1.6	180	2.0	1,200	1,200	280	15	12	150	55
60	1.1	1.3	15	1.6	180	2.0	800	800	280	15	12	150	55
60	1.0	1.2	13	1.6	180	2.0	800	800	280	10	12	150	55
70	1.5	1.6	17	2.2	400	2.2	1,200	1,200	320	30	15	175	65
95	1.6	1.8	20	2.1	280	2.6	1,200	1,200	355	15	19	200	75
90	1.6	1.7	20	2.1	260	2.6	1,200	1,200	340	15	16	200	75

[a] The allowances, expressed as average daily intakes over time, are intended to provide for individual variations among most normal persons as they live in the U.S. under usual environmental stresses. Diets should be based on a variety of common foods in order to provide other nutrients for which human requirement shave been less well defined. See text for detailed discussion of allowances and of nutrients not tabulated.

[b] Weights and heights of reference adults are actual medians for the U.S. population of the designated age, as reported by NHANES II. The use of these figures does not imply that the height-to-weight ratios are ideal.

[c] Retinol equivalents. 1 retinol equivalent = 1 µg retinol or 6 µg β-carotene.

[d] As cholecalciferol. 10 µg cholecalciferol = 400 iu of vitamine D.

[e] a-Tocopherol equivalent. 1 mg d-a tocopherol – 1 a-TE.

[f] 1 ND (niacin equivalent) is equal to 1 mg of niacin or 60 mg of dietary tryptophan.

Appendix 24-B: Estimated Sodium, Chloride, and Potassium Minimum Requirements for Healthy People

Age	Weight (kg)[a]	Sodium (mg)[a,b]	Chloride (mg)[a,b]	Potassium (mg)[c]
Months				
0–5	4.5	120	180	500
6–11	8.9	200	300	700
Years				
1	11.0	225	350	1,000
2–5	16.0	300	500	1,400
6–9	25.0	400	600	1,600
10–18	50.0	500	750	2,000
>18[d]	70.0	500	750	2,000

[a] No allowance has been included for large, prolonged losses from the skin through sweat.

[b] There is no evidence that higher intakes confer any health benefit.

[c] Desirable intakes of potassium may considerably exceed these values (~3,500 mg for adults).

[d] No allowance included for growth. Values for those below 18 years assume a growth rate at the 50th percentile reported for males and females by the National Center.

Appendix 24-C: Estimated Safe and Adequate Daily Dietary Intakes of Selected Vitamins and Minerals[a]

| Age Category | Age (years) | Vitamins | | Trace Elements | | | | |
		Biotin (mg)	Pantothenic Acid (mg)	Copper (mg)	Manganese (mg)	Fluoride (mg)	Chromium (mg)	Molybdenum (mg)
Infants	0–0.5	10	2	0.4–0.6	0.3–0.6	0.1–0.5	10–40	15–30
	0.5–1	15	3	0.6–0.7	0.6–1.0	0.2–1.0	20–60	20–40
Children and	1–3	20	3	0.7–1.0	1.0–1.5	0.5–1.5	20–80	25–50
Adolescents	4–6	25	3–1	1.0–1.5	1.5–2.0	1.0–2.5	30–120	30–75
	7–10	30	4–5	1.0–2.0	2.0–3.0	1.5–2.5	50–200	50–150
	11+	30–100	4–7	1.5–2.5	2.0–5.0	1.5–2.5	50–200	75–250
Adults		30–100	4–7	1.5–3.0	2.0–5.0	1.5–4.0	50–200	75–250

[a] Because there is less information on which to base allowances, these figures are not given in the main table of RDA and are provided here in the form of ranges of recommended intakes.

[b] Since the toxic levels for many trace elements may be only several times usual intake, the upper levels for the trace elements given in this table should not be habitually exceeded.

Appendix 24-D: Median Heights and Weights and Recommended Energy Intake

Category	Age (years) or Condition	Weight (kg)	Weight (lb)	Height (cm)	Height (in)	REE[a] (kcal/day)	Multiples of REE	Average Energy Allowance (kcal)[b] Per kg	Average Energy Allowance (kcal)[b] Per day[c]
Infants	0.0–0.5	6	13	60	24	320		108	650
	0.5–1.0	9	20	71	28	500		98	850
Children	1–3	13	29	90	35	740		102	1,300
	4–6	20	44	112	44	950		90	1,800
	7–10	28	62	132	52	1,130		70	2,000
Males	11–14	45	99	157	62	1,440	1.70	55	2,500
	15–18	66	145	176	69	1,760	1.67	45	3,000
	19–24	72	160	177	70	1,780	1.67	40	2,900
	25–50	79	174	176	70	1,800	1.60	37	2,900
	51+	77	170	173	68	1,530	1.50	30	2,300
Females	11–14	46	101	157	62	1,310	1.67	47	2,200
	15–18	55	120	163	64	1,370	1.60	40	2,200
	19–24	58	128	164	65	1,350	1.60	38	2,220
	25–50	63	138	163	64	1,380	1.55	36	2,200
	51+	65	143	160	63	1,280	1.50	30	1,900
Pregnant	Trimester 1								+0
	Trimester 2								+300
	Trimester 3								+300
Lactating	1st 6 Months								+500
	2nd 6 Months								+500

[a] Resting energy expenditure; calculation based on FAO.
[b] In the range of light to moderate activity, the coefficient of variation is ±20%.
[c] Figure is rounded.

Appendix 24-E: Clinical Signs Associated with Nutrition Deficiencies

Body Area	Normal Appearance	Clinical Signs	Nutritional Deficiency Indicated
Hair	Shiny, firm, not easily plucked	Hair dull and dry, lack of shine, thinness and sparseness, depigmentation, straightness of previously curly hair, easy pluckability	Protein-calorie; kwashiorkor or marasmus
Face	Uniform skin color, smooth, healthy appearance, no swelling	Depigmentation, skin dark over cheeks and eyes, moon face, scaling of skin around nostrils, nasolabial seborrhea	Protein-calorie, protein Riboflavin or niacin, pyridoxine
Eyes	Bright, clear, shiny, healthy pink moist membranes, no prominent blood vessels	Pale conjunctiva Bitot's spots, night blindness, conjunctival and corneal xeroxis (drying), keratomalacia, redness and fissuring of eyelid corners (angular palpebritis)	Anemia: iron; folate, Vitamins A or B_{12} Riboflavin, pyridoxine, niacin
Lips	Smooth, not chapped	Redness and swelling of mouth or lips, especially at corners (cheilosis), angular stomatitis, angular scars	Riboflavin, niacin, iron, pyridoxine
Mouth		Ageusia, dysgeusia	Zinc
Tongue	Deep red, not smooth or swollen	Glossitis, scarlet and raw magenta tongue	Niacin, folate, riboflavin, iron, vitamin B_{12}, nicotinic acid
Teeth	Bright, no cavities, no pain	Pitted, grooved teeth, missing teeth or erupting abnormally, gray or black spots (flurosis), cavities, mottled enamel	Vitamin D, fluoride Poor hygiene, lack of fluoride, excess fluoride
Gums	Healthy red, do not bleed, not swollen	Spongy, bleeding gums, swelling	Ascorbic acid (vitamin C)
Glands	Face not swollen	Thyroid enlargement, parotid enlargement	Iodine; starvation: protein-calorie
Skin	No signs of rashes, swelling, dark or light spots	Dryness (keratosis), sandpaper feel (follicular hyperkeratosis), petechial ecchymoses Red, swollen pigmentation of exposed areas (pellagrous dermatosis), flakiness, lack of fat under skin, scrotal and vulvar dermatosis	Vitamin A or essential fatty acids Ascorbic acid and vitamin D, nicotinic acid and tryptophan Kwashiorkor, essential fatty acids, riboflavin

Body Area	Normal Appearance	Clinical Signs	Nutritional Deficiency Indicated
Nails	Firm, pink	Spoon shaped nails (koilonychia)	Iron
Muscles and skeletal system	Good muscle tone, some fat under skin, can walk or run without pain	Muscle wasting Knock knees or bow legs, thoracic rosary, Musculoskeletal hemorrhage	Starvation, kwashiorkor, marasmus; vitamin D, ascorbic acid
Gastrointestinal system	No palpable organs or masses	Hematomegaly (fatty infiltration)	Protein
Cardiovascular system	Normal heart rhythm, no murmur, normal blood pressure for age	Cardiac enlargement, tachycardia	Thiamine
Nervous system	Psychological stability, normal reflexes	Psychomotor changes, mental confusion, sensory loss, motor weakness, loss of vibration, loss of ankle movement, knee jerks, calf tenderness	Kwashiorkor (protein); thiamine, nicotinic acid, vitamin B_{12}

Index

therapeutic modalities, team approach,
　　390–391
vitamin intake, 399
synthetic dietary supplements, metabolic
　　effect, 393

O

Obesity, binge-eating disorder, 14
Obsessive compulsive, anorexia nervosa, 8
Obsessiveness, 43
　　Maudsley Obsessional-Compulsive Inventory,
　　　　47
　　need for control, 45
Operant conditioning, 265
Orange dance (contact movement therapy), 370
Osteoporosis, 56
　　anorexia nervosa, 8
Ovarian volume, 53
Overgeneralization, 275
Over-protectiveness, 169
　　anorexia nervosa, 166
　　bulimia nervosa, 10, 170

P

Parasympathetic nerves, 124–125
Parental conflicts, child's involvement in, 166
Parents, *see also* Family
　　prevention of eating disorders, 245–246
Pathophysiology, eating disorders, 49–56
Peer relationships, 214
Perfectionism, 374, 44–45
　　anorexia nervosa, 5
　　binge-eating disorder, 14
　　described, 44
　　eat disorders risk factor, 218
　　Multidimensional Perfectionism Scale, 47
　　socially prescribed, 44
Peripheral nervous system, 120
　　parasympathetic branch, 124–125
Personal mission statement, constitution, 303
Personality traits, *see also* Risk factors
　　predisposition to eating disorders, 43
Physical abnormalities, 50
Physical abuse, 203
Physical fitness, 328
　　body composition, 330
　　cardiorespiratory standards, 328
　　exercise risks for children, 333
　　flexibility, 332
　　guidelines, 339
　　muscular strength and endurance, 329
Pituitary, reduced size, 54
PNS, *see* Peripheral nervous system
Positive punishment, 267
Positive reinforcement, 265
Potassium, minimum requirements, 398
Power and self-esteem, 284
Preadolescents, dieting and weight concerns, 242
Precede model, 232

Predisposing factors, 232
Prevention, 56
　　affective education model, 230–231
　　Bloom's model, 240
　　body esteem activity for children, 255
　　community role, 250
　　comprehensive intervention model, 231–232
　　eating disorders compared to substance abuse,
　　　　228
　　Eating Smart, 235
　　education, 225–236, 254–259
　　factors associated with eating disorders in
　　　　children, 211–221
　　health belief model, 232
　　health care providers' role, 250–251
　　information model, 229–230
　　learning strategies, 233
　　levels of, 226, 227
　　models, 229
　　obstacles for programs, 227
　　parents' and caregiver's role, 245–246
　　precede model, 232
　　primary, 226–229, 240
　　programs, 228, 233
　　school personnel role, 247, 248
　　school-based programs, 234–236
　　self-esteem activity for children, 255
　　social cognitive theory, 232–233
　　social influence resistance model, 231
　　stress, 244, 255
　　target age for programs, 227
　　teachers and coaches, role in, 247
　　Teaching Kids to Eat and Love Their Bodies
　　　　Too!, 235
　　teaching long-term vs. short-term
　　　　consequences, 230
　　Weigh-to-Eat program, 235
　　West Virginia Health Schools Program, 250
Problem solving, 299
　　increasing skills, 303
Prompting, behavior modification, 268
Protein starvation, 390
Psychological characteristics, 60
Psychological characteristics of eating disorders,
　　43
Puberty, body image during, 189
Puberty, *see also* adolescence, 212
　　peer relationships, 214
　　dieting, 212
Punishment, 266
Purging
　　anorexia nervosa, 5
　　bulimia nervosa, 9
　　cardiovascular problems resulting from, 52
　　dental problems caused by, 53
　　electrolyte abnormalities as result of, 51
　　expression of rebellion, 207

Q

Q-EDD, 79–82